The Economics of Health and Healthcare

The Economics of
Health and Healthcare

Edited by Bella Moody

hayle
medical

New York

Hayle Medical,
750 Third Avenue, 9ᵗʰ Floor,
New York, NY 10017, USA

Visit us on the World Wide Web at:
www.haylemedical.com

ISBN: 978-1-63241-626-1

Cataloging-in-Publication Data

The economics of health and healthcare / edited by Bella Moody.
    p. cm.
Includes bibliographical references and index.
ISBN 978-1-63241-626-1
1. Medical economics. 2. Medical care, Cost of. 3. Medical care. 4. Health. I. Moody, Bella.
RA410 .E26 2019
338.4--dc23

Table of Contents

Preface

The world is advancing at a fast pace like never before. Therefore, the need is to keep up with the latest developments. This book was an idea that came to fruition when the specialists in the area realized the need to coordinate together and document essential themes in the subject. That's when I was requested to be the editor. Editing this book has been an honour as it brings together diverse authors researching on different streams of the field. The book collates essential materials contributed by veterans in the area which can be utilized by students and researchers alike.

The branch of economics which studies the issues related to the efficiency, value, behaviour, and effectiveness in the production and consumption of health and healthcare is known as health economics. It involves the study of the functioning of the healthcare systems and the health affecting behaviors. The maintenance and improvement of health by preventing, diagnosing and treating illness, injuries, and diseases is called health care. Government intervention, barriers to entry, asymmetric information, and the presence of a third-party agent are some of the main factors which distinguish health economics from other related branches. In healthcare, the physician is the third-party agent, who is responsible for making purchasing decisions including the prescription of medicines, tests and surgery. This book studies, analyzes and upholds the pillars of the economics of health and healthcare and its utmost significance in modern times. It explores all the important aspects of health economics and healthcare in the present day scenario. Students, researchers, experts and all associated with health economics and healthcare will benefit alike from this book.

Each chapter is a sole-standing publication that reflects each author's interpretation. Thus, the book displays a multi-facetted picture of our current understanding of application, resources and aspects of the field. I would like to thank the contributors of this book and my family for their endless support.

Editor

On the interdependence of ambulatory and hospital care in the German health system

Tugba Büyükdurmus[1,2,3,4] (iD), Thomas Kopetsch[5], Hendrik Schmitz[2,6] and Harald Tauchmann[2,3,7]*

Abstract

For some considerable time now the interface between ambulatory and hospital care has been mooted as a cause of inefficiencies in the German health system and there have been calls for a softening of the strict separation between the two sectors. This debate emphasizes the need for detailed empirical information on the interdependence between the two sectors. Using extensive administrative data at the level of the 412 German counties for the years 2007 to 2009 and a simultaneous equation model which allows the numbers of ambulatory and hospital cases to be mutually interdependent, we examine the connection between ambulatory and hospital specialist care separately for ten medical specialties. The results show that the interdependence of ambulatory and hospital services is far from homogeneous. The relationship depends, on the one hand, on the specialty and, on the other, on the direction of the effect observed. This heterogeneity needs to be taken into account for cross-sector needs-based planning.

Keywords: Health care, Ambulatory care, Hospital care, Medical specialities, Instrumental variables

Background

Despite the aging society and the connected increase in demand for health services which in principle accompanies it, the German hospital market is still conspicuous for its overcapacities [1]. An international comparison shows that only Austria has a higher hospital bed density than Germany. While in Sweden 2.1 beds in acute hospitals for every 1000 inhabitants must suffice, in Germany there are 5.7 [2]. One reason for the overcapacities originates from progress in medical technology. Services which previously had to be performed in hospitals can now increasingly be carried out on an ambulatory basis. This is particularly true of Germany where, in contrast to most other countries, a recognised and accepted feature of the health-care system means that specialist medical services can be performed both on an ambulatory basis by office-based doctors and on an inpatient basis by specialist physicians working in hospitals.

For some considerable time now problems associated with this dual provision of medical care have been the subject of extensive debate in Germany, with the controversy focussing on the interface between the ambulatory and the hospital sectors. The loudest calls are for care to be reorganised to avoid this strict separation which manifests itself in the German health service not only in two completely different remuneration systems for ambulatory and inpatient services but also in two different planning regimes. While hospital planning is the prerogative of the 16 German states, there exists a separate system of needs-based planning for ambulatory medical practices with rules set at the federal level. In their present form these two planning systems are mutually incompatible. To quote but one example: planning in the hospital sector is by beds while in the ambulatory sector the planning unit is the individual doctor. During the drafting of the Statutory Health Insurance Structure of Services Act (2012) the idea of overcoming this incompatibility with cross-sectoral needs-based planning was suggested. Although in the end no such system was introduced, the recently added paragraph §90a in the German *Sozialgesetzbuch*, allows for a joint committee to be formed to submit recommendations on cross-sector healthcare issues.

*Correspondence: harald.tauchmann@fau.de
[2]CINCH - National Research Center for Health Economics, Essen, Germany
[3]RWI - Leibniz-Institut für Wirtschaftsforschung, Essen, Germany
Full list of author information is available at the end of the article

For the implementation and the functioning of a cross-sector needs-based planning it is essential to have information about the linkage between the provision of services in the two sectors, ambulatory and hospital. Only with this knowledge can a functioning cross-sector planning system be devised. The linkage between the provision of services in the ambulatory and hospital sectors of the health service is therefore the subject of this article.

To date there have been only few international studies which examine the connection between the ambulatory and hospital sectors. For most countries this is because their medical services are structured differently. For example, in some countries with what is known as the GP or Gatekeeper Model access to medical services is restricted by law. In this model the GP has the task of piloting the patient through the health service, authorising treatment by an office-based specialist or in hospital. This implies a purely complementary relationship between the two sectors. In the literature, this healthcare structure has been critically analysed both in respect of countries which are subject to these restrictions (cf. for example [3, 4]) and with a view to the introduction of this model in Germany (cf. for example [5, 6]).

In addition, there are some studies which analyse the relationships between GPs and the different specialists in both the public and the private sectors. An analysis of Italian data by Atella and Deb [7], for instance, finds a significant substitutive relationship between utilization in the two sectors. The relationships are estimated with the help of a simultaneous equation system. This is based on the assumption that GP consultations have an influence on the numbers of the specialists' cases, but not the other way around. It is also assumed that the case numbers of the specialists in the public system have an effect on those of their colleagues in the private system but not vice versa.

A study by Adhikari [8] which concentrates on the relationship between ambulatory and hospital medical services to treat visceral leishmaniasis in Australia, provides evidence of a substitutive relationship between the two sectors. In the study, the elasticity of demand is first calculated separately for each sector. Subsequently, the relationship between the sectors is analyzed on basis of cross price elasticity. Another study by Fortney et al. [9] presents results from a natural experiment at the U.S. Department for Veterans Affairs, in which primary care services were increased in some districts but not in others. They look at the relationship between the utilization of GP services and those of ambulatory and hospital specialists. Taking into account the interdependence of the utilization of GP and all other medical services the study identifies a substitutive relationship between GP and office-based specialist care. However, the relationship between ambulatory and inpatient specialist services is neglected.

Kopetsch [10] examines the relationship between the ambulatory and hospital services provided in Germany in the year 2000, using data at the county level for the states of Bavaria, North Rhine-Westphalia and Saxony. Since the relationship varies by medical speciality, the analysis is carried out separately for ten groups of specialists. For this, he estimates an equation in which the ambulatory case numbers per inhabitant and further control variables explain the number of the hospital cases per inhabitant. Potential endogeneity problems in the study are not dealt with. The empirical analysis finds a complementary relationship for the specialities dermatology, ENT, paediatrics and orthopaedics while no significant relationship between ambulatory and hospital cases is detected for the other specialities.

Another strand of the literature discusses whether the parallel provision of services by the two sectors can be considered an important cause of inefficiencies and waste of resources (cf. for example [11–14]). On the one hand, a structure which duplicates specialists can lead to vertical competition between the office-based specialists and the hospitals. In the absence of incentives this competition can be counterproductive since the services are not delivered where they can be performed most cost-effectively. On the other hand, unnecessary costs may be incurred for repeated examinations if ambulatory specialist treatment leads to hospitalization. Looking at the service event in the ambulatory and hospital sectors, most German and international studies concentrate on potential inefficiencies at the interface between the two sectors. Himmel et al. [15], for example, examined the problem of the flow of information between hospitals and GPs and the consequent discontinuity of care. In order to test this, the authors concentrated on the medication administered on admission to hospital and provided considerable evidence of changes in the prescriptions during the stay in hospital. Hach et al. [16] show that hospitalization neither saves the ambulatory follow-up treatment nor is accompanied by a reduction in medication.

There are also some studies, which concentrate on the re-hospitalization rates as an important indicator of inefficiency between the two sectors. Therefore, the impact of transitional care interventions compared to standard hospital discharges are analyzed. As an example Weinberger et al. [17] studied the effect of such an intervention, which was designed to increase access to primary care after hospitalization. However, they found that the veterans in the intervention group had significantly higher rates of re-hospitalization and if readmitted also longer stays in hospital than veterans in the control group. On the other hand a study by Coleman et al. [18] found significant reductions in re-hospitalization rates and also lower mean hospital costs for for the patients in the intervention group. Despite of contrary findings regarding to care transition and rehospitalization, it confirms once more that it is worth to analyze the interface of the two sectors.

It is important to note that the studies cited above focus on very specific aspects of the interdependence of ambulatory and hospital care for which the nature of the interplay between the two sectors might be quite different. In other words, one may well find a complementary relationship for one specific situation and a substitutive relationship for the other.

The present analysis takes broader perspective, unlike the majority of the existing studies, we use administrative data that comprehensively covers the provision of inpatient and ambulatory care in Germany. The present paper expands the empirical evidence on the interdependence between the two sectors in Germany, focussing on how the provision of services in one sector relates to utilization in the other. It should be noted, however, that the present paper is only an exploratory study and cannot say anything about possible channels for positive or negative relationships between utilization in different sectors. Nor can the paper make a statement on efficiency in the system, as both individual level data and data on health outcomes are missing. Yet the results could serve as a starting point to dig deeper into potential reasons for the found relationships.

The results show a significant negative relationship for paediatrics and dermatology, with more specialist ambulatory cases leading to fewer hospital admissions. Considering the reversed direction, however, i.e. the impact of additional hospitalizations on the number of ambulatory cases, a significant positive connection can be observed for orthopaedics, gynaecology and otorhinolaryngology (ENT), with more hospital cases leading to additional ambulatory cases and a significant negative relationship for internal medicine. Furthermore we report a significant positive effect of GP cases on surgery and orthopaedic cases in hospital and also a significant positive relationship between ENT and GP cases for the reversed direction. Considering an increase in the number of all specialist cases the results show a significant decrease of GP cases and except for internal medicine and surgery, the same connection can be observed for the opposite direction.

The results of this study highlight the importance of a disaggregation of the data for the individual medical specialities, as they reveal a clear heterogeneity in the interdependences between the sectors. The relationship depends, on the one hand, on the medical speciality and, on the other, on the direction of the influence observed. Any possible cross-sector needs-based planning should take these linkages into account.

Data and descriptive analysis

In the course of the analysis data from different sources are linked. The first of the two most important data sources is the accounting data of the KBV (National Association of Statutory Health Insurance Physicians), which contains in detail the ambulatory case numbers per medical speciality. This administrative data covers all infomation of utilization of medical services by members of the German statutory health insurance system, i.e. 90% of the population.[1] The case numbers are aggregated at the level of the 413 counties (412 after two counties merged in 2009). Since this information is used to calculate the quarterly remuneration of the statutory health insurance doctors, these data can be assumed to be highly accurate as they are thoroughly checked for both administrative and computational errors. The cases per county refer to the patients' place of residence rather than place of treatment. There are the separate case numbers for GPs and various specialities.

The second important source, the DRG statistics, provide details of the hospital cases, which are also based on the patients' place of residence. This source is also a full survey of all cases in Germany. To provide an initial overview, we first examine purely descriptively the relationship between the utilization of ambulatory and hospital services in the years 2007, 2008 and 2009. A key aspect of the analysis is that the various medical specialties differ in their care structures and technical facilities, and thus also in the extent to which medical progress has made it possible to shift services into the ambulatory sector. The pattern of interdependences between the sectors may therefore be specific to each speciality and is, in consequence, analysed separately for each of ten specialist fields. Both data sources allow separate empirical analyses for ten specialities: ophthalmology, surgery, internal medicine, gynaecology, dermatology, ENT, paediatrics, neurology, orthopaedics and urology. Due to the special role which they can play in the utilization of specialist services, GPs are also included in the study. Table 1 gives an overview of the mean average values of the case numbers per county for the years 2007 to 2009 combined.

Detailed descriptive statistics on the utilization of services can be found in the Appendix. They show that there is variation in the utilization of services not only between the regions but also from year to year. However, there is no systematic pattern of the relationship between ambulatory and hospital cases per speciality over time.

The heterogeneity between the counties can be clearly recognised. The average number of hospitalizations is up to seven times higher in some regions. In the ambulatory sector the average case numbers are in some regions up to eleven times higher than in regions with the lowest number of specialist cases. To illustrate the considerable regional variation Fig. 1 takes orthopaedics and ENT as examples of ambulatory and hospital cases. The gradient of the regression lines shows the respective direction of the correlation over all counties. Here the differences

Table 1 Descriptive statistics: utilization of services

	Hospitalizations per 100.000 SHI insurees			Ambulatory cases per 1.000 SHI insurees		
	Mean	Min	Max	Mean	Min	Max
GPs				2,708	1,391	3,669
Ophthalmology	413	155	1,042	409	214	793
Internal Medicine	8,919	5,596	14,847	383	180	866
Paediatrics	1,475	1,076	2,679	373	121	684
Surgery	5,943	4,292	10,538	191	66	428
Urology	926	604	1,581	153	69	378
Orthopaedics	979	575	1,753	315	144	755
Gynaecology	2,930	2,177	5,449	635	315	1,606
ENT	822	466	1,234	237	101	424
Neurology	1,051	590	2,102	181	61	545
Dermatology	266	164	488	273	69	784
Observations	1.238			1.238		

between the various medical specialities become apparent. While there is a positive correlation between hospital and ambulatory utilization in ENT the correlation in orthopaedics is negative. To provide a comprehensive summary of all medical specialities, the correlations of the case numbers in the two sectors are presented in Table 2.

Overall it becomes clear that the direction of the relationship crucially depends on the speciality. While for ophthalmology, internal medicine, surgery, urology, gynaecology, ENT and neurology there is a positive correlation, the correlation is negative in paediatrics, orthopaedics and dermatology. With the exception of neurology and dermatology, all correlations are significant.

However, the predominantly positive correlations still do not allow for drawing conclusions regarding a complementary relationship between ambulatory and hospital services. With a bivariate approach a positive correlation is to be expected everywhere since the average state of health of the respective population of the counties should be reflected in both measures. Counties with healthier inhabitants should in principle make fewer claims upon both ambulatory and hospital services. Equally, the demand for both types of medical service should be higher in counties with less healthy inhabitants.

Further control variables

An important measure for determining the level of regional utilization is the need for medical services in a given region. It is therefore essential to control for variations in population structure and the state of health in each county. To capture the average state of health in a county we use both average life expectancy and the 'RSA risk factor' devised by the Federal (Social) Insurance Office (*Bundesversicherungsamt* - BVA). The RSA risk factor is a measure of the average morbidity in a county. Used to calculate the compensatory transfers to those statutory health insurance funds whose membership evinces a higher risk structure, it summarizes as an index the morbidity of each county measured in terms of 80 important illnesses. This is a particularly attractive variable because it is objective, measuring the state of health as determined by doctors. At the same time, it is comprehensive and - like the dependent variables - probably highly accurate, as the information it provides determines the actual flow of money from the Risk Structure Compensation Scheme to the SHI funds.

In addition to health status, two other factors are relevant to our analysis. These are health behaviour and the

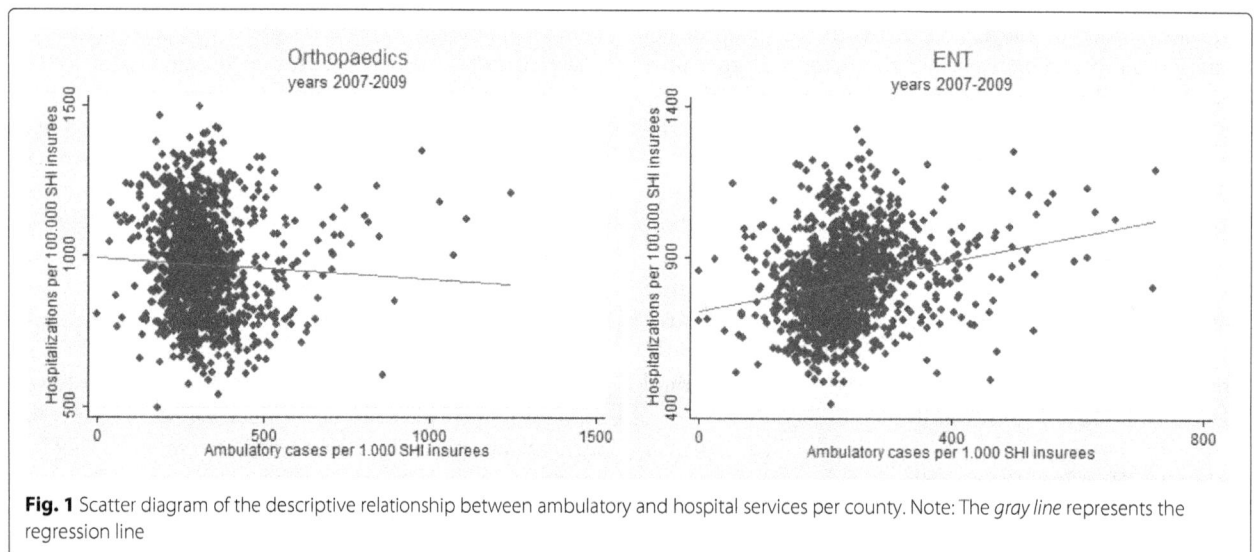

Fig. 1 Scatter diagram of the descriptive relationship between ambulatory and hospital services per county. Note: The *gray line* represents the regression line

Table 2 Correlations of the case numbers in the two sectors

	Correlation coefficient Total
Ophthalmology	0,2022*
Internal Medicine	0,0823*
Paediatrics	-0,1083*
Surgery	0,0567*
Urology	0,2553*
Orthopaedics	-0,1275*
Gynaecology	0,2415*
ENT	0,2257*
Neurology	0,0246
Dermatology	-0,0329

*Significant at the 5% level

efficiency of the individual's own health production, as proposed by [19]. It is well-known, for instance, that levels of education and income correlate positively with healthy behaviour. To capture these factors, we use corresponding variables from the INKAR database maintained by the Federal Office for Building and Regional Planning (BBR) for 2007 and 2009.[2] As there are no data available for 2008, we take the simplifying assumption that these structural variables remain constant over the short time span

of two years. Specifically we take the average net monthly household income, the unemployment rate, the number of regional centres, the proportion of highly qualified and low-skilled workers, the shares of single-person households and immigrants, and the number of long-term care recipients per 10,000 inhabitants.

To measure the influence of environmental conditions, we take the annual average level of particulate matter pollution (PM10) [3] recorded at over 400 measuring stations distributed across Germany and published by the Federal Environment Agency (*Umweltbundesamt*). An algorithm has been used to translate the data to the county level. An overview of all control variables and their descriptive statistics can be found in Table 3.

Methods

Any empirical analysis that is concerned with the interdependence of outpatient and inpatient care faces two methodological challenges. On the one hand, genuine interaction between the provision of services in the two sectors must be separated from correlation due to unobserved heterogenity, which might be an issue in the present data. In their analyses of the same data both Augurzky et al. [20] and Kopetsch and Schmitz [21] demonstrated that a large proportion of the regional variation in hospitalizations and physician consultations

Table 3 Descriptive statistics: control variables

	Mean	Std. Dev.	Min	Max
Health status				
Male life expectancy	77,077	1,460	72,200	81,100
Female life expectancy	82,103	1,020	77,900	84,900
RSA Risk Factor	1,009	0,071	0,847	1,204
Structural variables				
Proportion of population				
with SHI in %)	87,694	5,079	65,522	97,895
Long-term care recipients				
(per 10.000 population)	278,140	60,120	145,000	512,000
Unemployment rate in %	9,203	4,464	2,300	24,200
Net monthly household income	1.500,098	201,088	1.090,000	2.585,000
Number of large regional centres	0,401	0,564	0,000	4,000
Number of medium regional centres	2,219	2,149	0,000	11,000
Highly qualified workers in %	4,168	3,294	0,600	29,700
Low-skilled workers in %	14,400	4,825	6,400	39,500
Single-person households in %	36,290	4,379	20,400	55,800
Immigrants in %	7,152	4,536	0,700	25,200
Pollutants				
Particulate matter (PM 10)	19,737	6,112	0,000	31,000

could be explained by observable differences in demographic structures and state of health. Nevertheless, a considerable part of the variation at county level remained unexplained and may have been caused by specific unobserved health or preference differences between the counties which could not be controlled for.

On the other hand, the interaction between two endogenous measures has to be considered. Utilization in the two sectors thus represents both an explanatory variable and a variable, which has to be explained. The analysis therefore requires the estimation of a simultaneous equation model whose parameters can only be identified with the help of instrument variables.

Finally, in any given region the supply of general practitioners (GPs) could play a role in the relationship between ambulatory and hospital cases, too. GPs typically refer their patients to office-based specialists, but will on occasion arrange for them to be admitted directly to hospitals. GP behaviour which differed regionally in this regard or regional variation in GP densities would thus impact on the linkage under examination.

In principle, there are two simple but contrasting hypotheses concerning the interplay of office- and hospital-based specialist care.

First hypothesis (substitutes) It seems natural to regard ambulatory and hospital services as mutually substitutive. If medical services which can be rendered on either an ambulatory or an inpatient basis are performed by an office-based doctor, no hospitalization is required. The higher the physician density of the specialty or the higher the ambulatory cases, the lower the hospital cases in the region. Conversely, after a hospital stay the need for medical services should have been met without the need for corresponding ambulatory treatment. We hypothesize that this relationship exists for opthalmology, internal medicine, surgery, orthopaedics, neurology and dermatology. Our intuition is that this is due to the fact that several of the provided medical services in this diciplines can be performed on both ambulatory and hospital basis. An example for a medical service which is characteristic as a service that can be performed on ambulatory or hospital basis is cataract surgery.

Second hypothesis (complements) It can also be argued that a complementary relationship exists. If, in a given region, ambulatory specialist treatment frequently leads to a hospital referral, and hospital stays necessitate ambulatory after-care, the result will be a positive correlation between office- and hospital-based specialist treatment. We expect a complementary relationship for paediatrics, urology, gynaecology and ENT. These medical specialities distinguish themselves from the other disciplines due to fact that several medical services can only be performed

at a hospital while others can be carried out either at a hospital or on an ambulatory basis. Services which are characteristic for requiring a hospital stay are for example abdominal hysterectomy, thyroid surgery or an cochlear implant in case of deafness. This services are usually diagnosed by office-based doctors and require an admisssion to hospital, because of limitations in the ambulatory sector. There are different explanations for a complementary relationship.

1. A low density of specialists in the ambulatory care could increase the number of patients an individual doctor has to treat in a given period of time and consequently less diseases can be diagnosed due to less thorough examinations. Conversely, a high density of specialists allows the individual physician to spend more time with each patient. In this case more diseases could be diagnosed, which might lead to more hospital admissions.
2. Given a fixed treatment time per patient, a low physician density in a region would lead to less ambulatory cases or patients per office-based physician and thus to fewer hospital admissions than in an area with a higher physician density.
3. A high density of specialists in the ambulatory sector indicates high competition between the physicians. In this case the physician would rather refer the patient to a hospital than to another office-based doctor, as otherwise there would be the risk of the patient not returning to the referring physician. This argument also holds for GPs.

However, these attempted explanations show that the relationship may depend on the direction of the influence observed. This implies that in the present analysis the terms complements and substitutes are not used in accordance with their strict definitions used in microeconomic theory. There, two production factors can either be substitutes or complements but not both simultaneously. Deviating from this classical definition, here by complementary is meant that an increase in the number of cases in one sector results in an increased number of cases in the other, while substitutivity means that a reduced number of cases is the consequence. Rather than identifying the channels through which ambulatory and hospital cases influence each other, our contribution consists of illustrating the heterogeneity in the interdependence between the sectors over the various medical disciplines. This study is to be seen as a basis for further research, which needs to take the found linkages into account to organize a well-functioning cross-sector needs-based planning.

To explain the relationship between ambulatory and hospital case numbers, the following system of equations is formulated and estimated for each speciality separately:

$$HC_{ij} = \alpha_1 X_i + \beta_1 HBD_{ij} + \gamma_1 AC_{ij} + \delta_1 GPC_i + \varepsilon_{1ij} \quad (1)$$
$$AC_{ij} = \alpha_2 X_i + \beta_2 PD_{ij} + \gamma_2 HC_{ij} + \delta_2 GPC_i + \varepsilon_{2ij} \quad (2)$$
$$GPC_i = \alpha_3 X_i + \beta_3 GPD_i + \gamma_3 HC_{ij} + \delta_3 AC_{ij} + \varepsilon_{3ij} \quad (3)$$

where HC_{ij} denominates the number of hospital cases in speciality j per 100.000 inhabitants in county i[4], AC_{ij} the number of ambulatory cases in speciality j per 1.000 inhabitants in county i, GPC_i the number of GP cases per 1.000 inhabitants in county i and the X_i vector of control variables which contain, among other things, the average state of health in the county i. HBD_{ij} is the hospital bed density (beds per 100,000 inhabitants) in speciality j, PD_{ij} the physician density in speciality j and GPD_i is the GP density per 1,000 inhabitants in county i.

The equation system (1) to (3) thus allows ambulatory and hospital specialist utilization to be mutually interdependent. The GP care can be seen as both preceding and subsequent area. Thus the case numbers of GP care can also be influenced by specialist care. The particular aim of the analysis is the estimation of the coefficients γ_1 and γ_2, which model the nature of the interaction between hospital and ambulatory care, whereby positive values indicate a complementary and negative values a substitutive relationship.

We estimate the Eqs. (1) to (3) together with a three-stage least squares estimator (3SLS). For this the endogenous regressors HC_{ij}, AC_{ij} and GPC_i in the equation system (1) to (3) are instrumented. Specifically they are explained by all exogenous variables in the equation system and the fitted values are used as regressors in the second stage. The correlations between the error terms of the three equations are then estimated from the residuals of this regression and used in the third stage of the estimation to increase the precision of the estimation results by a generalized least square estimation.

Variables measuring the supply and exclusion restrictions
The utilization of services is closely linked to the supply in each of the sectors. A lack of availability in one sector could, in different regions, cause more services to be performed by specialists in the other. The analysis must therefore also consider the regional supply of hospital beds and office-based doctors.

In order to identify the model, we use exclusion restrictions. For instance the physician density (PD_{ij}) directly affects the specialist cases (AC_{ij}) but is excluded from Eq. (1). Thus, we assume that the physician density does not have an own effect on hospital cases once the supply of hospital beds and the specialist and GP cases are

controlled for. Note that this does not rule out that physician density indirectly affects hospital cases via specialist case. The same holds for the GP density (GPD_i).

Vice versa, hospital bed density (HBD_{ij}) and GP density GPD_i are assumed not to have an own effect on specialist cases once specialist physician density as well as hospital and GP cases are controlled for. Thus, they are excluded from Eq. (2). Using similar arguments, we exclude HBD_{ij} and PD_{ij} from Eq. (3).

When utilizing medical services patients do not respect county borders. In order to model the regional supply of ambulatory treatment facilities actually available to patients more accurately, we therefore define the catchment area for each county as including not only that county itself but also all surrounding counties whose central point is no more than a 30-minute drive from the central point of the first county. By doing so, we obtain the physician density for a regional area which is of greater relevance for utilization patterns than the "county" as a purely administrative unit. The bed density (beds per 100,000 inhabitants) as a measure of the regional supply of hospital treatment facilities is determined for a geographical area which can be covered by car within 60 minutes. This takes account of the fact that patients are willing to cover longer distances to reach hospitals than to consult office-based doctors. The underlying data for this are provided by the Directory of Hospitals and Prevention or Rehabilitation Facilities [22].

Results
Table 4 offers an overview of the average supply in the two sectors. Here, the previously mentioned, striking heterogeneity in the services available in the two sectors can be observed as well.

Table 5 show the results of the three-stage least square estimation for each speciality. Each of the ten columns refers to a regression with a different speciality. Besides the three regressors of prime interest to us, all control variables mentioned above were included in the regression and are to be found in the Appendix.

Where hospitalizations serve as a dependent variable (Eq. 1), we obtain for paediatrics and dermatology a substitutive while for the other specialities there is no significant connection. Examining the estimated effect of GP cases on the number of hospital cases reveals a significant complementary relationship for surgery and orthopaedics. While for no other specialty a significant connection is apparent, the sign of the estimated coefficients points in the same direction, with the exceptions of ophthalmology, ENT, neurology and dermatology. Yet for the latter three, the coefficient is almost zero. Disregarding statistical significance, for the majority of specialties the pattern points to extensive utilization of GP's

Table 4 Descriptive statistics: supply of ambulatory and hospital services

	Mean	Std. Dev.	Min	Max
Supply of hospital services per 100.000 inhabitants within a radius of 60 minutes				
Bed density in ophthalmology	6,571	2,593	0,000	13,544
Bed density in internal medicine	192,611	30,886	97,041	306,750
Bed density in paediatrics	24,496	6,676	6,465	56,350
Bed density in surgery	133,667	19,133	72,922	253,616
Bed density in urology	18,935	4,079	1,640	32,310
Bed density in orthopaedics	30,399	11,081	0,000	105,177
Bed density in gynaecology	45,311	6,114	26,798	62,291
Bed density in ENT	14,799	4,596	0,000	37,291
Bed density in neurology	26,648	8,763	0,000	82,163
Bed density in dermatology	6,332	3,987	0,000	24,234
Supply of ambulatory services per 1.000 inhabitants within a radius of 30 minutes				
Physician density for GPs	0,655	0,065	0,481	1,070
Physician density in ophthalmology	0,064	0,015	0,024	0,174
Physician density in internal medicine	0,108	0,039	0,015	0,323
Physician density in paediatrics	0,074	0,020	0,039	0,250
Physician density in surgery	0,056	0,020	0,015	0,199
Physician density in urology	0,033	0,008	0,013	0,076
Physician density in orthopaedics	0,064	0,018	0,018	0,149
Physician density in gynaecology	0,121	0,027	0,053	0,299
Physician density in ENT	0,047	0,013	0,015	0,134
Physician density in neurology	0,056	0,020	0,008	0,135
Physician density in dermatology	0,041	0,013	0,005	0,091
Observations		1.238		

Source: KHV, BAR (Federal Medical Register)

services increases the number of hospitalizations. One possible explanation is that more GP visits generate more opportunities for diagnosing diseases leading to hospital admissions. However, whether this interpretation is indeed correct could only be verified with the help of individual level data. The bed density and therefore the supply of hospital services has a positive influence on the hospital case numbers for all specialities. The service event in hospital care is therefore determined to a substantial degree on the supply side.

The results of the estimation of the equation with the ambulatory case numbers as a dependent variable (Eq. 2) indicate a significantly complementary relationship for orthopaedics, gynaecology and ENT. It is interesting that for some specialties more hospital cases lead to *more* ambulatory cases in these specialities whereas - looked at the other way around - more ambulatory cases lead to *fewer* hospital cases. There is therefore no clear interdependence between ambulatory and hospital cases here. This could be due to the fact that there are services in these specialities which are not feasible on an ambulatory basis and must therefore be performed in a hospital. Viewed the other way around, however, a hospital stay requires follow-up treatment in the ambulatory area and therefore manifests a complementary relationship. It should be noted, however, that most of the coefficients are not statistically significant.

Furthermore, all specialities are seen to have a substitutive relationship with the GP cases. Unlike specialist care in the hospital sector, more GP consultations do not lead to more cases for office-based specialists. Comprehensive GP care seems to obviate treatment by office-based specialists in many cases across all specialities. This result

Table 5 Regression results for Eqs. (1), (2) and (3)

	Ophthalmology	Internal medicine	Paediatrics	Surgery	Urology
Hospitalizations (1)					
Specialist Ambulatory Cases	0,251 (0,30)	-0,746 (0,81)	-0,751* (0,33)	-0,918 (1,47)	1,660 (1,66)
GP Cases	−0,151 (0,10)	0,082 (0,53)	0,160 (0,13)	1,966*** (0,52)	0,200 (0,29)
Bed Density	8,972*** (1,78)	14,882*** (1,08)	6,794*** (1,09)	12,009*** (1,26)	10,503*** (1,61)
Specialist Ambulatory Cases (2)					
Specialist Hospitalizations	−0,349 (0,22)	-0,041** (0,01)	0,134 (0,10)	-0,024 (0,01)	0,043 (0,05)
GP Cases	−0,301** (0,09)	−0,419*** (0,11)	−0,257*** (0,05)	−0,251*** (0,06)	−0,158*** (0,03)
Specialist Physician Density	1034,214** (318,21)	1193,020*** (204,96)	1150,209*** (205,80)	1062,275*** (207,65)	353,974 (275,68)
GP Cases (3)					
Specialist Hospitalizations	−0,576 (0,40)	−0,031 (0,02)	0,128 (0,25)	−0,047 (0,04)	0,199 (0,27)
Specialist Ambulatory cases	−1,139* (0,55)	0,152 (0,24)	−1,427*** (0,34)	−0,045 (0,54)	−3,958* (1,61)
GP	587,778***	833,681***	621,521***	852,000***	340,511
Physician Density	(153,70)	(123,07)	(131,93)	(150,49)	(232,39)

	Orthopaedics	Gynaecology	ENT	Neurology	Dermatology
Hospitalizations (1)					
Specialist Ambulatory Cases	−0,291 (0,27)	−0,107 (0,49)	0,834 (0,49)	−2,529 (1,66)	−0,189* (0,09)
GP Cases	0,185* (0,09)	0,271 (0,20)	−0,023 (0,12)	−0,062 (0,22)	−0,063 (0,04)
Bed Density	4,538*** (0,53)	10,526*** (2,27)	6,823*** (1,52)	4,529*** (0,98)	1,877*** (0,40)
Specialist Ambulatory Cases (2)					
Specialist Hospitalizations	0,174* (0,07)	0,320** (0,12)	0,255*** (0,06)	0,083 (0,07)	−0,200 (0,56)
GP Cases	−0,200*** (0,05)	−0,353** (0,13)	−0,137*** (0,03)	−0,124*** (0,03)	−0,306*** (0,06)
Specialist Physician Density	1097,432*** (193,76)	768,731* (314,89)	557,960** (204,31)	236,741* (106,28)	1214,036*** (339,65)
GP Cases (3)					
Specialist Hospitalizations	0,297 (0,21)	0,178 (0,23)	1,259** (0,45)	0,569 (0,33)	−0,797 (1,31)
Specialist Ambulatory Cases	−1,616*** (0,39)	−0,874* (0,42)	−3,759*** (1,00)	−4,453*** (1,30)	−1,339** (0,41)
GP	727,780***	646,518***	530,148**	451,625*	556,333***
Physician Density	(151,53)	(170,14)	(179,20)	(181,75)	(154,93)

Standard error in parentheses, * $p<0,10$,** $p<0,05$,*** $p<0,01$
Note: All above mentioned variables were controlled for. Full results can be found in the Appendix

clearly argues against the hypothesis of initial GP visits often resulting in treatment cascades involving numerous subsequent specialist visits. For all specialities except for urology the physician density has a significantly positive influence on the case numbers. The supply side thus also plays an important role for the service event in ambulatory care.

The results of Eq. 3, where GP cases function as a dependent variable, we found a complementary relationship to ENT hospitalizations. This might be due to follow-up treatment that must not necessarily performed by a specialist, such as wound care. In accordance with this result, we find a qualitatively equivalent pattern of results concerning the link between ENT specialist ambulatory cases and GP cases (Eq. 2). Except for internal medicine and surgery, we also observe a substitutive connection for all specialties, which indicates a competitive relationship between GPs and office-based specialists.

With the help of F tests we examine whether the relevant instruments contribute significantly to the explanation of the instrumented variables. Table 6 shows that the instruments for all specialities have a significant explanatory power with regard to the variation in the specialist cases and all F tests are clearly over the critical rule-of-thumb limit of 10. This implies that the estimation results of the three-stage least square estimation are not the product of weak instruments and make an interpretation possible.

All in all the results clearly suggest that, within the sector of ambulatory care, a substitutive relationship exists beween GPs and specialists visits. Our results are less clear with respect to the interaction of ambulatory and inpatient care. For several specialities no significant direct link in the number of cases is found in the data. Moreover, the few statistically significant effects are heterogeneous in their directions. All in all the results of this study highlight the importance of a disaggregation of the data for the individual medical specialities, as they reveal a

clear heterogeneity in the interdependences between the sectors.

Discussion

In Germany specialist care can be provided by both the ambulatory and the hospital sectors. The purpose of this study has been to examine the interdependencies between the two sectors. In doing so, we have taken account of the potential problem that the number of the specialist cases could be endogenous. That is to say, a complementary connection cannot be immediately inferred from a positive correlation, because in certain regions both ambulatory and hospital services could occur with particular frequency or infrequency due to unobserved factors, such as unobserved morbidity differences. Another problem with the potential to cause misleading interpretations of the correlation is that more hospital cases might also lead directly to more ambulatory cases.

The connections have been investigated by means of a simultaneous system of equations which not only controls for the regional differences in state of health and other structures but also takes into account the interdependent relationship between hospital and ambulatory cases. A strength of the study lies in its analysis of the treatments according to medical specialities, a procedure made possible by comprehensive administrative data sources. This differentiation by individual specialities clearly identifies relationships which would not be recognisable with less specific data, i.e. if ambulatory and hospital services were each treated as homogeneous goods. The heterogeneous basis of the analysis crystallises out the specific differences between the medical disciplines. It makes little sense to cast ophthalmological and gynaecological services together "into the same pot" since they are neither comparable nor mutually interchangeable. Finally, policy recommendations will also vary according to the speciality in question.

Table 6 F-Test of the instruments

	Ophthalmology	Internal medicine	Paediatrics	Surgery	Urology
Bed density for Specialists (radius 60)	$F(1,1219) = 52,77$ Prob > F = 0,0000	$F(1,1219) = 168,14$ Prob > F = 0,0000	$F(1,1219) = 16,67$ Prob > F = 0,0000	$F(1,1219) = 130,49$ Prob > F = 0,0000	$F(1,1219) = 77,68$ Prob > F = 0,0000
Physician density for Specialists (radius 30)	$F(1,1219) = 16,16$ Prob > F = 0,0001	$F(1,1219) = 35,30$ Prob > F = 0,0000	$F(1,1219) = 94,27$ Prob > F = 0,0000	$F(1,1219) = 50,94$ Prob > F = 0,0000	$F(1,1219) = 7,05$ Prob > F = 0,0080
Physician density for GPs (radius 30)	$F(1,1219) = 35,95$ Prob > F = 0,0000	$F(1,1219) = 47,74$ Prob > F = 0,0000	$F(1,1219) = 35,57$ Prob > F = 0,0000	$F(1,1219) = 51,39$ Prob > F = 0,0000	$F(1,1219) = 47,13$ Prob > F = 0,0000
	Orthopaedics	Gynaecology	ENT	Neurology	Dermatology
Bed density for Specialists (radius 60)	$F(1,1219) = 46,91$ Prob > F = 0,0000	$F(1,1219) = 42,29$ Prob > F = 0,0001	$F(1,1219) = 78,34$ Prob > F = 0,0000	$F(1,1219) = 42,12$ Prob > F = 0,0000	$F(1,1219) = 13,44$ Prob > F = 0,0003
Physician density for Specialists (radius 30)	$F(1,1219) = 78,28$ Prob > F = 0,0000	$F(1,1219) = 17,77$ Prob > F = 0,0000	$F(1,1219) = 64,05$ Prob > F = 0,0000	$F(1,1219) = 31,44$ Prob > F = 0,0000	$F(1,1219) = 51,03$ Prob > F = 0,0000
Physician density for GPs (radius 30)	$F(1,1219) = 31,51$ Prob > F = 0,0000	$F(1,1219) = 35,43$ Prob > F = 0,0000	$F(1,1219) = 47,25$ Prob > F = 0,0000	$F(1,1219) = 41,63$ Prob > F = 0,0000	$F(1,1219) = 42,36$ Prob > F = 0,0000

The results show a substitutive relationship for paediatrics and dermatology with more ambulatory cases leading to fewer hospital cases. If the perspective is reversed, however, and the focus is on how additional hospital cases influence case numbers in the ambulatory sector, a complementary relationship can be observed for orthopaedics, gynaecology and otorhinolaryngology (ENT). It is interesting that for some specialties more hospital cases lead to *more/fewer* ambulatory cases in these specialities whereas - looked at the other way around - more ambulatory cases lead to *fewer/more* hospital cases. Thus in this speciality there can be talk of neither a clearly substitutive nor an unambiguously complementary relationship. However, this interpretation mainly grounds in the point estimates as many of the estimated coefficients are not statistically significant.

The role played by general practice in all this is interesting. While GP consultations displace the services of ambulatory specialists across all disciplines, for hospital care the picture is different. Even it is just significant for surgery and orthopaedics the results indicate that additional cases for GPs seem to entail more hospital admissions for some specialities. Thus increasing the supply of GPs may well eliminate potentially superfluous specialist consultations, albeit at the price of raising the number of particularly cost-intensive hospitalizations. This might be due our theoretical argument of a substitutive relationship. The higher the competition between the physicians or the risk that a patient does not return to the referring physician the higher is the incentive to refer directly to the hospital.

On the other hand additional ambulatory cases in the specialities go along with smaller numbers of GP cases except for internal medicine.

The question as to whether ambulatory and hospital services complement or substitute each other depends, on the one hand, on the medical speciality and, on the other, on the direction of influence. Depending on the treatment needed, some patients can already be cared for entirely on an ambulatory basis or at least receive sufficient treatment from office-based doctors to avoid hospitalization. On the other hand, a hospital stay can necessitate intensive aftercare treatment which is then provided by office-based doctors. Accordingly, the interdependence of ambulatory and hospital cases can vary in its intensity and even direction.

Our paper has several limitations which are grounded in the availability of data and should be taken into account when implications are considered. Given that our data are aggregated on the county level, we cannot clearly say, in case of a complementary relationship, whether patients first see a GP or ambulatory specialist and then enter a hospital or whether it is the other way around. Moreover, a complementary relationship per se is not informative

about efficient or inefficient use of resources in the system. Positive relationships might either indicate that both sectors work well together, or hint at unnecessary duplications of services – and vice versa for substitutive relationships. Outcome data might be a way to evaluate this which, however, are not available in the present study.

Nevertheless, this exploratory study has its value in being a first starting point in a not well understood research area, and should be seen as a basis for digging deeper into the question of which deficits in the interplay of both sectors exist and how to improve the efficiency of health care provision in Germany. Heterogeneity in the interdependencies can also be identified on the aggregate level and the main policy implication is that this should be taken into account in cross-sector needs-based planning. This means, for example, that any reduction in capacity deemed necessary in the hospital sector should not be carried out indiscriminately across all medical specialities. Such cuts are better suited to departments whose services can be absorbed by the ambulatory sector than to those where they cannot.

Conclusions

Again, while this study cannot make a statement on the current state of efficiency in the interplay between both sectors, it should be the starting point for further analysis, which focusses on implementing a well-functioning cross-sector needs-based planning regime. Especially for analysis of the committees, which were formed in individual states in 2012, to submit recommendations on cross-sector healthcare issues.

Endnotes

[1] Just over 10% of the German population are privately insured.

[2] This database contains a total of some 500 indicators, based almost exclusively on official statistics, on topics such as population and social structure, the economy and employment, income and education, aggregated according to administrative areas (states, counties, local government districts). A precise description can be found at www.bbsr.bund.de.

[3] PM_{10} (Particulate Matter 10) is a commonly-used standard specifying the aerodynamic diameter from which particles count as particulate matter. In the case of PM_{10} particles with a size of up to 15 microns go into a weighting function, in which at a size of approx. 10 micron half the particles go in.

[4] Here and in the following "inhabitants" always means "statutorily insured inhabitants". The term has been abbreviated for the sake of simplicity.

Appendix

Table 7 Utilization of services (supplement to Table 1)

	Mean			Min	Max	Min	Max	Min	Max
	2007	2008	2009	2007	2007	2008	2008	2009	2009
Hospital cases per									
100.000 SHI population									
Ophthalmology	412	415	413	175	1118	164	1064	126	1023
Internal Medicine	8.720	8.952	9.084	5.564	14.233	2.967	14.973	5.409	15.335
Paediatrics	1.471	1.481	1.474	1.073	2.632	838	2.727	990	2.678
Surgery	5.804	5.962	6.062	4.049	10.054	3.088	10.703	3.932	10.856
Urology	910	931	938	601	1.532	371	1.535	464	1.677
Orthopaedics	947	985	1.006	495	1.713	536	1.798	600	1.763
Gynaecology	2.970	2.953	2.869	1.786	5.804	1.528	5.114	1.444	5.428
ENT	817	826	825	417	1.326	488	1.250	491	1.252
Neurology	1.016	1.045	1.092	558	2.055	397	2.169	614	2.082
Radiology	200	197	192	72	431	52	457	69	406
Dermatology	256	268	274	161	503	164	491	168	468
Ambulatory cases per									
1.000 SHI population									
General Practice	2.427	2.677	3.020	482	3.786	577	3.972	2.023	4.505
Ophthalmology	368	414	444	53	587	107	700	104	1.433
Internal Medicine	312	375	462	109	693	113	762	36	1.770
Paediatrics	303	461	355	28	480	65	722	59	961
Surgery	167	195	211	39	410	65	431	30	737
Urology	133	151	177	10	301	55	359	0	657
Orthopaedics	274	321	351	41	729	73	561	0	1.637
Gynaecology	564	647	693	149	859	152	967	100	3.551
ENT	214	240	257	14	417	73	461	0	722
Neurology	160	182	202	33	407	76	406	0	863
Radiology	148	233	288	9	509	93	544	0	1.879
Dermatology	245	278	295	65	546	81	457	0	1.544
N	413	413	412						

Source: DRG statistics, KBV

Table 8 Complete estimation results of the 3SLS: Eq. (1)

Specialist hospitalizations	Ophthalmology	Internal medicine	Paediatrics	Surgery	Urology
Specialist Ambulatory Cases	0,251 (0,30)	−0,746 (0,81)	−0,751* (0,33)	−0,918 (1,47)	1,660 (1,66)
GP Cases	−0,151 (0,30)	0,082 (0,81)	0,160 (0,33)	1,966*** (1,47)	0,200 (1,66)
Bed Density	8,972*** (1,78)	14,882*** (1,08)	6,794*** (1,09)	12,009*** (1,26)	10,503*** (1,61)
Male Life Expectancy	−13,322 (8,78)	−251,611*** (55,48)	−49,505*** (9,92)	−55,089 (51,37)	16,414 (23,11)
Female Life Expectancy	−13,904* (6,87)	−252,349*** (47,11)	−7,400 (10,23)	−60,530 (37,80)	−26,399** (8,51)
RSA Risk Factor	790,668*** (239,02)	9416,139*** (1217,78)	59,333 (234,30)	235,517 (1032,70)	16,951 (719,47)
Long−Term Care Recipients per 10.000 Population	−0,342*** (0,10)	3,882*** (0,73)	0,146 (0,14)	1,446* (0,58)	0,389** (0,13)
Unemployment Rate in %	−1,748 (3,57)	−57,284* (23,05)	−4,133 (4,96)	−10,953 (18,52)	1,093 (5,22)
Net Monthly Household Income	−0,026 (0,03)	−0,104 (0,23)	−0,133** (0,05)	0,256 (0,20)	0,070 (0,09)
Number of Large Regional Centres	26,504** (9,99)	−42,441 (72,12)	10,944 (15,06)	−178,167*** (53,27)	−4,221 (22,99)
Number of Medium Regional Centres	6,955*** (1,55)	56,546*** (11,04)	6,645** (2,08)	21,394* (8,94)	7,299*** (2,00)
Highly Qualified Workers in %	5,269* (2,31)	2,472 (15,94)	13,874*** (2,65)	0,411 (11,04)	−0,910 (4,60)
Low−Skilled Workers in %	−2,810 (1,52)	11,982 (10,86)	0,056 (2,08)	0,250 (8,55)	−1,716 (1,83)
Single−Person Households in %	1,040 (2,07)	−36,929*** (10,63)	−9,376*** (1,66)	−1,579 (5,67)	−5,070* (2,57)
Immigrants in %	−0,933 (2,45)	67,813*** (11,09)	10,472*** (1,83)	31,241*** (8,60)	5,143 (5,34)
Particulate Matter (PM 10)	−0,575 (0,93)	1,047 (6,42)	−3,085* (1,26)	−2,290 (4,08)	0,724 (1,20)
Year 2007	−97,177 (65,13)	−341,588 (343,76)	41,458 (84,38)	971,194** (344,37)	158,788 (234,79)
Year 2008	−62,836* (30,63)	−78,042 (191,63)	126,807*** (30,33)	642,815*** (184,00)	94,521 (126,57)
Constants	2210,626** (728,98)	36963,049*** (5216,84)	5895,104*** (840,37)	6794,790 (4629,84)	657,202 (1990,99)
N	1238	1238	1238	1238	1238
Specialist Ambulatory Cases	−0,291 (0,27)	−0,107 (0,49)	0,834 (0,49)	−2,529 (1,66)	−0,189* (0,09)
GP Cases	0,185* (0,09)	0,271 (0,20)	−0,023 (0,12)	−0,062 (0,22)	−0,063 (0,04)
Bed Density	4,538*** (0,53)	10,526*** (2,27)	6,823*** (1,52)	4,529*** (0,98)	1,877*** (0,40)
Male Life Expectancy	−33,468*** (7,99)	28,139 (16,89)	−23,392* (11,13)	−38,480* (16,05)	−13,574*** (2,93)
Female Life Expectancy	−17,195* (7,42)	−1,670 (14,56)	4,022 (6,38)	−49,471*** (10,52)	0,148 (2,39)

Table 8 Complete estimation results of the 3SLS: Eq. (1) *Continued*

Specialist hospitalizations	Orthopaedics	Gynaecology	ENT	Neurology	Dermatology
RSA Risk Factor	266,322 (186,38)	−1927,010*** (331,36)	28,083 (183,55)	1737,440* (696,28)	420,579*** (69,43)
Long−term Care Recipients per 10.000 Population	0,351** (0,11)	−0,023 (0,25)	0,543*** (0,09)	−0,047 (0,27)	0,067 (0,04)
Unemployment Rate in %	−9,086** (3,02)	16,902* (7,75)	−3,725 (2,89)	−13,861* (6,14)	−3,579** (1,33)
Net Monthly Household Income	0,132*** (0,03)	−0,347*** (0,08)	−0,059* (0,03)	−0,021 (0,07)	0,023* (0,01)
Number of Large Regional Centres	−4,828 (9,79)	−16,837 (21,50)	24,910* (12,05)	35,340 (26,27)	3,563 (4,09)
Number of Medium Regional Centres	10,657*** (1,77)	1,623 (3,63)	4,543** (1,55)	5,120* (2,46)	0,829 (0,55)
Highly Qualified Workers in %	0,213 (2,40)	30,002*** (7,32)	2,149 (2,08)	1,580 (3,03)	5,730*** (1,03)
Low−skilled Workers in %	−4,231* (1,67)	12,114*** (3,35)	2,948* (1,50)	4,016 (3,68)	−3,712*** (0,56)
Single−Person Households in %	−0,587 (1,87)	4,102 (7,25)	−8,417*** (2,23)	6,293 (7,25)	−0,410 (0,64)
Immigrants in %	5,108*** (1,54)	12,239*** (3,50)	0,695 (1,61)	6,908*** (2,08)	1,481* (0,67)
Particulate Matter (PM 10)	−0,664 (0,83)	−2,693 (2,21)	0,430 (0,68)	−4,217 (2,59)	−0,917* (0,37)
Year 2007	64,083 (61,50)	200,153 (142,10)	2,554 (84,09)	−170,225 (184,27)	−56,515* (25,84)
Year 2008	65,479* (30,37)	143,838* (65,05)	−4,045 (41,37)	−64,197 (86,16)	−22,976 (12,86)
Constants	3928,720*** (716,27)	1463,968 (1615,06)	2220,432* (980,77)	6785,421*** (1693,01)	1139,500*** (316,57)
N	1238	1238	1238	1238	1238

Standard error in parentheses, * $p<0,10$,** $p<0,05$,*** $p<0,01$
Note: All above mentioned variables were controlled for. Full results can be found in the Appendix

Table 9 Complete estimation results of the 3SLS: Eq. (2)

Specialists ambulatory cases	Ophthalmology	Internal medicine	Paediatrics	Surgery	Urology
Specialist Hospitalizations	−0,349 (0,22)	−0,041** (0,01)	0,134 (0,10)	−0,024 (0,01)	0,043 (0,05)
GP Cases	−0,301** (0,09)	−0,419*** (0,11)	−0,257*** (0,05)	−0,251*** (0,06)	−0,158*** (0,03)
Specialist Physician Density	1034,214** (318,21)	1193,020*** (204,96)	1150,209*** (205,80)	1062,275*** (207,65)	353,974 (275,68)
Male Life Expectancy	−27,529** (8,62)	−56,462*** (12,14)	−6,735 (7,12)	−29,130*** (5,48)	−12,677*** (3,33)
Female Life Expectancy	1,893 (7,42)	−11,697 (9,98)	13,939** (5,31)	3,563 (4,89)	3,268 (3,42)
RSA Risk Factor	963,151** (293,05)	1374,248*** (292,08)	342,856** (105,36)	499,031*** (108,87)	384,871*** (85,45)
Long−Term Care Recipients per 10.000 Population	−0,185 (0,14)	0,102 (0,15)	−0,014 (0,08)	0,134 (0,07)	−0,054 (0,05)
Unemployment Rate in %	−10,135** (3,11)	−23,250*** (4,25)	−9,766*** (1,97)	−9,558*** (2,13)	−2,354 (1,29)
Net Monthly Household Income	−0,057 (0,03)	−0,162*** (0,04)	−0,071** (0,02)	−0,073** (0,02)	−0,048*** (0,01)
Number of Large Regional Centres	30,030* (12,01)	53,129*** (12,92)	25,673*** (6,70)	14,811* (6,72)	11,818** (4,31)
Number of Medium Regional Centres	1,734 (2,15)	3,204 (2,50)	0,044 (1,35)	1,700 (1,19)	0,177 (0,90)
Highly Qualified Workers in %	6,752** (2,47)	10,888*** (2,76)	−0,687 (2,11)	2,167 (1,37)	2,318* (0,96)
Low−Skilled Workers in %	0,025 (1,77)	−1,163 (2,22)	2,103 (1,23)	−0,495 (1,11)	0,455 (0,74)
Single−Person Households in %	5,869*** (1,23)	4,935** (1,72)	3,231* (1,46)	−0,274 (0,75)	1,283* (0,57)
Immigrants in %	−7,687*** (1,61)	−4,667* (2,24)	0,080 (1,37)	−2,726* (1,17)	−3,074*** (0,68)
Particulate Matter (PM 10)	−2,660*** (0,77)	−5,063*** (1,00)	−2,331*** (0,56)	−1,068* (0,50)	−0,554 (0,33)
Year 2007	−218,644*** (58,23)	−307,591*** (65,29)	−162,635*** (31,99)	−158,596*** (32,08)	−131,132*** (20,08)
Year 2008	−90,597** (33,17)	−128,691*** (36,82)	54,803** (19,07)	−62,213*** (18,68)	−70,303*** (11,68)
Constants	2473,987** (932,71)	6143,137*** (1190,85)	−61,622 (750,33)	2672,262*** (526,49)	988,383** (349,18)
N	1.238	1.238	1.238	1.238	1.238
Specialist Hospitalizations	0,174* (0,07)	0,320** (0,12)	0,255*** (0,06)	0,083 (0,07)	−0,200 (0,56)
GP Cases	−0,200*** (0,05)	−0,353** (0,13)	−0,137*** (0,03)	−0,124*** (0,03)	−0,306*** (0,06)

Table 9 Complete estimation results of the 3SLS: Eq. (2) *Continued*

Specialists ambulatory cases	Orthopaedics	Gynaecology	ENT	Neurology	Dermatology
Specialist Physician Density	1097,432*** (193,76)	768,731* (314,89)	557,960** (204,31)	236,741* (106,28)	1214,036*** (339,65)
Male Life Expectancy	−8,219 (5,49)	−27,768* (12,56)	−8,234* (4,02)	−5,971 (3,29)	−20,240* (9,27)
Female Life Expectancy	7,037 (5,41)	3,935 (12,45)	0,829 (3,48)	1,152 (4,29)	−3,750 (6,49)
RSA Risk Factor	314,001** (104,84)	812,547** (296,34)	176,453* (70,24)	309,764*** (84,15)	515,128* (248,76)
Long−Term Care Recipients per 10.000 Population	−0,130 (0,08)	0,231 (0,19)	−0,150* (0,06)	−0,165** (0,05)	−0,033 (0,10)
Unemployment Rate in %	−1,822 (2,01)	−16,971*** (5,07)	−1,541 (1,29)	−1,981 (1,21)	−9,565*** (2,87)
Net Monthly Household Income	−0,037 (0,02)	0,016 (0,07)	0,004 (0,02)	−0,039** (0,01)	−0,032 (0,03)
Number of Large Regional Centres	9,840 (6,82)	29,436 (16,41)	8,303 (4,79)	13,189** (4,05)	28,567*** (8,38)
Number of Medium Regional Centres	−3,122* (1,43)	2,186 (2,97)	−0,112 (0,88)	−0,717 (0,87)	0,237 (1,55)
Highly Qualified Workers in %	4,029** (1,49)	2,648 (5,40)	1,101 (1,02)	0,760 (0,92)	8,692** (3,21)
Low−Skilled Workers in %	2,121 (1,23)	−3,070 (2,99)	0,381 (0,82)	1,883* (0,73)	−1,545 (2,61)
Single−Person Households in %	4,448*** (0,86)	11,395*** (2,03)	4,792*** (0,71)	4,060*** (0,61)	4,092** (1,26)
Immigrants in %	−2,260 (1,18)	−8,041* (3,25)	−1,560* (0,72)	−0,813 (0,78)	−4,108* (1,79)
Particulate Matter (PM 10)	−1,374* (0,54)	−2,727 (1,39)	−0,584 (0,36)	−1,413*** (0,34)	−2,948*** (0,70)
Year 2007	−160,511*** (30,80)	−284,296*** (75,82)	−107,172*** (19,82)	−101,125*** (17,88)	−210,424*** (40,46)
Year 2008	−65,327*** (18,76)	−113,216* (44,71)	−46,860*** (11,71)	−45,597*** (10,69)	−91,659*** (22,99)
Constants	374,894 (538,55)	1473,006 (1294,81)	697,276 (376,95)	492,033 (402,82)	2609,837*** (745,61)
N	1.238	1.238	1.238	1.238	1.238

Standard error in parentheses, * $p<0,10$,** $p<0,05$,*** $p<0,01$
Note: All above mentioned variables were controlled for. Full results can be found in the Appendix

Table 10 Complete estimation results of the 3SLS: Eq. (3)

GP cases	Ophthalmology	Internal medicine	Paediatrics	Surgery	Urology
Specialist Hospitalizations	−0,576 (0,40)	−0,031 (0,02)	0,128 (0,25)	−0,047 (0,04)	0,199 (0,27)
Specialist Ambulatory Cases	−1,139* (0,55)	0,152 (0,24)	−1,427*** (0,34)	−0,045 (0,54)	−3,958* (1,61)
GP Physician Density	587,778*** (153,70)	833,681*** (123,07)	621,521*** (131,93)	852,000*** (150,49)	340,511 (232,39)
Male Life Expectancy	−73,708*** (12,65)	−75,607*** (13,71)	−51,278* (20,17)	−76,703*** (15,01)	−74,444*** (13,93)
Female Life Expectancy	7,028 (16,70)	4,682 (13,98)	28,698* (14,45)	8,096 (13,36)	17,241 (18,18)
RSA Risk Factor	2124,649*** (383,09)	1673,021*** (349,39)	1371,695*** (227,19)	1510,455*** (259,30)	1989,814*** (400,82)
Long−Term Care Recipients per 10.000 Population	−0,163 (0,29)	0,317 (0,20)	0,054 (0,21)	0,290 (0,21)	−0,130 (0,29)
Unemployment Rate in %	−26,618*** (3,99)	−24,958*** (4,57)	−27,944*** (3,63)	−28,589*** (4,31)	−18,148*** (5,14)
Net Monthly Household Income	−0,158* (0,06)	−0,138* (0,06)	−0,213** (0,07)	−0,158** (0,06)	−0,247** (0,08)
Number of Large Regional Centres	76,274*** (18,36)	56,228*** (16,54)	76,514*** (16,51)	61,814*** (15,05)	68,596*** (19,08)
Number of Medium Regional Centres	2,888 (4,46)	2,880 (3,47)	0,486 (3,70)	1,623 (3,49)	0,741 (4,71)
Highly Qualified Workers in %	12,158* (4,97)	4,342 (4,31)	4,580 (5,76)	5,831 (3,82)	10,937* (5,30)
Low−Skilled Workers in %	−4,294 (3,76)	−6,206* (2,88)	−1,475 (3,31)	−6,552* (3,04)	−0,330 (4,39)
Single−Person Households in %	4,429 (4,43)	−9,315** (3,25)	1,041 (4,04)	−6,593** (2,37)	3,622 (4,93)
Immigrants in %	−15,685*** (3,58)	−7,856** (2,68)	−6,661* (3,30)	−10,046*** (2,44)	−15,960*** (3,63)
Particulate Matter (PM 10)	−2,988 (1,95)	0,739 (1,81)	−3,422 (1,80)	−0,179 (1,48)	−2,067 (1,92)
Year 2007	−637,721*** (31,80)	−576,277*** (32,89)	−628,767*** (27,37)	−586,597*** (29,41)	−739,949*** (68,96)
Year 2008	−316,683*** (23,21)	−312,976*** (21,37)	−148,151*** (42,11)	−312,622*** (20,07)	−399,917*** (42,43)
Constants	6808,650*** (1247,22)	7204,256*** (1465,95)	3720,273 (2109,81)	7229,778*** (1447,05)	6118,658*** (1458,26)
N	1.238	1.238	1.238	1.238	1.238
Specialist Hospitalizations	0,297 (0,21)	0,178 (0,23)	1,259** (0,45)	0,569 (0,33)	−0,797 (1,31)
Specialist Ambulatory Cases	−1,616*** (0,39)	−0,874* (0,42)	−3,759*** (1,00)	−4,453*** (1,30)	−1,339** (0,41)
GP Physician Density	727,780*** (151,53)	646,518*** (170,14)	530,148** (179,20)	451,625* (181,75)	556,333*** (154,93)
Male Life Expectancy	−54,815*** (16,44)	−68,119*** (13,62)	−51,877** (17,10)	−44,313* (19,47)	−69,495*** (18,80)
Female Life Expectancy	16,669 (15,86)	10,755 (16,83)	8,224 (17,78)	18,368 (23,83)	2,214 (15,48)

Table 10 Complete estimation results of the 3SLS: Eq. (3) *Continued*

GP cases	Orthopaedics	Gynaecology	ENT	Neurology	Dermatology
RSA Risk Factor	1448,408***	1501,701***	1264,721***	1721,808**	1673,007**
	(265,12)	(368,27)	(264,22)	(661,84)	(513,41)
Long—Term Care Recipients per 10.000 Population	−0,100	0,321	−0,574	−0,713*	0,090
	(0,25)	(0,27)	(0,37)	(0,35)	(0,25)
Unemployment Rate in %	−19,411***	−30,104***	−15,279**	−15,843*	−27,920***
	(5,09)	(5,48)	(5,19)	(6,40)	(4,73)
Net Monthly Household Income	−0,150*	−0,122	−0,037	−0,235**	−0,119
	(0,07)	(0,11)	(0,08)	(0,08)	(0,07)
Number of Large Regional Centres	52,497**	66,471***	47,696*	79,434***	70,791***
	(17,75)	(19,28)	(21,61)	(23,87)	(17,62)
Number of Medium Regional Centres	−5,559	2,750	−1,995	−4,924	0,677
	(4,37)	(4,18)	(4,52)	(4,76)	(3,71)
Highly Qualified Workers in %	10,878*	9,807	5,665	4,339	17,526*
	(4,60)	(7,39)	(5,18)	(5,27)	(8,30)
Low—Skilled Workers in %	−1,281	−6,163	−2,909	6,216	−7,735
	(3,80)	(4,05)	(4,17)	(5,23)	(5,90)
Single—Person Households in %	4,837	6,460	18,482*	18,637**	2,506
	(3,59)	(6,70)	(7,23)	(6,47)	(3,88)
Immigrants in %	−9,329**	−12,246**	−11,197***	−8,582*	−10,296**
	(2,85)	(4,32)	(3,20)	(3,80)	(3,95)
Particulate Matter (PM 10)	−1,767	−2,564	−1,574	−5,803*	−4,060
	(1,68)	(2,11)	(1,91)	(2,71)	(2,09)
Year 2007	−661,415***	−656,445***	−686,662***	−702,031***	−635,668***
	(31,22)	(48,38)	(38,98)	(60,98)	(34,01)
Year 2008	−326,545***	−322,895***	−333,583***	−340,861***	−314,415***
	(22,87)	(27,16)	(26,65)	(32,32)	(22,89)
Constants	4492,968**	5784,788***	4400,430**	3203,080	7198,978***
	(1678,49)	(1554,32)	(1635,34)	(2502,86)	(1535,34)
N	1.238	1.238	1.238	1.238	1.238

Standard error in parentheses, * $p<0,10$,** $p<0,05$,*** $p<0,01$
Note: All above mentioned variables were controlled for. Full results can be found in the Appendix

Acknowledgements
The authors thank two anonymous referees, Aloys Prinz, and participants of the annual meeting of the health economics section of the German economic association for valuable comments that improved the paper considerably. We gratefully acknowlege financial support by the "Bundesministerium für Bildung und Forschung" (BMBF).

Authors' contributions
All authors mentioned above have read the manuscript and agreed to its content and are accountable for all aspects of the accuracy and integrity of the manuscript in accordance with ICMJE criteria that is: all authors (i) make substantial contributions to the acquisition of the data or its analysis and interpretation, (ii) participated in drafting and revising the article in a way which is critically for its important intellectual content, (iii) gave their final approval of the version which is resubmitted to Health Economics Review. All authors read and approved the final manuscript.

Competing interests
The authors declare that they have no competing interests.

Author details
[1]Universität Duisburg-Essen, Essen, Germany. [2]CINCH - National Research Center for Health Economics, Essen, Germany. [3]RWI - Leibniz-Institut für Wirtschaftsforschung, Essen, Germany. [4]Ruhr-Universität Bochum, Bochum, Germany. [5]Kassenärztliche Bundesvereinigung, Berlin, Germany. [6]Universität Paderborn, Paderborn, Germany. [7]Friedrich-Alexander-Universität Erlangen-Nürnberg, Findelgasse 7/9, 90402 Nürnberg, Germany.

References
1. Boris A, Rosemarie G, Sebastian K, Christoph MS, Hartmut S, Hendrik S, Stefan T. Krankenhaus Rating Report 2011: Die fetten Jahre sind vorbei-Executive Summary. RWI Materialien. #, 2011. RWI - Leibniz-Institut für Wirtschaftsforschung, Essen. URL: http://www.rwi-essen.de/media/content/pages/publikationen/rwi-materialien/M_67_Krankenhaus-Rating-2011.pdf.
2. OECD. Health Data 2009. 2009. OECD Publishing.
3. Malcomson JM. Health service gatekeepers. RAND J Econ. 2004;35(2): 401–21.
4. González P. Gatekeeping versus direct-access when patient information matters. Health Econ. 2010;19(6):730–54.
5. Garrido MV, Zentner A, Busse R. The effects of gatekeeping: A systematic review of the literature. Scand J Prim Health Care. 2011;29(1):28–38.
6. Brekke KR, Nuscheler R, Straume OR. Gatekeeping in health care. J Health Econ. 2007;26(1):149–70.
7. Atella V, Deb, P. Are primary care physicians, public and private sector specialists substitutes or complements? Evidence from a simultaneous equations model for count data. J Health Econ. 2008;27(3):770–85.
8. Adhikari, SR. An assessment of a substitute or complement for inpatient and outpatient care of visceral leishmaniasis in Nepal. J Vector Borne Dis. 2012;49(4):242–8.
9. Fortney JC, Steffick DE, Burgess JF, Maciejewski ML, Petersen LA. Are primary care services a substitute or complement for specialty and inpatient services? Health Serv Res. 2005;40(5 Pt 1):1422–42.
10. Kopetsch T. Der Zusammenhang zwischen dem Leistungsgeschehen im ambulanten und stationären Sektor des deutschen Gesundheitswesens: Eine empirische Untersuchung/The Relationship Between Service Events in the Ambulatory and Hospital Sectors of the German Health System: An Empirical Study. Jahrbücher für Nationalökonomie und Statistik / J Econ Stat. 2007;227(1):49–64.
11. Albrecht M, Freytag A, Gottberg A, Storz P. Effiziente Strukturen ärztlicher Versorgung. Der Urologe. 2007;46(8):844–50.
12. Sobhani B, Kersting T. Wettbewerb zwischen Ärzten und Krankenhaus–Krankenhäuser als Gewinner? Zeitschrift für Evidenz. Fortbildung und Qualität im Gesundheitswesen. 2009;103(10):666–9.
13. Voigt G. Wettbewerb zwischen niedergelassen Ärzten und Krankenhäusern–Konsequenzen für den niedergelassenen Arzt. Zeitschrift für Evidenz, Fortbildung und Qualität im Gesundheitswesen. 2009;103(10):662–5.
14. Busse R. Wettbewerb im Gesundheitswesen–eine Gesundheitssystemperspektive. Zeitschrift für Evidenz. Fortbildung und Qualität im Gesundheitswesen, Evidenz. 2009;103(10):608–15.
15. Himmel W, Kochen MM, Sorns U, Hummers-Pradier E. Drug changes at the interface between primary and secondary care. Int J Clin Pharmacol Ther. 2004;42(2):103–9.
16. Hach I, Maywald U, Meusel D, König JU, Kirch W. Continuity of long-term medication use after surgical hospital stay. Eur J Clin Pharmacol. 2005;61(5-6):433–8.
17. Weinberger M, Oddone EZ, Henderson WG. Does increased access to primary care reduce hospital readmissions? N Engl J Med. 1996;334(22): 1441–7.
18. Coleman EA, Parry C, Chalmers S, Min S-J. The care transitions intervention: results of a randomized controlled trial. Arch Intern Med. 2006;166(17):1822–8.
19. Grossman M. On the concept of health capital and the demand for health. J Polit Econ. 1972;80(2):223–55.
20. Augurzky B, Kopetsch T, Schmitz H. What accounts for the regional differences in the utilisation of hospitals in Germany? Eur J Health Econ. 2013;14(4):615–27.
21. Kopetsch T, Schmitz H. Regional variation in the utilisation of ambulatory services in Germany. Health Econ. 2014;23(12):1481–92.
22. Statistisches Bundesamt. Wiesbaden: Statistisches Bundesamt; 2011.

2

Effect of reducing cost sharing for outpatient care on children's inpatient services in Japan

Hirotaka Kato[1*] and Rei Goto[2]

Abstract

Background: Assessing the impact of cost sharing on healthcare utilization is a critical issue in health economics and health policy. It may affect the utilization of different services, but is yet to be well understood.

Objective: This paper investigates the effects of reducing cost sharing for outpatient services on hospital admissions by exploring a subsidy policy for children's outpatient services in Japan.

Methods: Data were extracted from the Japanese Diagnosis Procedure Combination database for 2012 and 2013. A total of 366,566 inpatients from 1390 municipalities were identified. The impact of expanding outpatient care subsidy on the volume of inpatient care for 1390 Japanese municipalities was investigated using the generalized linear model with fixed effects.

Results: A decrease in cost sharing for outpatient care has no significant effect on overall hospital admissions, although this effect varies by region. The subsidy reduces the number of overall admissions in low-income areas, but increases it in high-income areas. In addition, the results for admissions by type show that admissions for diagnosis increase particularly in high-income areas, but emergency admissions and ambulatory-care-sensitive-condition admissions decrease in low-income areas.

Conclusions: These results suggest that outpatient and inpatient services are substitutes in low-income areas but complements in high-income ones. Although the subsidy for children's healthcare would increase medical costs, it would not improve the health status in high-income areas. Nevertheless, it could lead to some health improvements in low-income areas and, to some extent, offset costs by reducing admissions in these regions.

Keywords: Heath insurance, Cost sharing, Childcare, Inpatient care, Outpatient care

JEL codes: I12, I18, J13

Background

Many countries have adopted patient cost sharing as a way to control medical expenditures. However, the effects of patient cost sharing are yet to be completely understood. In particular, research on health impacts, the distributional consequences of cost sharing, and whether cost sharing for certain services affects the use of other services is sparse [1].

Cost sharing for a service could affect the utilization of the service itself (own-price effect) as well as reduce the utilization of complementary services or increase that of substitute services (cross-price effect). Therefore, it is important to examine both the cross-price and own-price effect. To this end, health policy studies have long debated the relationship between outpatient and inpatient services. While some insist that expanded access to primary care can reduce admissions, leading to reduced healthcare costs [2], this argument was empirically denied by the results of the RAND Health Insurance Experiment (HIE) in the mid-1970s [3, 4]. Given that hospitalization and emergency department admissions

---

* Correspondence: kato.hirotaka.44u@st.kyoto-u.ac.jp
[1]Graduate School of Economics, Kyoto University, Yoshida-honmachi, Sakyo, Kyoto 6068501, Japan
Full list of author information is available at the end of the article

are common measures of health and health expenditures [5] and psychological biases are likely to cause patients to overweigh the immediate cost of an outpatient service relative to expected future health benefits and costs [6], it is of critical importance to empirically assess whether reduced cost sharing for outpatient care, which is often inexpensive compared to inpatient care, affects hospitalization. Nevertheless, few studies have been conducted on the cross-price effect of reducing cost sharing for outpatient care.

This study examines whether reducing cost sharing for outpatient care increases hospitalization. If outpatient and inpatient services are substitutes, expanded access to outpatient care through reduced cost sharing decreases the number of admissions. A plausible scenario is that a primary care doctor detects and successfully treats a condition that would result in hospitalization. In this case, a reduction in the number of admissions is attributed to the decrease in the number of emergency admissions and admissions due to diseases which can be managed in primary care. On the other hand, if outpatient and inpatient services are complements, expanded access to outpatient services increases the number of admissions. In this case, it is also plausible that visiting a primary care doctor results in a referral to a specialist in the hospital and a hospitalization for diagnosis or/and treatment. If this is true, the increase in the number of admissions is attributed to the expansion in the number of non-emergency admissions and admissions for diagnosis. Therefore, analysing both total admissions and admissions by type would help to more accurately reveal the relationship between inpatient and outpatient care.

Fortunately, we have an example of a suitable policy change to empirically investigate the cross-price effect. Japan's local governments have rapidly and independently expanded subsidies for child healthcare. They have raised the upper age limit for children to access healthcare services for free or at minimal user charges. About half of them allow children to access healthcare services for free, while the other half imposes user charges—500 JPY per month as of 1 April 2012 (100 JPY equals approximately 1 USD), for example. However, the upper age limit and timing of these changes widely vary by local government. Even within a single local government, the subsidy for inpatient and outpatient care is often changed at different times. This may create exogenous variations in cost-sharing schemes for children.

Analysis of a large amount of administrative admission data shows that the subsidy for outpatient care does not significantly affect the number of overall admissions across areas. However, the effect of the subsidy on outpatient care varies by region. The outpatient care subsidy reduces the number of overall admissions in low-income areas but has the opposite effect in high-income areas, suggesting that outpatient and inpatient care are substitutes in low-income areas and complements in high-income areas.

Literature review

The HIE is a well-known study on the effects of cost sharing on the utilization of healthcare services [3, 4]. The experiment showed a significant but modest effect in response to changes in cost sharing. In particular, children from low-income households showed decreased use of healthcare services as a result of cost sharing. However, cost sharing had no impact on the health status of the overall population. Recent empirical studies on the effect of price changes also confirmed the HIE's findings on the own-price effect and health impact [7–10].

On the other hand, studies on the cross-price effect have obtained mixed results. Chandra et al. [11] examined a policy change which raised cost sharing for office visits and prescribed drugs for Medicare beneficiaries, and found it to be associated with a decrease in prescribed drugs and an increase in hospital admissions. Trivedi et al. [12] focused on an increase in cost sharing for outpatient care in Medicare, and showed the rise in co-payments reduced outpatient visits but increased hospitalization and inpatient days. Chandra et al. [13] analysed the impact of raising cost sharing for low-income populations and reported that inpatient and outpatient services might be substitutes, although their result was not statistically significant. By contrast, the HIE showed reduced primary care was associated with lower spending on hospitalization [4]. The Oregon Medicaid experiment also revealed that the expansion of health insurance is associated with increased hospitalization [7]. Kaestner and Sassob [14] showed that greater outpatient spending leads to higher inpatient spending. Thus, the findings on the cross-price effect are inconsistent. Moreover, since the majority of studies focus on the elderly or adults, there is little evidence on the cross-price effect for children. To our knowledge, there is little research on this issue outside the United States.

In Japan, Takaku [15] conducted a study on the impact of medical subsidies for children, specifically the effect of expanded outpatient care subsidy, using data from a nationally representative questionnaire survey conducted by the Ministry of Health, Labour and Welfare (MHLW). He found that the subsidy improved subjective health measures but did not reduce hospitalization for pre-school children, whereas it had no effect on the subjective health measures or hospitalization for school-aged children.

We believe our study complements Takaku's [15] in two aspects. First, we use administrative admission data which cover large areas of Japan. Since Takaku [15] referenced the questionnaire survey, there is a possibility of measurement errors, such as those due to a recall bias. He focused on whether a respondent was hospitalized on the date of the survey to identify hospitalization status. Since this clearly excludes admissions before and after the survey, the use of administrative admission data can be meaningful. Second, this study examines whether the effects of the subsidy vary by regional average income. This is important because the HIE found differential effects of cost sharing.

Institutional setting

According to official reports, all local governments subsidize out-of-pocket payments for child healthcare in Japan [16–18]. Japan's local governments are composed of two tiers: prefectures and municipalities. Prefectures define the eligibility for the subsidy but almost all municipalities expand it. Therefore, the actual grant of the subsidy is determined by the latter. Children living in the municipality and within the age limit are granted the subsidy by their respective municipalities, although many municipalities have recently increased the eligible age [15].

The subsidized children can avail of healthcare services free of cost or must incur a minimal user charge (e.g. 500 JPY per month). Without the subsidy, preschool children bear 20% of their medical costs, and the others incur 30%. Evidently, the subsidy increases access to healthcare. Note that healthcare fees are determined by the central government, and the price of medical services is common across Japan. Since the public health insurance system in Japan covers a broad range of healthcare services and private use accounts for only about 1% of total expenditure [19], the subsidy really reduces the barriers to healthcare services.

The subsidy amount varies by government since the upper age limit considerably differs by municipality. For example, the upper age limit was 22 years in Minamifurano-cho, Hokkaido Prefecture, and 4 years in Naha-shi, Okinawa Prefecture. In addition, while some governments do not offer a subsidy to children from high-income households, others do not impose such income caps. Some governments require a minimal user charge, whereas others do not. Finally, selected governments adopt an in-kind transfer method, while others prefer a refund.

Data

The data used in this study were taken from the Diagnostic Procedures Combination (DPC) Program. The DPC Program is a per-diem payment system for acute inpatient care and now includes a large number of hospitals for acute inpatient care. In 2012, about 1750 acute care hospitals (about 480,000 beds) participated in the DPC Program, which accounted for about 53% of all acute care beds in Japan. The DPC data include diverse information such as primary diagnosis, comorbidities, severities, treatment, admission route, admission date, discharge data, admission purpose, date of birth, and zip code of a patient. We use the data for children aged 6–18 years and hospitalized between fiscal year (FY) 2012 and 2013, since most municipalities had already subsidized healthcare for children aged up to 6 years by 2012. Note that, in Japan, the fiscal year begins on 1 April and ends on 31 March.

DPC data used here were offered by some DPC hospitals. In this study, we examined the admissions of 977 DPC hospitals which continuously provided their data for our study periods to ensure that our findings are not the result of hospital composition changes. Our data accounted for about 56% of all DPC hospitals.

A feature of DPC data is that they can provide detailed clinical information on admissions, which allows us to distinguish between emergency and non-emergency admissions, and between admissions for diagnosis and for treatments. It is important to investigate emergency admissions because these are particularly related to health.

DPC data might lead to selection bias because DPC hospitals cover only around half of acute care beds in Japan. It is true that our data include fewer patients admitted to smaller hospitals because DPC hospitals tend to be larger hospitals. However, hospitals with paediatrics tend to be still larger hospitals. According to the Survey of Medical Institutions published by the Ministry of Health, Labour and Welfare in 2013 [20], 1978 (73%) out of all 2702 hospitals with paediatrics have more than 100 beds. Therefore, the potential bias from using DPC hospital data is less serious if we focus on admissions of children.

Information on subsidy methods implemented by local governments was obtained from official reports [16–18]. These reports provide data on the upper age limits for inpatient and outpatient care subsidies: whether a local government imposed an income cap and if it applied user charges every year on 1 April. However, the reports do not offer information on the reimbursement method adopted by each municipality.

Local governments which did not have any patient aged 6–18 years during the study period were omitted. A total of 278 municipalities changed the upper age limits for outpatient care subsidy, and 1047 municipalities did not increase the limit during FY 2012–2013. We estimated 366,566 inpatients from 1390 municipalities. Table 1 presents the backgrounds of the patients examined in this study.

Method

Municipalities have mainly expanded the upper age limits of subsidies for children. However, the age limit

Table 1 Patient backgrounds (all admissions)

	First	Median	Average	Third	N
Age	8	12	11.715	15	366,566
Male	0	1	0.575	1	366,566
Duration of stay	3	5	8.869	9	366,566
Admission cost (JPY)	16,190	158,860	349,666.66	367,917.5	366,566
Emergency admission	0	1	0.537	1	366,566

Notes: Male = 1 if the patient is male. Emergency admission = 1 if the admission is an emergency. *JPY* Japanese yen

and timing of expansion considerably differ by municipality. We utilize these differences to identify the impact of expanding outpatient care subsidy.

We first aggregate DPC data, which are patient-level data. Using the patients' zip codes, we identify the municipalities in which patients live. Then, we count the number of admissions for each municipality by fiscal year and create municipality-level panel data for two periods. Next, we estimate our regression model. Since the subsidy change occurs at the municipality level, this study conducts the analysis at the municipality level ×fiscal year. We treat the number of admissions in each fiscal year as the dependent variable and the upper age limits for outpatient care subsidies as of April 1 2012 and 2013 as key explanatory variables. We control for the upper age limits of inpatient care subsidies, income cap, user charge, and their regional income in each year. We also include time fixed effects and municipality-level fixed effects as explanatory variables. It is necessary that unobserved factors do not change during the specification period. However, considering that we examine the admissions of 2 years and there is no change in public healthcare fee during the period, we can assume that the important unobserved factors such as population structure and providers' behaviour to fee-schedule are fairly stable during this short period. In addition, since we focus on DPC hospitals, patients' choice between DPC and non-DPC hospitals should be stable during the study period. According to a public report [21], the numbers of DPC hospitals (1505 and 1496 in April 2012 and 2013, respectively), as well as those of DPC-hospital beds (479,539 and 474,981 in April 2012 and 2013, respectively), were stable during our study period. Furthermore, as mentioned, there was no change in the public fee during this period. Thus, the number of choice patients and the price, except the cost-sharing rate, were stable. Though we believe that the association between DPC and non-DPC hospitals, which affects the patients' choices, is stable, we cannot reject the possibility of biases caused by time-variant factors affecting choice between DPC and non-DPC hospitals. Because our dependent variable is the number of admissions, we adopt a generalized linear model (GLM) and assume

that the dependent variable follows a negative binomial distribution. Note that because the variance is not statistically equal to the average, we do not adopt a Poisson distribution.

It is highly likely that the effect of the subsidy varies by population group, as the HIE found heterogeneity by income and health status, and the effect of cost sharing was particularly strong among children from low-income groups. Therefore, by dividing our sample, we can examine whether the impact of reducing cost sharing varies by regional average income level of local governments. Areas whose regional average income is higher than the median regional average income are defined as high-income areas; otherwise, they are low-income areas. The regional average income of local governments is the municipal tax on per taxpayer's income in FY 2012. Tax information was obtained from the *Survey of Local Tax* published by the Ministry of Internal Affairs and Communications.

To more clearly reveal the relationship between inpatient and outpatient care, we investigate the effects of the subsidy for each admission type. We consider two routes of admissions, two groups of primary diagnosis, and two purposes of admissions, that is, emergency and non-emergency admissions, ambulatory care sensitive condition (ACSC) and non-ACSC admission, and diagnosis and non-diagnosis admissions.

This study adopts the concept of ACSC to identify admissions sensitive to outpatient care intervention. ACSCs, which have been developed and mainly used in the United States and the United Kingdom, are conditions for which hospital admissions could have been prevented through primary care interventions [22]. We adopt the definition presented in Table 2 as the set of ACSC admissions. In our data, the number of admissions for ACSCs is 64,772, which accounts for 17.7% of all admissions.

Finally, we restrict the analysis to admissions from May to September. Since we use data on the subsidy structure as of 1 April in each year, we do not have exact data on when municipalities raised the upper age limits. In other words, we cannot deny the probability that some municipalities changed their subsidy policies during FY 2012. To address this problem and focus on the period for which we clearly understand the subsidy structure, we omit the second half of the analysed fiscal years. In addition, because April is the first month of the fiscal year, many municipalities might change their subsidies on 1 April, and admissions immediately after the policy change might be biased. Therefore, we omit admissions in April and focus on those from May to September. Table 3 reports the number of admissions for low- and high-income areas.

Table 2 Diseases defined as ambulatory care sensitive conditions (ACSCs) and number of patients by disease

ACSCs	ICD 10 codes	N
Angina	I20, I24.0, I24.8, I24.9	64
Asthma	J45, J46	13,699
Cellulitis	L03, L04, L08.0, L08.8, L08.9, L88, L98.0	2738
Congestive heart failure	I11.0, I50, J81	171
Convulsions and epilepsy	G40, G41, R56, O15	9618
Chronic obstructive pulmonary disease	J20, J41, J42, J43, J47	3705
Dehydration and gastroenteritis	E86, K52.2, K52.8, K52.9	2746
Dental conditions	A69.0, K02, K03, K04, K05, K06, K08, K09.8, K09.9, K12, K13	273
Diabetes complications	E10.0–E10.8, E11.0–E11.8, E12.0–E12.8, E13.0–E13.8, E14.0–E14.8	918
Ear nose and throat infections	H66, H67, J02, J03, J06, J31.2	8167
Gangrene	R02	1
Hypertension	I10, I11.9	43
Influenza and pneumonia	J10, J11, J13, J14, J15.3, J15.4, J15.7, J15.9, J16.8, J18.1, J18	19,684
Iron-deficiency anaemia	D50.1, D50.8, D50.9	127
Nutritional deficiency	E40, E41, E42, E43, E55.0, E64.3	22
Other vaccine-preventable diseases	A35, A36, A37, A80, B05, B06, B16.1, B16.9, B18.0, B18.1, B26, G00.0, M01.4	687
Pelvic inflammatory disease	N70, N73, N74	335
Perforated or bleeding ulcer	K25.0–K25.2, K25.4–K25.6, K26.0–K26.2, K26.4–K26.6, K27.0–K27.2, K27.4–K27.6, K280–K282, K284–K286	318
Pyelonephritis	N10, N11, N12, N13.6	1456

Source: Purdy et al. [22]

Results

Table 4 presents the descriptive statistics. The ratio of the total number of admissions in low-income areas to that in high-income areas is about 1:6, which is similar to the ratio of the populations in both areas. In low-income areas, the number of ACSC admissions is greater, and admissions for diagnosis are fewer than those in high-income areas.

Since it is important to examine the cross- and own-price effects, we present the results for both. Table 5 presents the results for overall admissions, and Table 6, for the respective effects of the subsidy by admission type.

Total number of admissions

Column (1) in Table 5 shows the effect of raising the upper age limit for the subsidy on the overall number of admissions in the total area (low- and high-income areas), and columns (2) and (3) do so for low- and high-income areas, respectively. The row showing details on ln(upper age limit of outpatient care) presents the change in total admissions as a result of expanding the upper age limit for outpatient care subsidy (cross-price effect). We find that the estimate is not significant for the total area. However, the estimate varies by regional income level: it is significantly negative in low-income areas (−0.2) but significantly positive in high-income areas (0.07). That is, raising the upper age limit for the outpatient care subsidy from 12 to 15 years (25% increase) could decrease the number of admissions by 5% in low-income areas but increase it by 2% in high-income areas.

The row showing details on ln(upper age limit of inpatient care) indicates the change in the total number of admissions caused by an increase in the upper age limit for the inpatient care subsidy (own-price effect). The estimates of the own-price effect are not significant in all columns.

Admission by type

Next, we show whether the effect of the subsidy varies by admission type. Panel A in Table 6 shows the results for the sample of the total area, while Panel B and Panel C do the same for low-income areas and high-income areas, respectively. Columns (1) and (2) show the effects on emergency and non-emergency admissions. The

Table 3 Number of admissions in the total area, and low- and high-income areas

	Total area	Low-income areas	High-income areas
Total admissions	366,566 (100%)	56,280 (100%)	310,286 (100%)
Emergency admissions	196,943 (53.7%)	31,408 (55.8%)	165,535 (53.3%)
Non-emergency admissions	169,623 (46.3%)	24,872 (44.2%)	144,751 (46.7%)
ACSC admissions	64,772 (17.7%)	11,107 (19.7%)	53,665 (17.3%)
Non-ACSC admissions	301,794 (82.3%)	45,173 (80.3%)	256,621 (87.2%)
Admissions for diagnosis	24,760 (6.8%)	2767 (4.9%)	21,993 (7.1%)
Non-diagnosis admissions	341,806 (93.2%)	53,513 (95.1%)	288,293 (92.9%)
Admissions in May–September	169,481 (46.2%)	26,043 (46.3%)	143,438 (46.2%)

ACSC ambulatory care sensitive condition

Table 4 Descriptive statistics of estimation data

	N or median (% or IQR)		
	Total area	Low-income areas	High-income areas
Number of admission			
Total admission	37 (12–111)	22 (8–52)	80 (24–217)
Emergency admission	18 (5–57)	10 (3–27)	39 (10–118)
Non-emergency admission	17.5 (6–51)	10 (4–24)	39 (12–97)
ACSC admission	6 (1–19)	3 (1–9)	11 (3–38)
Non-ACSC admission	30 (10–90)	18 (7–43)	66.5 (19–177)
Admission for diagnosis	2 (0–7)	1 (0–3)	5 (1–14)
Non-diagnosis admission	35 (11–104)	20 (7–49)	73.5 (22–200)
Admissions from May–September	17 (5–52)	10 (4–23)	38 (10–104)
Upper age limit for inpatient care	15 (12–15)	15 (12–15)	15 (15–15)
Upper age limit for outpatient care	15 (8–15)	15 (6–15)	15 (9–15)
Income cap			
With income cap	619 (22.3%)	263 (18.9%)	356 (25.6%)
Without income cap	2161 (77.7%)	1127 (81.1%)	1034 (74.4%)
User charge			
Minimal user charge	1162 (41.8%)	578 (41.6%)	584 (42%)
Free of charge	1618 (58.2%)	812 (58.4%)	806 (58%)
Regional average income (million JPY per taxpayer)	2.67 (2.46–2.95)	2.46 (2.33–2.56)	2.95 (2.78–3.18)

Source: Data on subsidy methods (upper age limits, income cap, and user charge) were sourced from the Ministry of Health, Labour and Welfare [16–18]. Data on regional average income were sourced from *Survey of Local Tax* in 2012 and 2013 published by the Ministry of Internal Affairs and Communications. IQR stands for interquartile range. *ACSC* ambulatory care sensitive condition. *JPY* Japanese yen

estimates of ln(upper age limit of outpatient care) for non-emergency admissions are significantly positive in the total area and high-income areas, whereas in the low-income areas, the estimate for emergency admissions is significantly negative. The own-price effects are not significant in both columns.

Columns (3) and (4) report the effect on ACSC and non-ACSC admissions. With regard to the total area and high-income areas, raising the upper age limit for outpatient care significantly increases non-ACSC admissions. By contrast, in low-income areas, the subsidy for outpatient services significantly reduces ACSC admissions. The estimates for ln(upper age limit of inpatient care) of ACSC admissions are significantly positive in the total area and high-income areas.

Columns (5) and (6) present the effects on diagnosis and non-diagnosis admissions. The estimates of ln(upper age limit of outpatient care) for admissions for diagnosis are significantly positive in the total area and high-income areas, whereas those for non-diagnosis admissions are significantly negative in the low-income areas. All the estimates for ln(upper age limit of inpatient care) are not significant.

Column (7) reports the result of the analysis in which we count only the admissions from May to September. The estimates in Table 5 and column (8) of Table 6 are not markedly different. The point estimates of ln(upper age limit of outpatient care) are similar in both low- and high-income areas. In addition, the estimate in low-income areas is also significant; however, that for high-

Table 5 Results for the effect of raising the upper age limit on the number of admissions

	(1)	(2)	(3)
	Total area	Low-income areas	High-income areas
ln(upper age limit of outpatient care)	0.027 [0.032]	−0.200 [0.100]	0.071 [0.03]
ln(upper age limit of inpatient care)	0.028 [0.039]	0.100 [0.069]	0.015 [0.049]
N	2780	1390	1390
AIC	17,782.07	7750.513	10,012.18

Notes: Only coefficients of the main explanatory variable are reported. The dependent variable is the number of total admissions, and explanatory variables are the dummy variables for whether the local government imposed an income cap and whether it imposed a minimal user charge, regional average income, time fixed effects, and individual fixed effects. Robust standard errors are clustered at the municipality level and reported in brackets

Table 6 Effects of raising the upper age limit on the number of admissions by type

	(1)	(2)	(3)	(4)	(5)	(6)	(7)
	Emergency admission	Non-emergency admission	ACSC admission	Non-ACSC admission	Admission for diagnosis	Non-diagnosis admission	Restricted period
Panel A. Total area							
ln(upper age limit of outpatient care)	−0.018 [0.045]	0.079 [0.033]	−0.116 [0.08]	0.064 [0.023]	0.201 [0.048]	0.017 [0.033]	0.045 [0.043]
ln(upper age limit of inpatient care)	0.058 [0.051]	−0.008 [0.039]	0.201 [0.077]	−0.01 [0.038]	−0.071 [0.092]	0.035 [0.041]	0.006 [0.055]
N	2780	2780	2780	2780	2780	2780	2780
AIC	16,194.42	15,284.45	12,412.16	16,890.36	9032.104	17,784.96	15,290.78
Panel B. Low-income areas							
ln(upper age limit of outpatient care)	−0.249 [0.12]	−0.118 [0.096]	−0.506 [0.224]	−0.06 [0.07]	0.195 [0.273]	−0.212 [0.101]	−0.166 [0.081]
ln(upper age limit of inpatient care)	0.061 [0.089]	0.125 [0.07]	0.295 [0.158]	0.028 [0.059]	0.327 [0.239]	0.086 [0.073]	0.19 [0.108]
AIC	6624.11	6444.212	4964.5	7385.877	3453.593	7677.529	6597.879
Panel C. High-income areas							
ln(upper age limit of outpatient care)	0.031 [0.046]	0.098 [0.04]	−0.01 [0.078]	0.081 [0.024]	0.191 [0.048]	0.064 [0.03]	0.079 [0.044]
ln(upper age limit of inpatient care)	0.065 [0.064]	−0.034 [0.048]	0.186 [0.093]	−0.02 [0.047]	−0.166 [0.101]	0.031 [0.051]	−0.051 [0.06]
N	1390	1390	1390	1390	1390	1390	1390
AIC	9073.718	8462.417	7259.917	9481.202	5593.513	9968.935	8942.465

Notes: Only coefficients of the main explanatory variable are reported. The dependent variable is the number of admissions by type, and the explanatory variables are the dummy variables for whether the local government imposed an income cap and whether it imposed minimal user charges, regional average income, time fixed effects, and individual fixed effects. Robust standard errors are clustered at the municipality level and reported in brackets. ACSC ambulatory care sensitive condition income areas is not significant at the 5% level but is significant at the 10% level (Table 6).

Discussion

We find that the outpatient care subsidy does not have a significant impact in the total area. However, the effects vary by regional income level: while the outpatient care subsidy decreases the number of admissions in low-income areas, it increases those in high-income areas. In addition, as expected, when the subsidy reduces the number of admissions, the number of emergency and ACSC admissions decreases, and when it increases the number of admissions, those for non-emergency and admissions for diagnosis increase.

It may be not surprising that the own-price effect is not significant because our admission data constitute patients with acute conditions, whose demand for inpatient services is probably less sensitive to price change.

Our results lead us to conclude that outpatient and inpatient services are substitutes in low-income areas but complements in high-income ones. Thus, even within the same country and time period, the relationship between inpatient and outpatient services is sensitive to regional income level. This possibly explains why previous research on the relationship between inpatient and outpatient care presents mixed results.

In addition, we assess the impact of the subsidy. In high-income areas, despite the increase in admissions for diagnosis, the number of emergency admissions does not decrease. Since the number of emergency admissions has been used as a reliable and common measure of health [5], it appears that the recent dramatic expansions of the subsidy increase medical expenditures but may not improve the health levels of children in high-income areas. However, in low-income areas, the reduction of cost sharing for outpatient care decreases the number of admissions, including emergency admissions. Although the magnitude of the effect of the subsidy on hospitalization is not as large, this implies that reducing cost sharing for outpatient care provides some health improvements, and its cost could be somewhat offset by the declining number of admissions in low-income areas. In addition, it suggests that people in low-income areas may underuse outpatient care in the absence of the subsidy.

There are numerous reasons people with varying income levels are affected differently by cost sharing [13]. First, low-income groups may simply be more responsive because they face a greater budget constraint. Second, such groups may underestimate the marginal benefits of healthcare services and thereby, underuse them probably because of their lower education levels. Third, they are more likely to suffer from chronic illness. These reasons explain why regional income level strongly affects the relationship between inpatient and outpatient care.

The contributions of this study are as follows. First, this study adopted rich administrative admission data, making it possible to avoid biases from a questionnaire survey and to allow a more accurate estimation of admissions. Since the public health insurance system in Japan covers a broad range of healthcare services, the administrative data contain almost all information on inpatient care usage. In addition, because the data cover most areas in Japan, we could report results which are not specific to a municipality or health insurer. Second, this study focuses on children. Few studies conducted on the cross-price effect have done so from the viewpoint of child admissions. Since hospitalization is highly expensive and a reliable measure of health [5], and childhood health is known to have a long-term impact [23], the findings of this study are of critical importance. The results of the cross-price effects have implications for a more suitable cost-sharing design.

The policy implication of this study is as follows. The subsidy for outpatient care increases the usage of medical services but may not achieve apparent health improvement. However, the subsidy in low-income areas may improve children's health by reducing the number of emergency admissions and ACSC admissions. Hence, the current rapid expansion of subsidy for outpatient care in Japan cannot be supported. Eligibility of subsidy for outpatient care should be more carefully examined; provision of subsidy depending on the regional income level could be more efficient. Implementing this policy may be difficult if municipalities emulate other municipalities [24, 25], which could lead to excessive yardstick competition on generous cost-sharing and deteriorations of financial conditions of particular municipalities in financial difficulties. However, the central government in Japan has the power to control each municipality to a certain extent by monitoring the use of strategic subsidy. Thus, the central government may be able to reduce the problem arising from competition on cost-sharing rate among municipalities. Furthermore, it has already begun to pay more attention to cost-containment policy for healthcare. The central government could play an important role to more efficiently design the subsidy policy in the future.

However, our study is subject to certain limitations. First, our data consist of DPC hospitals treating acute patients. Therefore, we are not sure whether our results are applicable to non-acute patients although our data include non-emergency admissions and admissions for diagnosis as shown in Table 3. In addition, we cannot access the total impact on the utilization of outpatient care. Second, we cannot directly solve the potential endogeneity of policy change. Municipalities whose admissions tend to vary might raise the upper age limit of the subsidy. Because we do not have proper instrumental variables, we cannot completely address this problem. However, many municipalities have stated that the key objective of the subsidy is to prevent a decline in birth rate, and access to health care and low birth rate are administered by different sections in many municipalities. Therefore, this endogeneity is probably not a serious problem. Nevertheless, if municipalities decide their subsidies based on the decisions of other municipalities, the change in cost sharing is not independent, which may create a bias in our results. We do not overcome this potential problem.

Third, our results might be biased due to the confounding variables which cannot be controlled by fixed effects: we cannot completely control the bias arising from the change in the population or population structure which is associated with subsidy policy. For example, the subsidy policy could induce patient relocations: it is likely that parents with sick children move to an area whose government offers a larger subsidy. Patient relocation inevitably alters the population number and its structure, thereby affecting the number of admissions. Although the incentive to relocate may not be strong since the eligibility for the subsidy is temporary (as children will eventually outgrow the target age of subsidies (15)) and the relocation problem could not explain the decrease in the number of admissions in low-income areas, our results might be biased to some extent because of the above-mentioned problem.

Finally, as mentioned, the subsidy structure is not completely understood in this study. Owing to the lack of data, we are unaware of the exact time each government expanded its subsidy and of the reimbursement method (in-kind transfer or refund). Although this may cause biases, since the results of the restricted analysis do not markedly differ from the main findings, and the change in reimbursement methods does not completely explain why some admission types are affected and others are not, we believe that the biases do not fully erode the key conclusions of this study. However, it is desirable to more accurately understand the finer details of the subsidy policy. These issues will be addressed in future research.

Conclusions

We find that reduced cost sharing for outpatient care decreases the number of admissions in low-income areas, while it increases those in high-income areas. These results suggest that outpatient and inpatient services are substitutes in low-income areas but complements in high-income ones. Our study makes a significant contribution to the literature because research on cross-price effects is limited. Our findings expand our understanding of the relationship between inpatient and outpatient care, and show the importance of considering variation in the effects of cost sharing by subpopulation. This could help implement more effective health insurance design and policy.

Acknowledgements
We thank Professor Yasunaga and Dr. Matsui (The University of Tokyo) for providing us with data. We also thank Dr. Yuda (Chukyo University), and the participants of the conferences of the Japan Health Economics Association in Tokyo (2016) and of the Japan Economic Association in Nagoya (2016) for their valuable comments.

Funding
This research is funded by JSPS KAKENHI Grant Numbers 15 J03333 and 15 K03508, and grants from the Ministry of Health, Labour and Welfare, Japan (H27-Policy-Strategic-011), and Actualize Energetic Life by Creating Brain Information Industries of ImPACT program of Cabinet Office, Government of Japan.

Authors' contributions
HK contributed to all aspects of the study, including manuscript preparation and submission. RG worked on the design of, preparation for, and conduct of the study, as well as the interpretation of results, editing, and final approval of the manuscript. Both authors read and approved the final manuscript.

Competing interests
The authors declare that they have no competing of interests.

Author details
[1]Graduate School of Economics, Kyoto University, Yoshida-honmachi, Sakyo, Kyoto 6068501, Japan. [2]Graduate School of Business Administration, Keio University, Yokohama, Japan.

References
1. Kiil A, Houlberg K. How does copayment for health care services affect demand, health and redistribution? A systematic review of the empirical evidence from 1990 to 2011. Eur J Health Econ. 2014;15(8):813–28.
2. Rittenhouse DR, Shortell SM. The patient-centered medical home: will it stand the test of health reform? JAMA. 2009;301(19):2038–40.
3. Lohr KN, Brook RH, Kamberg CJ, Goldberg GA, Leibowitz A, Keesey J, et al. Use of medical Care in the Rand Health Insurance Experiment: diagnosis- and service-specific analyses in a randomized controlled trial. Med Care. 1986;24(9):S1–S87.
4. Newhouse JP, Insurance Experiment Group. Free for all?: lessons from the RAND health insurance experiment. 2nd ed: Harvard University Press; 1993.
5. Goldman DP, Joyce GF, Zheng Y. Prescription drug cost sharing: associations with medication and medical utilization and spending and health. JAMA. 2007;298(1):61–9.
6. Baicker K, Mullainathan S, Schwartzstein J. Behavioral hazard in health insurance. Q J Econ. 2015;130(4):1623–67.
7. Finkelstein A, Taubman S, Wright B, Bernstein M, Gruber J, Newhouse JP, et al. The Oregon health insurance experiment: evidence from the first year*. Q J Econ. 2012;127(3):1057–106.
8. Fukushima K, Mizuoka S, Yamamoto S, Iizuka T. Patient cost sharing and medical expenditures for the elderly. J Health Econ. 2016;45:115–30.
9. Han H-W, Lien HM, Yang T-T. Patient cost sharing and healthcare utilization in early childhood: evidence from a regression discontinuity design. 2016.
10. Shigeoka H. The effect of patient cost sharing on utilization, health, and risk protection. Am Econ Rev. 2014;104(7):2152–84.

11. Chandra A, Gruber J, McKnight R. Patient cost-sharing and hospitalization offsets in the elderly. Am Econ Rev. 2010;100(1):193–213.

12. Trivedi AN, Moloo H, Mor V. Increased ambulatory care copayments and hospitalizations among the elderly. N Engl J Med. 2010;362(4):320–8.

13. Chandra A, Gruber J, McKnight R. The impact of patient cost-sharing on low-income populations: evidence from Massachusetts. J Health Econ. 2014;33:57–66.

14. Kaestner R, Sasso ATL. Does seeing the doctor more often keep you out of the hospital? J Health Econ. 2015;39:259–72.

15. Takaku R. Effects of reduced cost-sharing on children's health: evidence from Japan. Soc Sci Med. 2016;151:46–55.

16. Ministry of Health, Labour and Welfare. Survey on the Medical Subsidy for Infants and Children in 2012 2013 [Available from: http://www.mhlw.go.jp/stf/houdou/2r9852000002xx3m.html.

17. Ministry of Health, Labour and Welfare. Survey on the Medical Subsidy for Infants and Children in 2013 2014 [Available from: http://www.mhlw.go.jp/stf/houdou/0000040997.html.

18. Ministry of Health, Labour and Welfare. Survey on the Medical Subsidy for Infants and Children in 2014 2015 [Available from: http://www.mhlw.go.jp/stf/houdou/0000078806.html.

19. Ministry of Health, Labour and Welfare. Survey on national health expenditure 2016 [Available from: http://www.mhlw.go.jp/toukei/saikin/hw/k-iryohi/14/.

20. Ministry of Health, Labour and Welfare. Survey of Medical Institutions. 2013.

21. Ministry of Health, Labour and Welfare. Size of DPC hospitals and that of hospitals participating in DPC survey 2014 [Available from: http://www.mhlw.go.jp/file/05-Shingikai-12404000-Hokenkyoku-Iryouka/0000041708.pdf.

22. Purdy S, Griffin T, Salisbury C, Sharp D. Ambulatory care sensitive conditions: terminology and disease coding need to be more specific to aid policy makers and clinicians. Public Health. 2009;123(2):169–73.

23. Currie J. Healthy, wealthy, and wise: socioeconomic status, poor health in childhood, and human capital development. J Econ Lit. 2009;47(1):87–122.

24. Besley T, Case A. Incumbent behavior: vote-seeking, tax-setting, and yardstick competition. Am Econ Rev. 1995;85(1):25–45.

25. Case AC, Rosen HS, Hines JR. Budget spillovers and fiscal policy interdependence. J Public Econ. 1993;52(3):285–307.

3

Medicare modernization and diffusion of endoscopy in FFS medicare

Lee R. Mobley[1*], Pedro Amaral[2], Tzy-Mey Kuo[3], Mei Zhou[1] and Srimoyee Bose[1]

Abstract

Objective: To examine how FFS Medicare utilization of endoscopy procedures for colorectal cancer (CRC) screening changed after implementation of the Medicare Prescription Drug, Improvement, and Modernization Act (MMA) in 2006, which provided subsidized drug coverage and expanded the geographic availability of Medicare managed care plans across the US.
Data Sources/Study Setting. Using secondary data from 100% FFS Medicare enrollees, we analyzed endoscopy utilization during two intervals, 2001-2005 and 2006-2009.

Study design: We examined change in predictors of county-level endoscopy utilization rates based on a conceptual model of market supply and demand with spillovers from managed care practices. The equations for each period were estimated jointly in a spatial lag regression model that properly accounts for both place and time effects, allowing robust assessment of changes over time.

Data collection/Extraction methods: All Medicare FFS enrollees with both Parts A and B coverage who were age 65+, remained alive and living in the same state over the interval were included in the analyses. The later interval used a new cohort defined the same as the earlier interval. 100% Medicare denominator files were also used, providing county of address to use for county-level aggregation. The outcome variable was defined as county-level proportion of enrollees who ever used endoscopy over the interval.

Principal findings: Endoscopy utilization by FFS Medicare increased, and became more accessible across the US. Medicare managed care plan spillovers onto FFS Medicare endoscopy utilization changed over time from a significant negative (restraining) effect in the early period to no significant effect by the later period.

Conclusions: The MMA eased budget constraints for seniors, making endoscopic CRC screening more affordable. The MMA policies also strengthened managed care business prospects, and enrollments in Medicare managed care escalated. The change in managed care spillover effects reflects the gradual acceptance of endoscopic CRC screening procedures, as they emerged as the gold standard during the period.

Background

Utilization of endoscopic procedures (colonoscopy, sigmoidoscopy) for colorectal cancer (CRC) screening is effective in preventing precancerous tumors from developing into cancer, however the utilization rate is lower than recommended guidelines [1–3]. In 2001, the Centers for Medicare and Medicaid Services (CMS) expanded Medicare coverage to cover colonoscopy for persons with average risk for CRC, in the face of an emerging body of cost-effectiveness research on endoscopy screening for

CRC and evidence recommending use of colonoscopy [4]. Over the next six years, utilization of colonoscopy diffused rapidly across FFS Medicare markets, and came to dominate the endoscopy services. At first, the expansion occurred in those markets with more favorable business prospects, and was slower to diffuse to minority-dominated areas [5]. Although the expansion in coverage for endoscopy helped improve uptake of endoscopic screening procedures, it still left the beneficiary facing substantial out-of-pocket copayments and facility fees, and utilization rates were suboptimal according to emerging screening guidelines.

In 2006, the implementation of the Medicare Prescription Drug, Improvement, and Modernization Act (MMA) offered subsidized prescription drug packages to seniors, available to

* Correspondence: lmobley@gsu.edu
[1]Georgia State University, 1 Park Place, Suite 700, Atlanta, GA 30304, USA
Full list of author information is available at the end of the article

both traditional fee-for-service (FFS) enrollees and managed care plan enrollees. The savings afforded by the drug plan coverage might have loosened budget constraints for many seniors, perhaps making the endoscopy copayments more affordable. Thus it is reasonable to expect that there might have been an increase in demand for endoscopic CRC screening after implementation of the MMA in 2006.

In addition, the MMA led to considerable expansion in the Medicare managed care program across the US. The Act renamed the Medicare + Choice program the Medicare Advantage (MA) program, and made it much more attractive to seniors by adding prescription drug coverage to all MA plans [6]. CMS also re-defined the so-called 'CMS Regions' into ten new areas configured to enhance expansion of MA plans into all areas of the US ([7]; CMS [8]). The Medicare managed care penetration rate increased from 15% in 2000 to 24% in 2010 and continued to increase thereafter [9]. Figure 1 shows the penetration by Medicare MA plans in 2005 (before The Act was implemented), and in 2015 (most recent data available) across the ten CMS regions.

Managed care plans have been reputed to disseminate best-practice guidelines and encourage use of preventative services with established cost-effectiveness evidence. Managed care penetration may have helped encourage the diffusion of colonoscopy as a CRC screening procedure. In 2008, colonoscopy was recommended as one of the primary colorectal cancer screening tests by the United States Preventive Services Task Force, following a systematic review of studies demonstrating colonoscopy as a cost-effective CRC screening procedure [10–12]. Since then one might expect that managed care practices would embrace and disseminate this information, resulting in an increase of colonoscopy utilization for CRC screening. Such a phenomenon may also spill over to non-managed care enrollees, as prior studies have shown managed care practices influence and spill over onto other market constituents, including Medicare FFS enrollees [13, 14]. For example, using data from 1999 and 2001-2006, two studies found modest spillover effects from MA penetration on FFS Medicare utilization of endoscopy for CRC screening [5, 15]. Therefore, it is reasonable to expect that the demand for endoscopic CRC screening increased for FFS Medicare enrollees through spillover effects from MA penetration after implementation of the MMA.

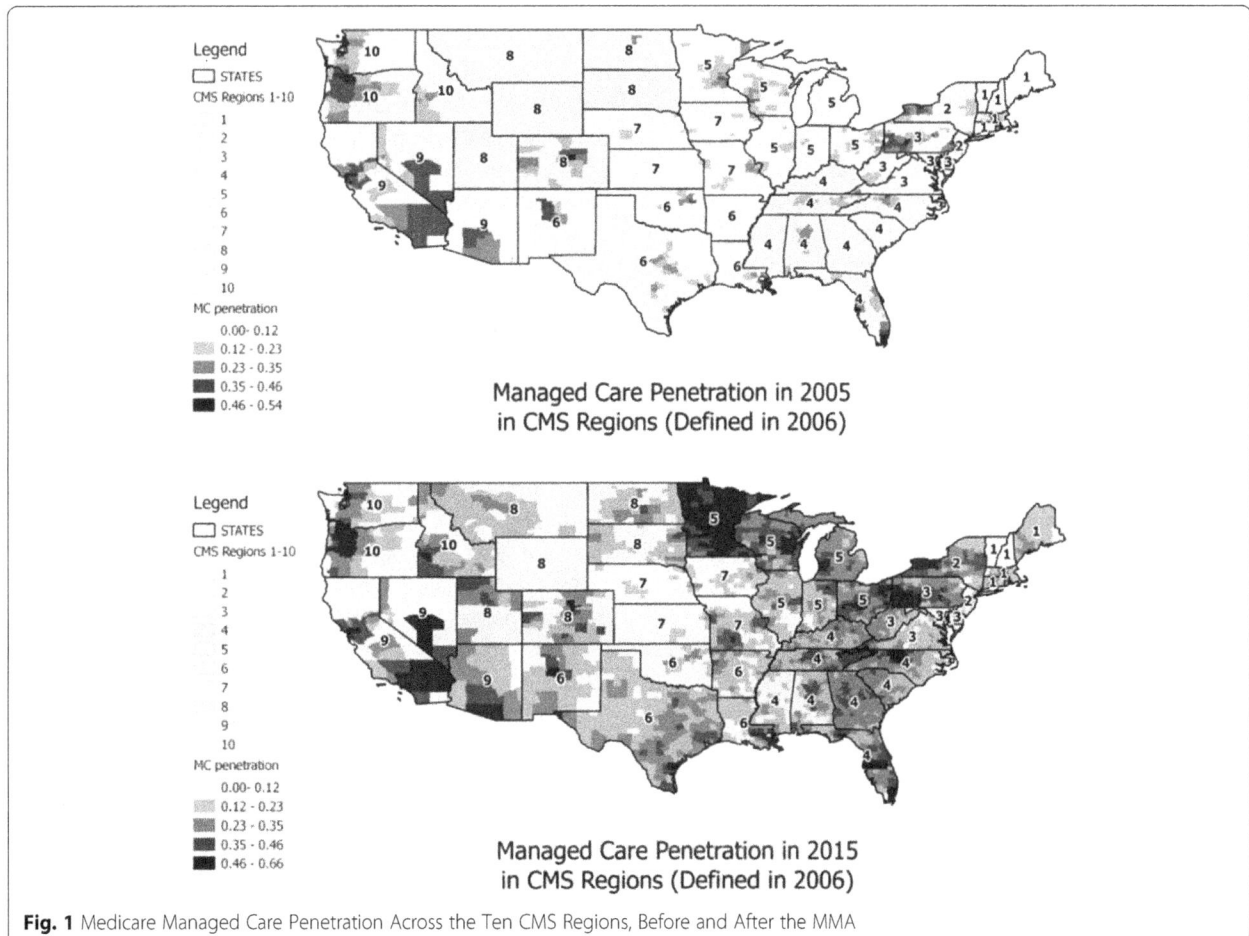

Fig. 1 Medicare Managed Care Penetration Across the Ten CMS Regions, Before and After the MMA

In this study, we exploited the natural experiment provided by the MMA implementation in 2006, to determine how the changes in market conditions during this decade predicted utilization of endoscopic CRC screening among the aged. The focus is on the traditional FFS Medicare enrollees for whom complete medical claims exist for study. Relaxation of personal budget constraints due to newly available subsidies, and market spillover effects emanating from managed care expansion are expected to increase both supply and demand for these services.

Methods
Conceptual model
We adapt the conceptual model used in published studies which included a comprehensive set of supply and demand factors that would determine the feasibility of establishing endoscopic CRC screening services in a given market [5, 16]. Acquisition of endoscopy equipment and the necessary training to use it will depend on the expected return on investment, which is a function of market conditions. Observed utilization rates will depend on various market factors, summarized in Table 1, which describes the variables we use to capture these aspects.

From the perspective of determinants of market potential, we use demographic factors defined for all Medicare eligibles (including those under age 65) from the Medicare denominator file to characterize the age distribution, race or ethnicity, and vulnerability in the Medicare population. Vulnerability is defined as eligibility for additional benefits to assist the low income (who may be dually eligible for Medicare and Medicaid benefits), the disabled, and those with end-stage renal disease (ESRD). This measure of vulnerability also captures some degree of medical need or comorbidity. Areas with higher percentages of vulnerable beneficiaries are not expected to be as manageable or as profitable for managed care plans that were reluctant to expand into all markets after experimental demonstrations by CMS offered substantial subsidies [17]. The acculturation, educational attainment, and area poverty variables capture aspects of demand for the services. The first two are defined for persons aged 65+, while area poverty is defined as average area poverty over two decades. Better educated elderly with good English language skills are expected to have a better grasp of the benefits and a greater demand for endoscopic screening. Persistently poorer areas are not expected to be attractive to entry by endoscopy providers. Market size, which affects the pace of return on investment, is reflected in population density and the percent of the population with Medicare Part A benefits. We surmise that the higher the percentage of the population with Medicare Part A benefits, the more important is Medicare as a demand segment in the market.

Health market conditions are reflected by the geographic density of endoscopy providers, measured as the average distance among FFS claimants to providers closest to their ZIP code of residence, and a competition index among endoscopy providers (an inverse Herfindahl index, where 0 = no competition and 1 = maximal competition). Another health market condition factor is the prevalence of Medicare managed care plans, which may have spillover effects on FFS enrollee utilization rates.

Managed care spillovers
There has been sustained interest over the years in the impacts of managed care plans on other market participants, the so-called 'spillover effects' of managed care. Defined as changes in financial incentives, physician practice patterns, costs, or the diffusion of new technology relative to what might occur in markets with little managed care influence - spillovers have been examined empirically for over twenty years [5, 13, 14, 18–24].

Changes in practice patterns for a substantial proportion of insured patients can spill over to people who are not insured by the managed care plans (including the FFS Medicare population) who are seen by the same physicians influenced by the managed care practices and protocols. Also, individuals not enrolled in managed care plans might compare prescribed treatment options with their peers who are enrolled in managed care plans. These behavioral spillovers among people and physicians ensure that managed care plans can impact the way medicine is practiced in their markets. With particular relevance to this study, managed care spillovers can impact adherence to CRC screening guidelines by patients, irrespective of whether they are enrolled in managed care plans.

To obtain robust and reliable estimates for these spillovers onto FFS Medicare utilization, empirical models must deal with sources of selection bias that could influence the estimates [5, 13]. Selection effects can be related to the relative generosity of MA plan versus FFS plan payment rates, the fact that wealthier elderly would have to give up supplemental coverage to enroll in managed care, the benefits to lower income elderly of obtaining 'free' Part B coverage by enrolling in managed care plans, and other socio-economic factors varying from place to place [5, 18, 25–27]. These socio-economic factors are expected to impact the demography of enrollment into MA plans, and the specifics of particular markets that MA plans may choose to enter. Factors among the Medicare population such as lower income or greater morbidity, age distribution, and racial or ethnic concentrations that vary from place to place are all factors that may have impacted where MA plans originally entered and attracted enrollees. After the MMA implementation in 2006, MA plans spread across the US to enter new markets not previously served, where spillover

Table 1 Market conditions fostering FFS Medicare utilization of endoscopy services, and variables used in modeling

	2001-2005		2006-2009		
	Mean	St. Dev	Mean	St. Dev	Source
Dependent Variable: Avg. Annual % Endoscopy Utilization	7.4	1.2	7.9	1.3	100% of traditional FFS Medicare endoscopy claims
Market Demographics of the Medicare population (%)					
Age < 65	16.9	6.1	18.4	6.1	100% Medicare denominator files, averages 2001-2005; 2006-2010
Age 65-74	44.5	3.7	43.5	3.9	
Age 75-84	28.6	3.6	27.2	3.5	
Age 85+	9.9	2.4	10.9	2.8	
Female	55.0	2.8	54.2	2.5	
Caucasian	90.6	13.2	90.2	13.5	
African American	7.3	12.7	7.5	12.9	
Hispanic	1.0	3.2	1.0	2.9	
Asian	0.3	0.8	0.3	1.0	
American Indian and other races/ethnicities	0.8	4.3	1.0	4.9	
Dual/ESRD/disabled benefits	20.9	10.7	27.9	10.6	
Acculturation and educational attainment of the market population, and area poverty:					
Persons Aged 65+ with little or no English language ability (2000)	14.3	14.7	14.3	14.7	US Census 2000; American Community Survey, 2006-2010; Census SAIPE
Persons aged 65+ with graduate or professional degrees (2000; 2006-2010)	4.4	2.8	5.7	4.0	
Average poverty in the area over the past 20 years (1990-2000; 1995-2005)	14.8	6.7	14.1	5.7	
Market size, which affects pace of return on investment:					
Population density (2000, 2005) per sq. mile	235.1	1661.8	242.8	1713.4	Area Health Resource Files
Percent of the population with Medicare Part A benefits (2001, 2006)	14.1	2.0	14.8	2.0	
Health market conditions:					
Prevalence of managed care plans: Medicare managed care penetration, lagged 1 year (2000, 2005)	4.9	9.7	4.6	8.4	RTI Spatial Impact Factor Database
Prevalence of endoscopy providers: average distance from FFS claimants to closest provider (2001, 2006)	10.4	8.8	11.7	9.2	
Competition among endoscopy providers (2001, 2006) index, where 1 = perfect and 0 = no competition	0.020	0.046	0.021	0.052	

effects might reach fertile new ground. So there are many reasons to expect changes over time in the ecological model of county-level utilization of endoscopic CRC screening by the FFS Medicare population.

Analysis samples, outcomes, and contextual factors

To examine how the MMA may have influenced endoscopic CRC screening utilization for the Medicare FFS enrollees, we constructed the population-based study sample in two cohorts based on the 100% FFS insured Medicare enrollees. First, we included the entire Medicare FFS population aged 65+ each year during 2001-2005, or 2006–2009. We then excluded all persons who did not have *traditional FFS Medicare coverage* (defined as both Parts A and B coverage for at least 11 months of the year) for all years in each interval. We excluded people who died or who moved to a different state during the interval, and a new cohort was derived using

these criteria for the second interval. Current CRC screening guidelines for persons of average risk from the USPSTF recommend fecal occult blood testing (FOBT) every year, sigmoidoscopy every 5 years, and colonoscopy every 10 years. We focus only on the diffusion of endoscopy services because they are costly to provide and their availability is expected to fluctuate with market conditions. Following the approach in a previous study, we focus on 'any utilization', rather than attempting to ascertain optimal utilization patterns for each beneficiary, which is beyond the scope of this paper [5]. Focusing on 'any utilization' allows us to ascertain availability and diffusion of the services as predicted by market influences.

We first created an indicator for whether or not an individual had *ever used either of the services* over the interval. Services were defined using a comprehensive list of medical procedure codes consistent with other studies of endoscopic technology utilization for CRC screening (G0104,G0105,G0121,44388-44397,45300, 45305, 45308, 45309, 45315, 45317, 45320, 45327,45330,45331, 45333-45335, 45338-45342, 45345, 45355, 45378-45387, 45391, 45392) [2, 5, 15]. Procedures include, among other things, 'screening with polyp removal and biopsy', which insurers view as 'diagnostic'. We include these because this more complex endoscopic procedure is prescribed by the endoscopy guidelines to meet the gold standard of screening for CRC. If the person used endoscopy more than once, the county of residence at first use was kept as the county of record for the analysis.

The sum of these person-level endoscopy utilization indicators by county is the numerator used in creating the county proportion of all traditional FFS Medicare enrollees (defined above) who had ever used one of the services over the interval. Because the early period is 1 year longer than the late period, and we desire a fair comparison of changes in utilization rates over time, we created the average annual utilization rate in each period by dividing the multi-year construct by the number of years it spanned. Thus the outcome variable of interest is the average annual utilization rate in the county for endoscopy services used during 2001-2005 or 2006-2009, among traditional FFS Medicare enrollees. The county-level proportion was defined separately for each county and time interval, and converted to a percentage for use in the analysis.

For the market contextual factors, we used 100% Medicare population demographic information from the Medicare denominator files to describe characteristics of beneficiaries, including age groups, sex, race or ethnicity, and vulnerability (Dual, disabled, ESRD) status. Averages over the intervals were used to represent these compositional factors. Other factors describing local market conditions were drawn from the U.S. Census and American Community Survey, the Area Health Resources Files, and the RTI Spatial Impact Factor database (see Table 1). These ecological variables together reflect aggregate market conditions in all counties across the continental United States, over the two time periods. Managed care penetration was defined for a one-year lag prior to each interval (2000 for 2001-2005; 2005 for 2006-2009) to reduce potential endogeneity. This variable was constructed from the CMS Geographic Service Area files, which provide the county number and proportion of enrollees in various types of plans (including managed care plans) by county.

Descriptive analyses

We calculated descriptive statistics for the variables we included in the statistical models, for the early (2001-2005) and late (2006-2009) periods, summarized in Table 1. In addition, we used mapping of the average annual utilization rates by county in each period to discern whether there was apparent diffusion of these services over the geography of the US (Fig. 2). Using the same cutpoints in the two figures allows a fair comparison over time of the average annual percent of FFS Medicare enrollees ever using these services each period. It is evident from a comparison of the two periods that average utilization increased over time and diffused or spread out over more geographic areas over time, as endoscopy became an accepted component of the gold standard for CRC screening.

Statistical analysis

To estimate the associations between ecological factors and market outcomes, and how these may have changed over time, the challenge is to simultaneously handle two data correlation issues: (1) adjacent county observations on the screening utilization outcome may be spatially correlated, and (2) the county observations themselves may be correlated over time. Both situations may lead to reduced efficiency and reliability of statistical inference, and the first may result in spatial multiplier bias. We use the spatial seemingly unrelated regression (SSUR) empirical model that deals with both of these aspects.

First, we expected to see evidence of statistically significant spatial autocorrelation. Spatial autocorrelation across adjacent areas in outcomes related to public goods or preventive health care services that are expensive to provide is well documented in the empirical literature [28–32]. Because the decision regarding whether to establish endoscopy services in a county may be affected by prevalence of these services in adjacent counties, we expect there will be spatially correlated errors in the ecological models. Ignoring this is equivalent to falsely assuming that observations (county utilization rates) are statistically independent, which is a standard assumption under ordinary least squares (OLS) regression. This can lead to either efficiency bias, parameter bias, or both [33]. Recent papers have shown that ignoring spatial spillovers can yield highly inflated estimates of the marginal impact of living in rural poverty on preventive care service utilization by the elderly, misleading antitrust prescriptions, and inflated estimates of managed care spillover effects [5, 31, 32]. These misspecification effects can be corrected using a spatial regression model.

The second problem facing the ecological model is the possibility that area rates may be correlated over time. Ignoring this source of similarity or redundancy in the data inflates statistical significance. To reliably ascertain whether observed changes in parameter estimates over time are statistically significant, it is important to use an estimation setup that pools the two time periods and allows the two cross-sectional equations to have correlated errors over time. Thus, in estimation, we need an empirical approach that can deal with both spatial and time

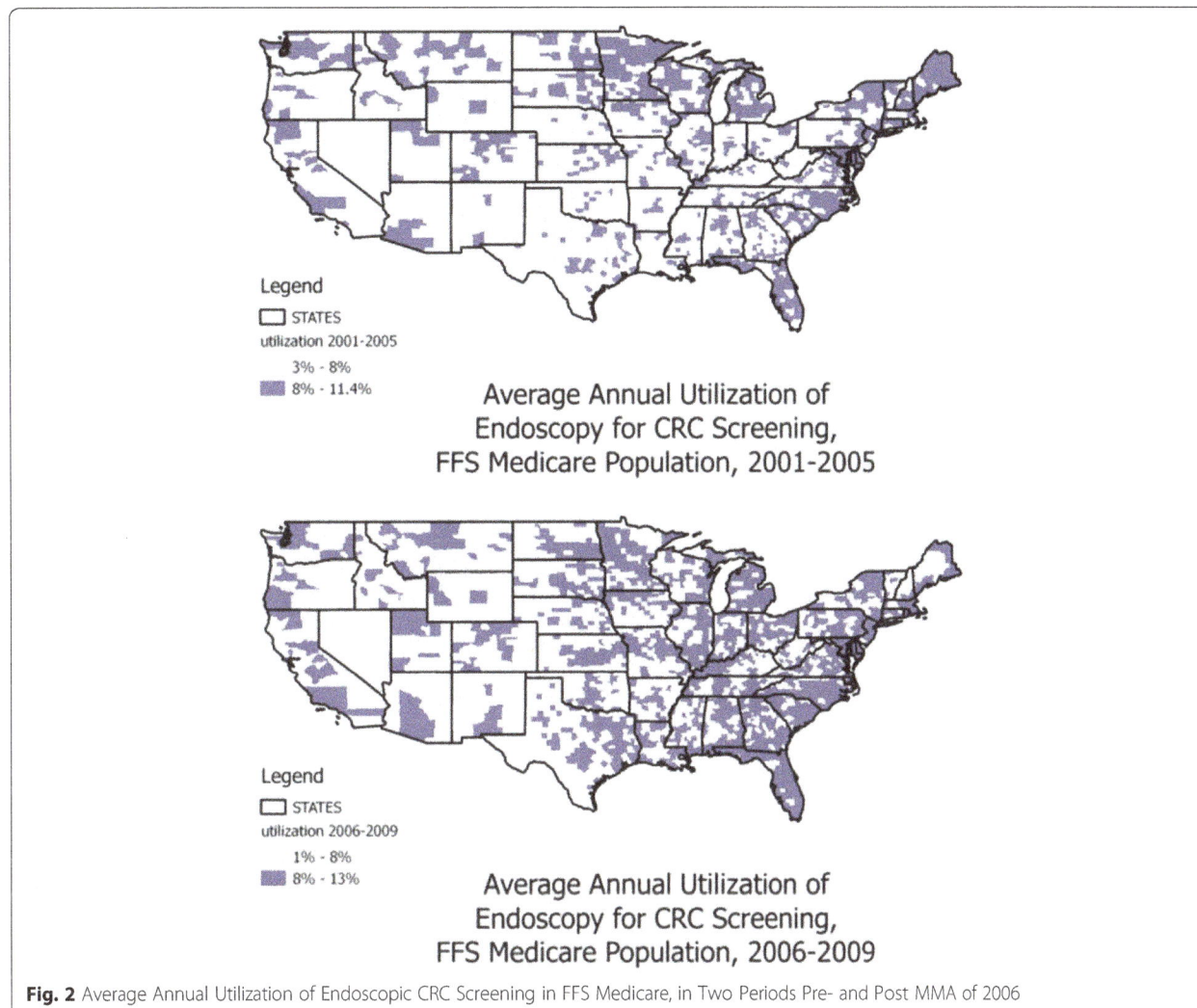

Fig. 2 Average Annual Utilization of Endoscopic CRC Screening in FFS Medicare, in Two Periods Pre- and Post MMA of 2006

correlation. We adopt the seemingly-unrelated regressions (SUR) approach pioneered by Zellner [34], and expanded to include spatial autocorrelation by Anselin [33]. We used the residuals from OLS regression as diagnostics to test for spatial correlation and determine the best spatial model to employ. We then estimated a spatial lag model specification to perform the spatial regressions over the early (2001-2005) and late (2006-2009) time periods, incorporated within a seemingly unrelated regression (SUR) framework, which allowed us to pool the two equations over time [33, 35, 36]. All models were estimated using PySAL, a Python library for spatial analysis developed by the GeoDa Center for Geospatial Analysis and Computation [37]. The programming code for the spatial SUR models is now publicly available for general applications as part of PySAL, as described in a recent applied spatial econometrics textbook [36].

The spatial SUR (SSUR) model allows for spatially correlated error terms within each equation and across equations, with separate parameter estimates for each

time period. To assess diffusion effects, we performed parameter-specific Wald tests to test for the stability of parameters across time. The null hypothesis under the Wald test is that parameters are stable (do not change significantly) over time. When this hypothesis is rejected, we can conclude that a significant change over time occurred; these are indicated with asterisks on the variables named in Table 2. The PySAL software also provides a Lagrange Multiplier test to assess whether the SUR simultaneous-equation estimation significantly improves the efficiency of the effect estimates (relative to an unpooled model).

Results
Characteristics of the samples
Figure 2 shows the average annual utilization rates for the FFS Medicare cohorts defined for the two periods. Many counties show annual utilization rates of less the 8%. However, it is apparent when comparing the figures that utilization rates increased over time, increasing the

Table 2 Estimation results, using ordinary least squares and spatial seemingly unrelated regression models

	OLS Model, 2001-2005		OLS Model, 2006-2009		SSUR Model, 2001-2005		SSUR Model, 2006-2009	
	Coef.	$P > |t|$	Coef.	$P > |t|$	Coef.	$P > |t|$	Coef.	$P > |t|$
Age 65-74[a]	0.013	0.112	-0.019	0.123	0.012	0.077	-0.016	0.144
Age 75-84[a]	**0.059**	**0.000**	**-0.037**	**0.011**	**0.035**	**0.000**	**-0.042**	**0.002**
Age 85 + [a]	**-0.110**	**0.000**	**-0.182**	**0.000**	**-0.077**	**0.000**	**-0.185**	**0.000**
Female[a]	-0.002	0.850	**0.120**	**0.000**	-0.002	0.825	**0.121**	**0.000**
African American	**0.019**	**0.000**	**0.018**	**0.000**	**0.016**	**0.000**	**0.016**	**0.000**
Asian	-0.042	0.127	0.005	0.851	-0.022	0.358	0.020	0.430
Hispanic[a]	**-0.037**	**0.000**	-0.001	0.960	**-0.025**	**0.000**	0.002	0.877
all other[a]	**-0.016**	**0.001**	**-0.023**	**0.000**	**-0.012**	**0.004**	**-0.023**	**0.000**
Population density	0.000	0.989	0.000	0.481	0.000	0.979	0.000	0.539
Poor English	-0.002	0.079	**-0.004**	**0.028**	-0.002	0.087	**-0.003**	**0.031**
Graduate[a]	**0.087**	**0.000**	**0.035**	**0.000**	**0.065**	**0.000**	**0.023**	**0.000**
Importance Medicare[a]	**0.030**	**0.003**	**0.046**	**0.000**	**0.022**	**0.014**	**0.044**	**0.000**
Average Poverty	**-0.032**	**0.000**	**-0.026**	**0.001**	**-0.030**	**0.000**	**-0.019**	**0.009**
Distance endoscopy	**-0.026**	**0.000**	**-0.021**	**0.000**	**-0.021**	**0.000**	**-0.017**	**0.000**
Dual/ESRD/disabled[a]	**-0.024**	**0.000**	**-0.041**	**0.000**	**-0.021**	**0.000**	**-0.043**	**0.000**
MA plan penetration	**-0.005**	**0.009**	-0.004	0.182	**-0.007**	**0.000**	-0.004	0.073
Competition endoscopy	**1.325**	**0.007**	**1.073**	**0.041**	**1.342**	**0.002**	**1.083**	**0.031**
Spatial lag[a]					0.029	0.000	0.019	0.000

Numbers highlighted in bold indicate statistically significant estimates in each model
[a]indicates a significant Wald test of parameter stability over time

geographic coverage of counties with more than 8% average annual utilization.

Table 1 summarizes the set of supply and demand conditions used in the regression modeling. Sample statistics show means and standard deviations for the county-level data, as well as data sources. The average annual endoscopy utilization among the traditional Medicare enrollees increased slightly over time, from 7.4 to 7.9 percent. The average percentage across counties of all Medicare beneficiaries in the youngest and the oldest age groups increased, and the percentage of vulnerable people eligible for extra benefits (DUAL, disabled, ESRD) increased from 20.9 to 27.9 percent. The percentage of over age 65 with graduate or professional degrees increased slightly, as did population density, and the percent of the Medicare Part A coverage market increased from 14.1 to 14.8. All health market conditions, including MA plan penetration were fairly stable.

Estimates from multivariate analyses

Table 2 presents the results from both ordinary least squares (OLS) and SSUR regressions. The SSUR models include a spatial lag parameter in addition to other coefficient estimates. The results are very similar across the model types, where statistically significant results for each model are highlighted in bold font (Table 2). For both models, the Lagrange Multiplier test (not shown)

allowed us to conclude that the SSUR model improved efficiency significantly as compared to an unpooled model, and parameter-specific Wald tests found many significant changes in parameters over time, as indicated by superscripted lowercase letter a. The significance of changes over time were consistent across the OLS and the spatial lag regressions. The spatial lag estimate is fairly small but statistically significant; the small lag effect is consistent with the similarity of estimates across the OLS and SSUR models.

First we discuss the demographic characteristics of the Medicare population, and how these are associated with the average annual endoscopy utilization rates in the counties they represent. Places with higher percentages of older Medicare populations saw lower screening rates, and they dropped significantly over time. Places with higher percentages of Medicare-eligible females had significantly higher rates in the later period, climbing from no difference in rates in the early period. Places with higher percentages of African Americans had higher rates in both periods. Places with higher percentages of Hispanics had lower rates in the early period, but no difference in the later period. Places with higher percentages of 'all other' populations (these are dominated by American Indian enclaves) exhibited significantly lower rates and these declined even more over time. Places with a higher percentage of vulnerable eligibles had significantly lower rates, and this disparity increased significantly over time.

Next we discuss market contextual factors. Places with higher percentages of elderly with graduate or professional degrees had higher utilization rates, but this disparity decreased significantly over time. Places with higher importance of Medicare in the market exhibited higher rates, and this disparity increased significantly over time. Places with higher average poverty exhibited lower rates, but this disparity did not change over time. Places with greater distance to endoscopists exhibited lower rates, and this remained steady over time. Places with a more competitive endoscopy environment exhibited significantly higher rates, and this was stable over time. Places with higher MA plan penetration saw significantly lower screening rates in the early period, but this disparity became statistically weaker by the later period and the change over time was not statistically significant.

Discussion

This study demonstrated there was an increase in endoscopy utilization among FFS Medicare after implementation of the MMA. However, the increase was not uniform across geography and various contextual and compositional market factors predicted the observed changes in utilization noted over time. Disparities (lower utilization rates) for places with higher percentages of Medicare eligible women and Hispanics decreased over time. Disparities (lower utilization rates) for places with higher percentages of 'other' races or ethnicities – dominated by American Indian enclaves - increased over time. Places with the highest percentages of older age groups saw significant declines over time in their screening rates, which is appropriate as screening guidelines suggest cessation of screening after age 75 because risks may outweigh benefits. Places with higher percentages of vulnerable beneficiaries exhibited lower screening rates that became even lower over time, which suggests a widening disparity over time for this more vulnerable group who may have greater difficulty undergoing the procedure and/or greater risk of complications from the procedure. Overall, the changing composition of the Medicare eligible population helped predict the net effects of supply and demand interaction on area utilization rates.

The spatial lag parameter was statistically significant and positive, suggesting that endoscopists establishing services in one county were aware of competitors in nearby counties. However, this effect diminished significantly over time, reflecting the fact that utilization tended to be geographically concentrated in the early period and became less concentrated over time as the endoscopy services diffused to underserved and new market areas (Fig. 2).

Turning to contextual market factors, Managed care spillovers were significant and negative in the early

period, but became weaker and statistically insignificant over time. The significantly negative spillover effect in the earlier period is consistent with findings from an earlier paper that looked at colonoscopy and sigmoidoscopy separately. That paper found that managed care spillovers were significantly negative for colonoscopy, but significantly positive for sigmoidoscopy - the older, simpler, less risky and less costly procedure [5]. During the early period, following expansion of Medicare coverage for colonoscopy in 2001, the newer colonoscopy service diffused and came to dominate FFS Medicare endoscopy markets by 2005. The national guidelines had not yet been established during the early period, although cost-effectiveness evidence was mounting in favor of a combined use of the two endoscopy procedures, culminating in a complex screening protocol established as the gold standard in 2008 [11]. Findings here suggest that the managed care spillover seemed to have restraining influences on colonoscopy utilization at first, but this gradually diminished as the procedure gained medical acceptance over the period, and by the later period, exhibited no significant spillover effects.

During the time of this study (2001-2009), a substantial out-of-pocket copayment was required for endoscopic CRC screening. With the implementation of the MMA in 2006, subsidized coverage for prescription drugs would perhaps relax budget constraints for seniors, making such copayments more affordable, and increase utilization rates. Also, with drug coverage available in all MA plans, enrollments escalated and MA plans moved into previously underserved Medicare markets (Fig. 1). With this expansion, dissemination of best practices regarding endoscopic CRC screening might have spread into these newer, less urban markets. Such dissemination could be accompanied by spillover effects encouraging the use of endoscopy for CRC screening by FFS Medicare enrollees in those markets. With both effects in play, we expected to see an increase in utilization rates by FFS Medicare insureds over time, and an increasing MA spillover onto the FFS Medicare beneficiaries over time.

Conclusions

The data show that annual utilization rates of endoscopy among FFS Medicare enrollees did increase over time, and findings suggest that managed care spillover effects did increase over time (from retraining to non-restraining). This is great news, because as shown in Fig. 2, overall utilization rates are low, and much improvement is needed in many areas of the country to encourage these recommended gold-standard CRC screening services. These findings suggest that policies such as those enacted in the Affordable Care Act of 2010 - which prohibited copayments for CRC screening by endoscopy for enrollees in private insurance or Medicare - are expected to result in higher rates of screening uptake, which would be an important topic for a future study.

Abbreviations
CMS: Centers for medicare and Medicaid Services; CRC: colorectal cancer; ESRD: end stage renal disease; FFS: fee for service; MA: Medicare Advantage; MMA: Medicare Modernization Act; OLS: ordinary least squares; SSUR: spatial seemingly unrelated regressions; USPSTF: United Stated Preventive Services Task Force

Funding
Agency for Healthcare Research and Quality, R01 grant (1R01HS021752).

Authors' contributions
LRM led the work and manuscript development, and wrote the first and final drafts. PA wrote the programming code and did the SSUR regression analyses. SB, LRM and T-MK performed analyses in STATA to assess the sufficiency of instrumental variables. T-MK and MZ developed the CMS data from the raw claims extracts into the county-level files. All contributed to the draft manuscript revisions to develop the final manuscript. All authors read and approved the final manuscript.

Competing interests
The authors declare that they have no competing interests.

Author details
[1]Georgia State University, 1 Park Place, Suite 700, Atlanta, GA 30304, USA. [2]Cedeplar - Universidade Federal de Minas Gerais, Belo Horizonte, Brazil. [3]University of North Carolina, Chapel Hill, USA.

References
1. Klabunde C, Lanier D, Meissner H, Breslau E, and Brown M. Improving Colorectal Cancer Screening Through Research in Primary Care Settings. Medical Care, 2008;46(9)(Suppl 1): S1–S4.
2. Schenck AP, Peacock SC, Klabunde CN, Lapin P, Coan JF, Brown ML. Trends in Colorectal Cancer Test Use in the Medicare Population, 1998–2005. Am J Prev Med. 2009;37(1):1–7.
3. Shapiro J, Seeff L, Thompson T, Nadel M, Klabunde C, Vernon S. Colorectal Cancer Test Use from the 2005 National Health Interview Survey. Cancer Epidemiol Biomarkers Prev. 2008;17(7):1623–30.
4. Zauber AG. Cost-Effectiveness of Colonoscopy. Gastrointest Endosc Clin N Am. 2010;20(4):751–70.
5. Mobley L, Subramanian S, Koschinsky J, Frech HE, Clayton L, Anselin L. Managed care and the diffusion of endoscopy in fee-for-service Medicare". Health Serv Res. 2011;46(6):1905–27.
6. Megellas, Michelle M. Medicare Modernization: The New Prescription Drug Benefit and Redesigned Part B and Part C. Proceedings (Baylor University. Medical Center) 19.1 (2006): 21–23. Print. Available online February 2016: http://www.ncbi.nlm.nih.gov/pmc/articles/PMC1325278/
7. Federal Register 2004. "Medicare Program; Medicare Prescription Drug Benefit", available online March 2016: https://www.cms.gov/Medicare/Prescription-Drug-Coverage/PrescriptionDrugCovGenIn/downloads/CMS-4068-F3Column.pdf
8. CMS Regions 2006. Available online March 2016: https://innovation.cms.gov/initiatives/regional-innovation-network/. Accessed 01 Mar 2017.
9. Neuman T, Casillas G, Jacobson G (2015). Medicare Advantage and Traditional Medicare: Is the Balance Tipping? Kaiser Family Foundation (KFF) Issue Brief: October 2015. Available online: http://files.kff.org/attachment/issue-brief-medicare-advantage-and-traditional-medicare-is-the-balance-tipping
10. Pignone M, Saha S, Hoerger T, Mandelblatt J. Cost-effectiveness analyses of colorectal cancer screening: a systematic review for the U.S. Preventive Services Task Force. Ann Intern Med. 2002;137(2):96–104.
11. USPSTF. Screening for colorectal cancer: U.S. Preventive Services Task Force recommendation statement. Ann Intern Med. 2008;149(9):627–37.
12. Whitlock EP, Lin JS, Liles E, Beil TL, Fu R. Screening for Colorectal Cancer: A Targeted, Updated Systematic Review for the U.S. Preventive Services Task Force. Ann Intern Med. 2008;149(9):638–58.
13. Baker L. Managed care spillover effects. Annu Rev Public Health. 2003;24(1): 435–56.
14. Miller RH, Luft HS. Managed care plan performance since 1980: a literature analysis. JAMA. 1994;271:1512–9.
15. Koroukian S, Litaker D, Dor A, Cooper G. Use of Preventive Services by Medicare Fee-for-Service Beneficiaries Does Spillover From Managed Care Matter?". Med Care. 2005;43(5):445–52.
16. Tangka F, Molinari N, Chattopadhyay S, Seeff L. Market for Colorectal Cancer Screening by Endoscopy in the United States. Am J Prev Med. 2005;29(1):54–60.
17. Pope G, Greenwald LM, Kautter J, Olmstead EA, Mobley LR. Medicare preferred provider organization demonstration: Plan offerings and beneficiary enrollment. Health Care Financ Rev. 2006;27(3):96–109.
18. Afendulis C, Chernew M, and Kessler D. The Effect of Medicare Advantage on Hospital Admissions and Mortality. NBER Working Paper No. 19101, Issued in June 2013. Available online March 2016: http://www.nber.org/papers/w19101.
19. Baicker K, and Robbins J. Medicare Payments and System-Level Health-Care Use: The Spillover Effects of Medicare Managed Care. Am J Health Economics, Fall 2015, Vol. 1, No. 4, 399-431
20. Baker L, Corts K. HMO penetration and the cost of health care: market discipline or market segmentation?". Am Econ Rev. 1996;86(2):389–94.
21. Basu J. "Preventable hospitalizations and Medicare managed care: a small area analysis. Am J Manag Care. 2012;18(8):e280–90.
22. Bian J, Dow WH, Matchar DB. Medicare HMO penetration and mortality outcomes of ischemic stroke". Am J Manag Care. 2006;12(1):58–64.
23. Glied S, Zivin J. How do doctors behave when some (but not all) of their patients are in managed care?". J Health Econ. 2002;21(2):337–53.
24. Volpp K, Buckley E. The effect of increases in HMO penetration and changes in payer mix on in-hospital mortality and treatment patterns for acute myocardial infarction". Am J Manag Care. 2004;10(7 Pt 2):505–12.
25. Atherly A, and Thorpe KE. 2005. Value of Medicare Advantage to Low-Income and Minority Medicare Beneficiaries. Atlanta, GA: Emory University Rollins School of Public Health. Available online June 2016 at: c0540862.cdn.cloudfiles.rackspacecloud.com/Ken_Thorpe_MA_Report.pdf
26. Chovan C, and Lemieux J. 2005. Low-Income and Minority Beneficiaries in Medicare Advantage Plans, 2002. AHIP Center for Policy and Research, available online June 2016 at the archive: http://health-equity.pitt.edu/245/1/Low-Income_and_Minority_Beneficiaries_in_Medicare_Advantage_Plans%2C_2002.pdf
27. McGuire T, Newhouse J, Sinaiko A. An Economic History of Medicare Part C". Milbank Quarterly. 2011;89(2011):289–332.
28. Brueckner J. Testing for strategic interaction among local governments: The case of growth controls. J Urban Econ. 1998;44(3):438–67.
29. Brueckner J. Strategic interaction among governments: An overview of empirical studies. Int Reg Sci Rev. 2003;26(2):175–88.
30. Brueckner J, Saavedra L. Do local governments engage in strategic property-tax competition?". Natl Tax J. 2001;54:203–29.
31. Mobley LR, Root ED, Anselin L, Lozano-Gracia N, and Koschinsky J. 2006. Spatial Analysis of Elderly Access to Primary Care Services. International Journal of Health Geographics, 5, epub May 15, 2006.
32. Mobley LR, Frech H, Anselin L. Spatial Interaction, Hospital Pricing and Hospital Antitrust. Int J Econ Bus. 2009;16(1):1–17.
33. Anselin L. Spatial Econometrics: Methods and Models. Dordrecht: Kluwer Academic; 1988.
34. Zellner A. An Efficient Method of Estimating Seemingly Unrelated Regressions and Tests for Aggregation Bias. J Am Stat Assoc. 1962;57:348–68.
35. Anselin L. Spatial dependence and spatial structural instability in applied regression analysis. J Regional Sci. 1990;30:185–207.
36. Anselin L, Rey S. Modern Spatial Econometrics in Practice. GeoDa Press LLC. 2014. ISBN-10: 0986342106. ISBN-13: 978-0986342103.
37. Rey S, Anselin L. PySAL, a python library of spatial analytical methods. Rev Reg Stud. 2007;37(1):5–27.

4

Economic conditions, hypertension, and cardiovascular disease: analysis of the Icelandic economic collapse

Kristín Helga Birgisdóttir[1*], Stefán Hrafn Jónsson[2] and Tinna Laufey Ásgeirsdóttir[1]

Abstract

Previous research has found a positive short-term relationship between the 2008 collapse and hypertension in Icelandic males. With Iceland's economy experiencing a phase of economic recovery, an opportunity to pursue a longer-term analysis of the collapse has emerged. Using data from a nationally representative sample, fixed-effect estimations and mediation analyses were performed to explore the relationship between the Icelandic economic collapse in 2008 and the longer-term impact on hypertension and cardiovascular health. A sensitivity analysis was carried out with pooled logit models estimated as well as an alternative dependent variable. Our attrition analysis revealed that results for cardiovascular diseases were affected by attrition, but not results from estimations on the relationship between the economic crisis and hypertension. When compared to the boom year 2007, our results point to an increased probability of Icelandic women having hypertension in the year 2012, when the Icelandic economy had recovered substantially from the economic collapse in 2008. This represents a deviation from pre-crisis trends, thus suggesting a true economic-recovery impact on hypertension.

Keywords: Prolonged exposure, Crisis, Economic conditions, Economic downturn, Hypertension, Iceland

Background

The link between business cycles and health has been studied to a considerable extent. The Great Recession has sparked interest and opportunities to pursue this line of research further. The Icelandic economic collapse is already established as a favorable treatment [1–13] due to the clear before and after contrast that results from a collapse that can be pinpointed almost to a specific date; October 6th 2008 when Iceland's Prime Minister announced the risk of national bankruptcy [14]. Subsequently, the Icelandic economy contracted by 6.6% in 2009 and 4.1% in 2010 and was among the hardest hit in the world [15]. Thereafter, the Icelandic economy experienced substantial recovery, so much so, that it received international attention as one of Europe's top performers [16–21].

Up until the early 2000s, Iceland's economy was export-driven, with fishing and aluminum smelting serving as the main industries, but after the deregulation of Icelandic banks the country's financial sector expanded in a major way, with the three biggest commercial banks in Iceland growing to almost 10 times the size of the Icelandic economy. This led to a bubble that was primed to pop when international short-term funding dried up [22]. For a country the size of Iceland, with a population of 330,000, the impact of the economic collapse was widely felt; people's savings vanished with the crash of the Icelandic stock market (of which the three biggest commercial banks comprised more than half of listed stocks) [23–25], monthly unemployment tripled and remained high compared to the pre-crisis long-term unemployment rate of around 2.5–3% [26] (Fig. 1), and real wages plummeted [27] (Fig. 2).

Not all medical conditions are theoretically likely to be affected by external factors, for example various genetic diseases. Cardiovascular events have however been shown to be responsive to such factors, for example stressful circumstances such as war [28, 29] and earthquakes [30–32], as well as important sporting events which might trigger emotional stress [33–37]. For this reason, cardiovascular outcomes have been of interest in

* Correspondence: khb6@hi.is
[1]Faculty of Economics, University of Iceland, Oddi v/Sturlugotu, 101 Reykjavik, Iceland
Full list of author information is available at the end of the article

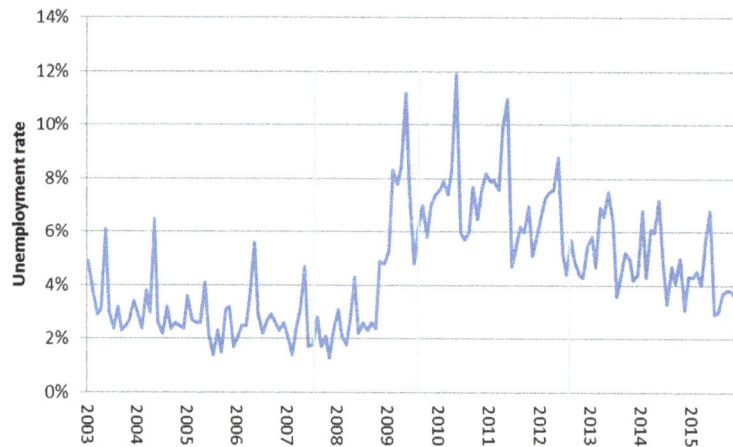

Fig. 1 Monthly unemployment rate in Iceland January 2003-December 2015. Source: Statistics Iceland. Accessed October 17th 2016 from: http://px.hagstofa.is/pxen/pxweb/en/Samfelag/Samfelag__vinnumarkadur__vinnumarkadur/VIN00001.px/table/tableViewLayout1/?rxid = 07c0d8b2-a5b9-4bc0-a75c-a40e871fd831. Notes: Vertical lines refer to the timing of 1st, 2nd, and 3rd waves of data collection for the survey data used here

the health and business cycle literature (see for example studies by Gerdtham and Ruhm [38], Ruhm [39], Ruhm [40], Ruhm [41], Neumayer [42], Tapia Granados and Ionides [43]). It seems a priori plausible that as large a business cycle event as the economic collapse in Iceland would affect hypertension and cardiovascular diseases in Icelanders. Although effects of business cycles on health could be the greatest at the extremes of the cycle, it is possible that some health effects take time to present themselves, as explored for total mortality in Ruhm [44] and Stuckler et al. [45], as well as other diseases, such as cardiovascular diseases in Gerdtham and Ruhm [38] and Ruhm [41]. The immediate effects of the Icelandic economic collapse on health have been studied to some extent, but a chance to examine longer-term effects for

comparison is gradually emerging as time passes. We focus first and foremost on longer-term effects on hypertension, one of the most important risk factors for cardiovascular diseases [46–49] and the leading preventable risk factor for premature death worldwide [50, 51], but also examine cardiovascular disease for completeness, thus following up on a previously published analysis of short-term effects on those outcomes [7].

Both the short and longer-term impacts of economic conditions on cardiovascular disease are unclear, due to the multitude of determinants of cardiovascular health. Some are known to get more favorable during times of economic hardship, such as smoking and alcohol misuse [1–3, 6, 44, 52, 53] and others are known to become less favorable, such as psychological morbidity [5]. Similarly

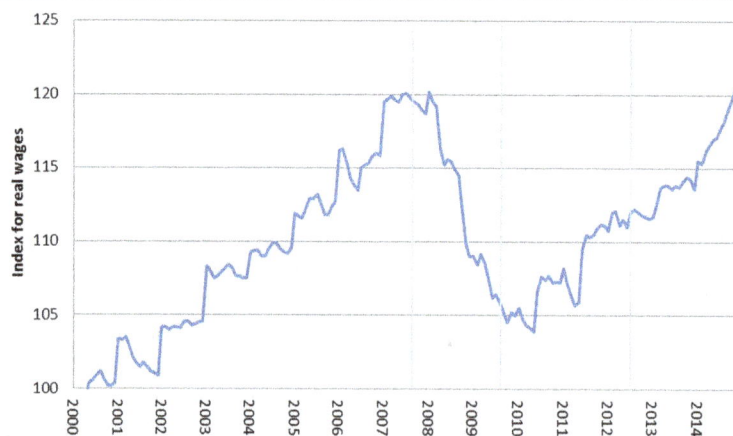

Fig. 2 Monthly index for real wages in Iceland January 2003-December 2015. Source: Statistics Iceland. Accessed October 17th 2016 from: http://px.hagstofa.is/pxen/pxweb/en/Efnahagur/Efnahagur__thjodhagsreikningar__efnahagslegar_skammtimatolur/THJ00117.px/table/tableViewLayout1/?rxid = 07c0d8b2-a5b9-4bc0-a75c-a40e871fd831. Notes: Base level of 100 is set in the year 2000. The index refers to the change in the wage index deflated by the CPI converted to mid-month figures. Vertical lines refer to the timing of 1st, 2nd, and 3rd waves of data collection for the survey data used here

the determinants of cardiovascular health include both long-term determinants that make the individual more vulnerable, as well as short-time stressors [54–56], making it important to examine effects with a different time lag. Aside from the factors mentioned, unemployment and income are examined here as possible mediators in the relationship, as they have been found to be positively associated with cardiovascular mortality and morbidity [57–62], possibly through changed behavior and consumption patterns. As the literature has moved towards more detailed exploration of possible mechanisms underlying the relationships explored, we follow that direction in our mediation analysis. Overall, the empirical framework for our study stems from the pioneering work of Grossman [63, 64], as well as on the Grossman-derived demand for health behaviors as described in work by Xu and Kaestner [65].

The relationship between economic downturns and cardiovascular health is complicated and results have been mixed across settings (the interested reader is referred to the extensive supplementary online literary review by Asgeirsdottir et al. [7]). This study adds to the growing literature in various ways. Firstly, it does so by examining the longer-term effects in a follow-up study to Asgeirsdottir et al. [7], which looked into the short-term effects. Secondly, nationally representative, individual-level data are used, where the same Icelanders have partaken in a survey before and after the economic downturn, as opposed to aggregate data which have been dominant in the field. This allows us to study possible individual-level mediators in the relationship between the economic crisis and cardiovascular health, i.e. to assess the extent to which heterogeneously felt effects of the crisis explain the effects of the economic-recovery indicator. Similar to the way that Asgeirsdottir et al. [3] expanded on the short-term results of Asgeirsdottir et al. [2] on health behaviors, this paper expands on the short-term results of Asgeirsdottir et al. [7] on hypertension and cardiovascular diseases, largely following the methodology of those studies. Thirdly, an unusually comprehensive dataset on hypertension and cardiovascular morbidity is utilized, whereas the previous literature has, due to data restrictions, mostly studied mortality.

Methods
The data used here is the lifestyle survey "Heilsa og líðan Íslendinga" (Health and well-being of the Icelandic population) carried out by the Icelandic Public Health Institute in 2007 and 2009 and then Icelandic Directorate of health in 2012, providing data from periods of economic boom, bust, and recovery. The survey contains questions regarding health and lifestyle, as well as demographics, labor participation, and income.

A stratified random sample of 9807 individuals 18–79 years old was drawn. In 2007 9711 individuals received questionnaires with a response rate of 60.9%, or 5909 returned questionnaires. The 2009-sample included 5294 of the original individuals who had agreed to be contacted again. For the 2009 survey the response rate was 69.3%, or 4092 individuals. In 2012 the sample of original participants who had agreed to be contacted for follow-up studies consisted of 3.659 individuals. The response rate was 88.5%, or 3238 individuals, corresponding to 33.0% of the original sample. Additionally, in 2012 a sample of 3506 new subjects was added. The sampling method for the new entrants was comparable to the ones of the original sample in 2007, thus providing cross-sectional data across 2007 and 2012, in addition to the panel of same individuals answering in those years. In our main analysis using fixed-effect models and in the sensitivity analysis using panel data we use a balanced panel of only those who answered questionnaires from all three years. Answers from the new participants in 2012 were however only used in an alternative analysis (results found in the supplementary online material) where the cross-sectional aspects of the data were taken advantage of.

We perform two analyses, using the panel data. Methodologically, each one has its pros and cons, but together they provide a more comprehensive picture than each individual method. For our main analysis we estimate individual fixed-effects models, as is frequently done when panel data are available. These models implicitly control for all unobserved time-invariant individual heterogeneity. Additionally, they account for cross-period correlation in standard errors. An argument against using fixed-effects models in our analyses is a possible bias in the measurement of the coefficient we are most interested in measuring, the recovery indicator, as reported and explained in Asgeirsdottir et al. [7] with a detailed mathematical rationalization of the choice for a pooled model in their supplementary online material. Their explanation applies here as well. Therefore, in our sensitivity analysis we perform an additional analysis, with pooled logit models. In addition, we use a different variable to gauge health of participants, i.e. the use of prescription medication. One would expect the correlation between a diagnosis of a disease and the use of prescription medication for that disease to be high, but in our data, that is not the case; the highest correlation coefficient found in the data is 0.658 for hypertension. Hence, we feel that a sensitivity analysis using prescription medication as a proxy for health is in order. Furthermore, we perform an attrition analysis to address the concern of possible attrition bias (results available in the supplementary online material).

Due to deliberate oversampling of older age groups and those living outside the capital area, sample weights are included in all estimations. When sample weights are used, the sample is representative of the Icelandic population in 2007 [66].

In Tables 1 and 2 unadjusted summary statistics are reported for males and females in the full panel data sample. To inspect the statistical significance of the differences in each variable between waves, t-tests were carried out and corresponding p-values reported in the same tables. The summary statistics only represent the raw data for participants in the final sample and do not expose any crisis effect since important factors have not been controlled for.

Dependent variables

The dependent variables used are: hypertension; coronary thrombosis; coronary disease; stroke; and cardiovascular disease, and a binary variable indicating whether participants had any cardiovascular disease (CVD), i.e. coronary thrombosis, coronary disease, or stroke. Hypertension is the main outcome variable, but following Asgeirsdottir et al. [7] variables regarding cardiovascular health were included for completeness although the low number of observations for those outcomes leads to unreliable results. The response options in 2007 and 2009 were: "yes, have got it now"; "have had it before but not now"; "no, have never had it". In the 2012 survey the response categories where changed so they became: "yes, have got it now"; "do not have it now, but had it within the last 12 months"; "do not have it now, but had it more than 12 months ago"; "no, have never had it". If respondents answered "yes, have got it now", they were also asked if a doctor had diagnosed them with the medical condition in question. A binary variable for the outcomes was constructed, taking into account the altered answering arrangement between waves, taking the value 1 if respondents marked both "yes, have got it now" for the relevant cardiovascular condition and if the medical condition in question was diagnosed by a doctor, but 0 otherwise. Due to few observations of coronary thrombosis, coronary disease, and stroke, a binary variable was created indicating if an individual reported having any cardiovascular disease (coronary thrombosis, coronary disease, or stroke). As can be seen in the summary statistics in Tables 1 and 2, the difference between 2007 and 2012 in the prevalence of both hypertension and cardiovascular diseases, is statistically significant for both genders.

In the sensitivity analysis we use binary variables for participants' prescription medication use as dependent variables. Responses to questions on medication use for both hypertension as well as cardiovascular and cholesterol diseases were used. The variables take the value 1 if respondents answered positively to having taking such medication in the last 2 weeks, but 0 otherwise.

As we follow subjects over time in this analysis, preexisting trends in the health outcomes present a potential methodological challenge in our study. Data on trends in hypertension and cardiovascular morbidity in Iceland is not available, but in an attempt to take this informally into account, figures from Iceland relating to the prevalence of these medical conditions were inspected, in addition to our sensitivity analyses using participants' use of prescription medication as dependent variables. Specifically, aggregate data from Landspitali University Hospital from 2000 to 2014 on the prevalence of hypertension in all patients suffering from cardiovascular diseases were inspected (Fig. 3), as well as consumption of drugs for the blood and blood-forming organs, and cardiovascular system in Iceland [67] (Fig. 4). Furthermore, aggregate mortality rates due to circulatory diseases in Iceland and other countries [68] were examined (Fig. 5). Research on current and predicted hypertension prevalence is available for other countries, which find generally unchanged prevalence in most countries, although awareness and treatment of the disease is improving, thus leading to better hypertension outcomes [69–74]. A similar pattern is found between males and females when examining the prevalence of patients suffering from cardiovascular diseases, but not a specific time trend over the period as a whole (see Fig. 3). From 2000 to 2005 a near doubling of the prevalence (in absolute terms) is found followed by a substantial decline after the economic collapse in 2008. A clear upward trend in usage of the drugs is evident in the years and decades prior to the crisis. In the case of cardiovascular drugs, a peak was reached in 2008, followed by a rather steep decline until 2011, and during the economic recovery usage levelled off. Usage of drugs for blood and blood-forming organs was relatively even in the boom years (2004-2007) and during the crisis (2008–2010), with an increase during the economic recovery (2011–2012) (see Fig. 4). Mortality rates due to circulatory diseases are distinctly downward trending both before and throughout the study period (see Fig. 5); a similar trend can be seen in other Western countries which experienced the Great Recession to varying degrees (UK, USA, Germany, Norway, and Denmark). Although these numbers do not represent the impact of the economic crisis and recovery on hypertension and cardiovascular diseases, they do provide a context to interpret our results. This context is important as we are examining a single economic fluctuation. Although that fluctuation presents an important research opportunity, due to the exceptionally large changes in conditions over a short time period that are likely to overshadow other societal events occurring at the same time, we cannot rule out that normal fluctuations affect the results with this research design.

Control variables

Depending on estimation model, either only age squared or both age and age squared are used as controls in continuous form. Five dummy variables are used for marital

Table 1 Full panel data sample summary statistics: males answering both waves

Variable	2007			2012			t-test
	Mean	SD	N	Mean	SD	N	p-value
Age	55.075	14.893	1501	60.075	14.893	1501	0.0000
1 if hypertension	0.218	0.413	1460	0.259	0.438	1438	0.0086
1 if coronary thrombosis	0.019	0.137	1458	0.030	0.171	1431	0.0598
1 if coronary disease	0.029	0.168	1451	0.051	0.221	1422	0.0022
1 if stroke	0.004	0.064	1466	0.004	0.065	1433	0.9685
1 if cardiovascular disease	0.041	0.197	1502	0.061	0.239	1502	0.0125
No. of children	2.594	1.563	1482	2.692	1.533	1490	0.0840
1 if rural	0.382	0.486	1494	0.387	0.487	1487	0.7436
1 if married	0.703	0.457	1479	0.707	0.455	1472	0.8107
1 if cohabiting	0.124	0.330	1479	0.117	0.321	1472	0.5285
1 if single or in a relationship	0.116	0.320	1479	0.094	0.292	1472	0.0524
1 if divorced	0.035	0.184	1479	0.043	0.202	1472	0.2837
1 if widowed	0.022	0.146	1479	0.039	0.195	1472	0.0050
1 if educ1[a]	0.295	0.456	1498	0.295	0.456	1498	
1 if educ2[a]	0.292	0.455	1498	0.292	0.455	1498	
1 if educ3[a]	0.182	0.386	1498	0.182	0.386	1498	
1 if educ4[a]	0.138	0.345	1498	0.138	0.345	1498	
1 if educ5[a]	0.091	0.288	1498	0.091	0.288	1498	
1 if hypertension medication	0.219	0.414	1440	0.310	0.463	1447	0.0000
1 if cholesterol medication	0.148	0.355	1454	0.224	0.417	1466	0.0000
1 if circulatory disease medication	0.054	0.226	1465	0.068	0.252	1463	0.1033
Body Max Index (BMI)	27.410	4.243	1472	27.506	3.808	1478	0.5194
1 if underweight	0.003	0.052	1472	0.002	0.045	1478	0.7012
1 if optimal weight	0.272	0.445	1472	0.262	0.440	1478	0.5435
1 if overweight	0.519	0.500	1472	0.520	0.500	1478	0.9447
1 if obese	0.207	0.405	1472	0.216	0.412	1478	0.5358
1 if non smoker	0.829	0.377	1468	0.876	0.330	1470	0.0004
1 if daily smoker	0.137	0.344	1468	0.091	0.288	1470	0.0001
1 if weekly smoker	0.016	0.124	1468	0.017	0.129	1470	0.7747
1 if seldom smoker	0.018	0.134	1468	0.016	0.127	1470	0.6683
1 if non drinker	0.114	0.318	1469	0.144	0.351	1475	0.0149
1 if daily drinker	0.028	0.165	1469	0.029	0.168	1475	0.8396
1 if frequent drinker	0.338	0.473	1469	0.296	0.457	1475	0.0142
1 if seldom drinker	0.378	0.485	1469	0.372	0.483	1475	0.6965
1 if rare drinker	0.142	0.349	1469	0.159	0.366	1475	0.1787
Perceived Stress Scale (PSS)	7.154	1.757	1446	7.468	1.695	1428	0.0000
1 if unemployed	0.027	0.161	1457	0.037	0.189	1449	0.1079
1 if much better financial status[b]	0.017	0.128	1446	0.017	0.128	1440	0.9884
1 if considerably better financial status[b]	0.126	0.332	1446	0.120	0.325	1440	0.6397
1 if somewhat better financial status[b]	0.214	0.410	1446	0.210	0.408	1440	0.8296
1 if similar financial status[b]	0.508	0.500	1446	0.501	0.500	1440	0.6830

Table 1 Full panel data sample summary statistics: males answering both waves *(Continued)*

1 if somewhat worse financial status[b]	0.082	0.275	1446	0.095	0.294	1440	0.2251
1 if considerably worse financial status[b]	0.036	0.186	1446	0.042	0.200	1440	0.4277
1 if much worse financial status[b]	0.017	0.130	1446	0.014	0.117	1440	0.4612
Real income[c]	5.869	3.136	1445	4.558	2.340	1449	0.0000
Work hours	5.815	4.868	1386	4.976	4.844	1327	0.0000

Summary statistics only represent the data and do not display any crisis effect. Means are unweighted. *P*-values are from *t*-test for differences in means between 2007 and 2012

[a]Education level is represented by dummy variables: educ1 represents primary or lower level secondary education; educ2 stands for vocational master or journeyman certificate; educ3 stands for high school or equivalent; educ4 stands for technical graduate or undergraduate degree; educ5 stands for master's degree or a Ph.D

[b]Perceived financial status represents respondents' own perception of their families' financial status relative to other families

[c]Real income is reported at 2012 price level in millions of Icelandic kronas (ISK)

status; married; cohabitating; divorced; widowed; and single or in a non-cohabitating or non-marital relationship, which is used as the benchmark variable for marital status. A variable for the number of children was used in continuous form. A binary variable indicates whether an individual lived in an urban (an area of more than 5000 inhabitants) or rural area. As can be seen in Tables 1 and 2 demographics are relatively stable across waves.

Answering options were added on the questionnaire in 2009 regarding the education of respondents, and therefore it is not clear that changed answers between 2007 and 2009 reflect added education during that time, or that respondents found a more suitable answering option that fitted their educational status. Due to the greater detail in answering options a new time-invariant variable for education was constructed using the educational level in 2012 as a base, but imputations from 2009 to 2007 were used when answers were missing. Owing to the increased clarity of the educational question this is deemed the best option, and justified as variability in education is small over such a short time span. Education is thus rather being used as a control for a wider reaching social status. However, this variable is only used in the logit regression since a time-invariant variable cannot be included in the fixed-effects models. As the fixed-effects capture inherently what our education variable measures, it can be emitted from the fixed-effects models without harming the analysis. Five dummy variables were constructed for education; *educ1* represents those who finished primary or lower level secondary education and is use as benchmark in the analyses; *educ2* those who finished a vocational master or journeyman certificate; *educ3* those who finished high school or equivalent; *educ4* those who finished a technical graduate or undergraduate degree; and *educ5* those who had finished a master's degree or a Ph.D.

Exposure

Exposure to certain economic conditions is measured with time indicators. Due to the follow-up nature of this study, as an expansion of previous work on the short term effects of the collapse, the key independent variable *t2012* is a dummy for the time of the economic recovery during the third wave of data collection. Additionally, the time variable *t2009* captures the short-term exposure of the participants in our sample, but as noted earlier, the short-term impact on hypertension and cardiovascular disease was previously reported on in the literature [7]. Both variables, *t2009* and *t2012*, take the value 1 for the respective years, but zero otherwise. By including both time variables in all estimations, the year 2007 is used as a reference against the short-term and longer-term exposure of participants to the economic crisis.

Mediators

The purpose of the mediation analysis is to attempt to disentangle the individual-level impact of the crisis on the possible mediating factors rather than to obtain unbiased estimates of the impact of each pathway. As this is an extension of previous work by Asgeirsdottir et al. [7], we conduct our mediation analysis in a similar way. The body mass index (BMI) is used to proxy overall body composition. BMI is calculated by dividing an individual's weight in kilograms by the square of their height in meters. Four dummy variables corresponding to the four BMI categories were constructed (<18.5 is underweight; 18.5–24.9 is optimal and used as the benchmark; 25–29.9 is overweight; ≥30 indicates obesity). Four dummy variables representing smoking behaviors are: *daily smoker*; *weekly smoker*; *seldom smoker* for those who report smoking less than once a week; *non-smoker* is the benchmark for smoking behavior. While the unadjusted t-tests in Tables 1 and 2 show mostly a non-significant statistical difference between years in health behaviors, i.e. smoking and alcohol consumption, a reduction in daily smokers and increase in non-smokers for both genders is notable.

Five dummy variables represent alcohol consumption in the last 12 months. The variables are: *daily drinker*; *frequent drinker* for those who answered to having at

Table 2 Full panel data sample summary statistics: females answering both waves

Variable	2007			2012			t-test
	Mean	SD	N	Mean	SD	N	p-value
Age	52.057	16.190	1736	57.057	16.190	1736	
1 if hypertension	0.234	0.423	1690	0.293	0.455	1667	0.0001
1 if coronary thrombosis	0.005	0.073	1688	0.009	0.092	1646	0.2685
1 if coronary disease	0.016	0.126	1674	0.026	0.160	1631	0.0411
1 if stroke	0.002	0.049	1683	0.004	0.060	1645	0.5033
1 if cardiovascular disease	0.019	0.137	1736	0.030	0.171	1736	0.0369
No. of children	2.572	1.550	1727	2.701	1.468	1717	0.0121
1 if rural	0.355	0.479	1704	0.347	0.476	1689	0.6214
1 if married	0.591	0.492	1711	0.584	0.493	1705	0.6647
1 if cohabiting	0.151	0.358	1711	0.129	0.335	1705	0.0669
1 if single or in a relationship	0.120	0.326	1711	0.104	0.305	1705	0.1246
1 if divorced	0.061	0.239	1711	0.070	0.256	1705	0.2573
1 if widowed	0.077	0.267	1711	0.113	0.317	1705	0.0003
1 if educ1[a]	0.454	0.498	1730	0.454	0.498	1730	
1 if educ2[a]	0.034	0.182	1730	0.034	0.182	1730	
1 if educ3[a]	0.210	0.408	1730	0.210	0.408	1730	
1 if educ4[a]	0.218	0.413	1730	0.218	0.413	1730	
1 if educ5[a]	0.083	0.275	1730	0.083	0.275	1730	
1 if hypertension medication	0.219	0.414	1672	0.293	0.455	1676	0.0000
1 if cholesterol medication	0.078	0.268	1689	0.134	0.341	1692	0.0000
1 if circulatory disease medication	0.017	0.130	1688	0.030	0.170	1679	0.0157
Body Max Index (BMI)	27.278	5.378	1683	27.448	4.988	1691	0.3419
1 if underweight	0.005	0.073	1683	0.006	0.077	1691	0.8262
1 if optimal weight	0.380	0.485	1683	0.352	0.478	1691	0.1008
1 if overweight	0.358	0.479	1683	0.374	0.484	1691	0.3333
1 if obese	0.257	0.437	1683	0.268	0.443	1691	0.4839
1 if non smoker	0.803	0.398	1676	0.853	0.355	1690	0.0001
1 if daily smoker	0.157	0.364	1676	0.116	0.320	1690	0.0005
1 if weekly smoker	0.015	0.121	1676	0.014	0.116	1690	0.7492
1 if seldom smoker	0.026	0.158	1676	0.018	0.132	1690	0.1155
1 if non drinker	0.155	0.362	1697	0.180	0.384	1692	0.0542
1 if daily drinker	0.015	0.123	1697	0.009	0.097	1692	0.1229
1 if frequent drinker	0.199	0.399	1697	0.180	0.384	1692	0.1598
1 if seldom drinker	0.402	0.491	1697	0.391	0.488	1692	0.4823
1 if rare drinker	0.229	0.420	1697	0.241	0.428	1692	0.4136
Perceived Stress Scale (PSS)	7.374	2.009	1668	7.852	1.705	1640	0.0000
1 if unemployed	0.293	0.169	1671	0.033	0.179	1684	0.5134
1 if much better financial status[b]	0.010	0.101	1641	0.011	0.102	1618	0.9670
1 if considerably better financial status[b]	0.090	0.286	1641	0.092	0.289	1618	0.8032
1 if somewhat better financial status[b]	0.190	0.392	1641	0.193	0.395	1618	0.7756
1 if similar financial status[b]	0.521	0.500	1641	0.498	0.500	1618	0.1916

Table 2 Full panel data sample summary statistics: females answering both waves *(Continued)*

1 if somewhat worse financial status[b]	0.124	0.329	1641	0.143	0.350	1618	0.1093
1 if considerably worse financial status[b]	0.052	0.223	1641	0.047	0.212	1618	0.4755
1 if much worse financial status[b]	0.012	0.110	1641	0.015	0.121	1618	0.5131
Real income[c]	3.799	2.446	1647	3.389	1.898	1629	0.0000
Work hours	4.514	4.119	1592	4.085	4.127	1569	0.0035

Summary statistics only represent the data and do not display any crisis effect. Means are unweighted. *P*-values are from *t*-test for differences in means between 2007 and 2012
[a]Education level is represented by dummy variables: educ1 represents primary or lower level secondary education; educ2 stands for vocational master or journeyman certificate; educ3 stands for high school or equivalent; educ4 stands for technical graduate or undergraduate degree; educ5 stands for master's degree or a Ph.D
[b]Perceived financial status represents respondents' own perception of their families' financial status relative to other families
[c]Real income is reported at 2012 price level in millions of Icelandic kronas (ISK)

least one drink 1–4 times a week; *seldom drinker* for those who answered having a drink 1–3 times a month or at least one drink 7–11 times in the last 12 months; *rare drinker* stands for those who had a drink 1–6 times in the last 12 months; *non-drinker* for those not having had an alcoholic drink in the last 12 months is the benchmark variable for alcohol consumption.

A short form of the Perceived Stress Scale (PSS) was used, consisting of four questions that measure to which degree situations in one's life are conceived as stressful [75]. Five answering options for each question, translate to an overall score range from 0 to 16, with 16 representing the highest level of stress. Unadjusted stress levels increased significantly between the years for both genders (Tables 1 and 2).

The variable *work hours* refers to time spent on paid work. A question on hours spent each week on paid work had thirteen categories, ranging from 0 to over 60 hours per week. The midpoint of each category was used to ease readability of the estimated coefficients of work hours; the variable was scaled to working hours per day (assuming 5 working days per week) in continuous form. A dummy variable for unemployment was also used.

The variable *annual income* refers to the respondents' complete income before taxes. Ten answering options were available, from less than 900 thousand Icelandic kronas (ISK) annually to more than 8.4 million ISK annually. The midpoint of each category was used as continuous, with a top of 9.0 million ISK used for the highest category. Inflation between the years 2007 and 2009 was 27.05%, between 2007 and 2012 it was 42.73%. Amounts were set to the 2012 price level. Real income decreased by a statistically significant amount between 2007 and 2012 for both males and females.

Seven dummy variables were constructed from the equal amount of response categories for perceived relative financial status in society based on answers to the question "In a financial sense, how well or badly off do you consider your family to be relative to other families in Iceland?" A perceived similar financial status relative to other Icelandic families is used as the benchmark variable in the mediation analysis.

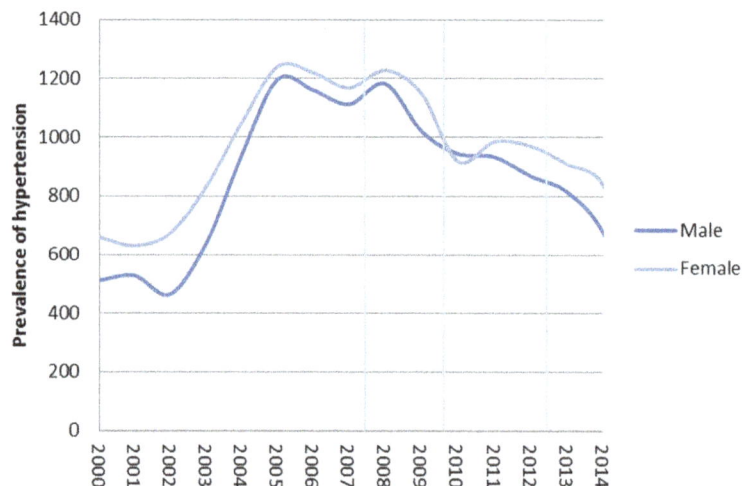

Fig. 3 Prevalence of hypertension among patients with cardiovascular diseases in January 2000-December 2014. Source: Landspitali University Hospital. Notes: Vertical lines refer to the timing of 1st, 2nd, and 3rd waves of data collection for the survey data used here. The prevalence of hypertension is reported in absolute terms

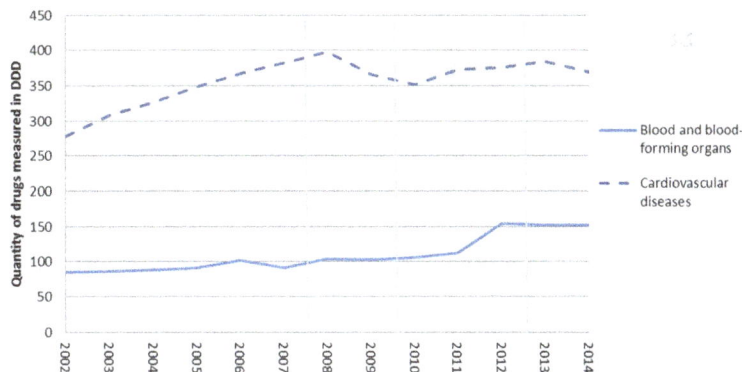

Fig. 4 Usage for medication for cardiovascular diseases and blood and blood-forming organs in 2000-2014. Source: Statistics Iceland. February 6th 2017 from: http://px.hagstofa.is/pxen/pxweb/en/Samfelag/Samfelag__heilbrigdismal__heilbrigdisthjonusta/HEI08101.px/table/tableViewLayout1/?rxid = b55fddaf-5d24-4e01-885f-299513510b32. Notes: Vertical lines refer to the timing of 1st, 2nd, and 3rd waves of data collection for the survey data used here. The quantity of drugs is shown in defined daily dose (DDD) per 1000 inhabitants. DDD is according to WHO standard of each year

Estimations

In our main analysis, fixed-effects models are used to estimate the relationship between the timing of responses and the dependent variables, with the recovery indicator *t2012* capturing the impact of the economic recovery compared to the pre-crisis. As fixed-effects logit models did not suit the data due to a big proportion of the sample having no within-individual variation leading to many observations being dropped, we estimate linear probability fixed-effects models instead, using the estimation equation:

$$H_{it} = \alpha + t2012_{it}\beta_1 + t2009_{it}\beta_2 + X_{it}\beta_3$$
$$+ M_{it}\beta_4 + v_i + e_{it}$$

$$(1)$$

Where α is a constant term, H is a health outcome for individual i at time t, *t2012* and *t2009* are indicators for long-term and short-term exposure to the economic

crisis, making β_1 our main coefficient of interest, X contains demographic variables including age, marital status, number of children, and residency, M are possible mediating factors that are only included in the mediation analysis, v is a term for individual fixed effects, and e is the disturbance term.

In the sensitivity analysis, pooled logit models are estimated. Similar to our main analysis the key variable is the recovery indicator, *t2012*. Results are reported as marginal effects calculated after logit regressions and all analyses are performed separately for males and females. To account for individual heteroscedasticity, standard errors are clustered on individuals in the logit regressions.

In the mediation analysis, one possible mediating factor was added at a time to the base models in order to assess the extent to which changes in each factor can explain changes in the recovery indicator, being observant of both mediating and possibly suppressing roles of those variables in the causal path between the independent and

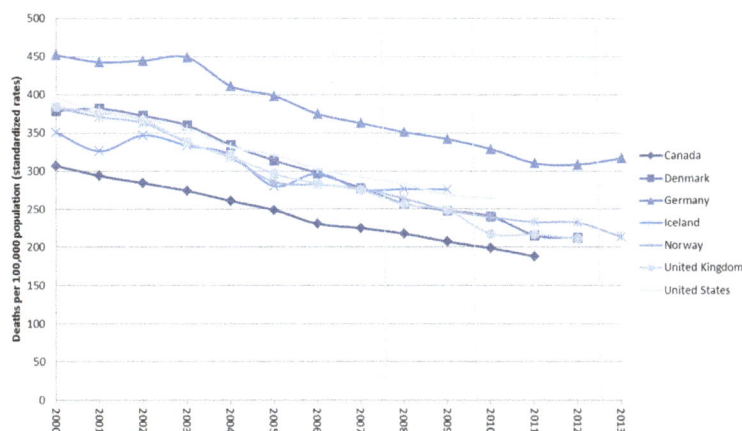

Fig. 5 Aggregate standardized mortality rates due to circulatory diseases in 2000-2013. Source: OECD. August 11th 2015 from: http://stats.oecd.org/index.aspx?DataSetCode = HEALTH_STAT. Notes: Vertical lines refer to the timing of 1st, 2nd, and 3rd waves of data collection for the survey data used here

dependent variable [76, 77]. In an alternate mediation model, an interaction term of the possible mediating factor and the recovery indicator was also included in the mediation analysis to account for the possibility of moderated mediation, i.e. that the strength of the mediated relationship is contingent on the value of the recovery indicator [78–80]. For the sake of brevity, the results from the alternate mediation model are only included in the supplementary online material. Mediation tests using uncontrolled models were performed to test the significance of mediators. A Sobel-Goodman test [81] was performed, both with and without alterations to fit logit models, as described by Mackinnon and Dwyer [82], yielding almost identical results.

Stata 13.1 was used for all statistical computations. The study was approved by the Directorate of Health (1311268/5.6.1/gkg), the Ethics Board of Iceland (07-081, 09-094 and 12-107) and the Data Protection Authority of Iceland (S4455).

Results

Very few observations of coronary thrombosis, coronary disease, and stroke led to imprecise estimates which did not show statistically significant effects in the recovery indicators, except for coronary diseases in females using fixed-effects and in males using pooled cross-sectional estimations (results shown in the supplementary online material). Results for the variable cardiovascular disease, representing all of the three related variables, are thus reported. Tables 3 and 4 show the results from the mediation analysis (for both genders), with the recovery indicator, $t2012$, reported as our main independent variable (full results from the base analysis are reported in the supplementary online material). Tables 5 and 6 for the pooled logit model in the sensitivity analysis are comparable to Tables 3 and 4 for the fixed-effects models. Figures 6 and 7 reveal the differences in the results for the recovery indicator, $t2012$, and indicator for short-term exposure, $t2009$, between the estimation models used. The figures show point estimates from regressions as well as 90% confidence intervals.

Fixed effects

A statistically significant (at the 10% level) negative relationship between the recovery indicator and hypertension in males was found, but a statistically -significant relationship was not found for cardiovascular diseases. For females, the recovery indicator is statistically significant for both hypertension and cardiovascular diseases (at the 5 and 1% level respectively), but the sign of the coefficient is not the same; a positive relationship is found between the recovery indicator and hypertension, but a negative relationship when cardiovascular diseases are explored. Point estimates for the recovery indicator

reveal a decreased probability for females of having cardiovascular disease during the economic recovery by 4.14 percentage points compared to pre-crisis (Table 4). For hypertension, our estimates point to an increased probability of having hypertension during the economic recovery by 7.39 percentage points compared to pre-crisis for females (Table 4), but a decrease of 4.69 percentage points for males (Table 3).

In the mediation analysis for hypertension in males, the recovery indicator was consistently negative, and statistically significant with the addition of every mediator except BMI and unemployment. For females, the same consistency was found, with the recovery indicator remaining positive and statistically significant with the addition of all mediators except BMI. The addition of possible mediators resulted in both a reduction and an increase in the coefficient for the recovery indicator, $t2012$, leading to the conclusion that some of the possible mediators serve as mediators and some as suppressors, although generally not confirmed with mediation tests ($p > 0.1$). For convenience, we guide the reader through one mediator (unemployment) for hypertension in females and one suppressor (stress) (see Table 4). The coefficient for the recovery indicator in the base model is indicated at the top of the table (0.0739). When income is added to the model, the recovery indicator is reduced (0.0661) by 10.55%, which indicates that changes in unemployment explain 10.55% of the recovery effect on hypertension in females. Smoking, BMI, alcohol consumption, and a person's perception of their financial status in society are also identified as mediators, albeit to a very limited extent and, except in the case of smoking, not confirmed with mediation tests ($p > 0.1$). The increased probability of females having hypertension between 2007 and 2012 seems suppressed by changes in stress and according to the mediation analysis hypertension would have increased by 17.86% more than current estimates suggest if no changes in stress would have occurred between waves. The other variables that were identified as suppressors for hypertension in females were working hours and income.

Sensitivity analysis – pooled logit model estimations

No statistically significant recovery effect was linked to cardiovascular diseases for either gender. However, a statistically significant effect at the 10% level was found for hypertension in females. Point estimates for the recovery indicator reveal an increased probability of having hypertension during the economic recovery by 2.58 percentage points compared to pre-crisis. A statistically significant relationship was not found for males.

In the mediation analysis for hypertension, the recovery indicator was never statistically significant for males (Table 5), but for females (Table 6) it was significant for

Table 3 Mediation analysis - males: Linear probability fixed-effects estimates

Dependent variable	Hypertension			Cardiovascular Disease		
	dy/dx	Robust SE		dy/dx	Robust SE	
Without mediators						
t2012	-0.0469	0.0284	*	-0.0092	0.0172	
BMI included						
t2012	-0.0468	0.0292		-0.0119	0.0177	
1 if underweight	-0.0112	0.0158		0.0096	0.0097	
1 if overweight	0.0044	0.0215		0.0083	0.0121	
1 if obese	0.0546	0.0426		0.0210	0.0182	
Alcohol included						
t2012	-0.0607	0.0292	**	-0.0093	0.0177	
1 if daily drinker	0.0537	0.1090		0.1070	0.0612	*
1 if frequent drinker	0.1300	0.0874		0.0928	0.0412	**
1 if seldom drinker	0.1100	0.0873		-0.0895	0.0412	**
1 if rare drinker	-0.0654	0.0808		0.0698	0.0373	*
Smoking included						
t2012	-0.0666	0.0275	**	-0.0137	0.0175	
1 if daily smoker	0.0556	0.0355		-0.0165	0.0166	
1 if weekly smoker	-0.0140	0.0240		-0.0476	0.0249	*
1 if seldom smoker	0.0134	0.0535		-0.0525	0.0250	**
Perceived status in society included						
t2012	-0.0605	0.0298	**	-0.0036	0.0178	
1 if much better	0.0260	0.0368		-0.0108	0.0208	
1 if considerably better	0.0143	0.0159		0.0181	0.0096	*
1 if somewhat better	-0.0011	0.0142		-0.0046	0.0080	
1 if somewhat worse	-0.0502	0.0244	**	0.0039	0.0072	
1 if considerably worse	-0.0769	0.0483		-0.0023	0.0190	
1 if much worse	-0.0695	0.0623		0.1330	0.0741	*
Stress included						
t2012	-0.0566	0.0300	*	-0.0022	0.0179	
pss	0.0063	0.0038	*	-0.0009	0.0018	
Unemployment included						
t2012	-0.0436	0.0296		-0.0073	0.0176	
1 if unemployed	0.0098	0.0451		-0.0097	0.0276	
Income included						
t2012	-0.0534	0.0285	**	-0.0148	0.0172	
real income	-0.0017	0.0038		0.0018	0.0015	
Working hours included						
t2012	-0.0726	0.0318	**	-0.0084	0.0193	
working hours per workday	-0.0016	0.0016		0.0005	0.0011	

Sample weights are applied. Covariates controlled for are number of children, marital status, residence, presciption mediation, and short-term crisis coefficient (t2009). *$p < 0.1$, **$p < 0.05$, ***$p < 0.01$

every addition of a mediator. For females the point estimates for the recovery indicator lowered with the addition of the variables representing health behaviors (BMI, alcohol consumption, and smoking) and the labor-market variables (unemployment, income, and working hours), with BMI mediating the largest effects out of the possible mediators studied (13.28%). However, stress and people's perception of their relative financial status in society led to

Table 4 Mediation analysis - females: Linear probability fixed-effects estimates

Dependent variable	Hypertension			Cardiovascular Disease		
	dy/dx	Robust SE		dy/dx	Robust SE	
Without mediators						
t2012	0.0739	0.0341	**	-0.0414	0.0145	***
BMI included						
t2012	0.0489	0.0326		-0.0391	0.0146	***
1 if underweight	0.0341	0.0352		-0.0068	0.0088	
1 if overweight	0.0222	0.0161		-0.0113	0.0094	
1 if obese	0.0283	0.0236		-0.0194	0.0117	*
Alcohol included						
t2012	0.0705	0.0347	**	-0.0434	0.0149	***
1 if daily drinker	-0.0239	0.0548		0.0152	0.0182	
1 if frequent drinker	-0.0610	0.0421		0.0106	0.0183	
1 if seldom drinker	-0.0461	0.0399		-0.0044	0.0178	
1 if rare drinker	-0.0408	0.0372		0.0032	0.0179	
Smoking included						
t2012	0.0730	0.0350	**	-0.0421	0.0149	***
1 if daily smoker	-0.0141	0.0349		0.0040	0.0069	
1 if weekly smoker	-0.0082	0.0452		0.0053	0.0062	
1 if seldom smoker	-0.0246	0.0348		0.0038	0.0036	
Perceived status in society included						
t2012	0.0632	0.0354	*	-0.0440	0.0149	***
1 if much better	-0.0034	0.0627		-0.0007	0.0050	
1 if considerably better	0.0184	0.0198		0.0025	0.0081	
1 if somewhat better	0.0095	0.0128		-0.0001	0.0047	
1 if somewhat worse	-0.0131	0.0145		-0.0050	0.0064	
1 if considerably worse	0.0335	0.0255		0.0084	0.0115	
1 if much worse	0.0537	0.0563		-0.0588	0.0548	
Stress included						
t2012	0.0871	0.0352	**	-0.0433	0.0151	***
pss	-0.0018	0.0034		0.0008	0.0017	
Unemployment included						
t2012	0.0661	0.0347	*	-0.0358	0.0123	***
1 if unemployed	0.0117	0.0247		0.0301	0.0166	*
Income included						
t2012	0.0808	0.0355	**	-0.0468	0.0161	***
real income	-0.0071	0.0038	*	0.0013	0.001	
Working hours included						
t2012	0.0874	0.0351	**	-0.0428	0.0154	***
working hours per workday	-0.0043	0.0016	***	-0.0006	0.0004	

Sample weights are applied. Covariates controlled for are number of children, marital status, residence, presciption medication, and short-term crisis coefficient (t2009). $*p < 0.1$, $**p < 0.05$, $***p < 0.01$

an increase in the recovery indicator, thus serving as suppressors in the relationship.

Results for the relationship between cardiovascular disease and the recovery indicator are reported in Tables 5 and 6 for males and females respectively. As expected, the precision of those measurements is low and the relationship is never found to be statistically significant, with or without mediators, for either gender.

Table 5 Pooled logit model estimations - Mediation analysis: males

Dependent variable	Hypertension			Cardiovascular Disease		
	dy/dx	Robust SE		dy/dx	Robust SE	
Without mediators						
t2012	0.0029	0.0119		0.0009	0.0023	
BMI included	ε	ε		ε	ε	
t2012	0.0049	0.0112		0.0012	0.0023	
1 if underweight						
1 if overweight	0.0497	0.0118	***	0.0005	0.0022	
1 if obese	0.2080	0.0315	***	0.0051	0.0046	
Alcohol included						
t2012	0.0021	0.0119		0.0009	0.0022	
1 if daily drinker	0.0555	0.0362		0.0225	0.0156	
1 if frequent drinker	0.0215	0.0165		0.0010	0.0030	
1 if seldom drinker	0.0403	0.0173	**	0.0003	0.0024	
1 if rare drinker	0.0348	0.0212		0.0057	0.0040	
Smoking included						
t2012	0.0024	0.0120		0.0012	0.0022	
1 if daily smoker	-0.0089	0.0147		0.0051	0.0036	
1 if weekly smoker	-0.0836	0.0148	***	-0.0068	0.0043	
1 if seldom smoker	0.0251	0.0440		-0.0058	0.0051	
Perceived status in society included						
t2012	0.0023	0.0120		0.0002	0.0022	
1 if much better	-0.0201	0.0322		-0.0072	0.0037	*
1 if considerably better	-0.0292	0.0137	**	0.0047	0.0035	
1 if somewhat better	-0.0033	0.0123		-0.0021	0.0024	
1 if somewhat worse	0.0124	0.0196		-0.0006	0.0029	
1 if considerably worse	0.0382	0.0327		0.0096	0.0062	
1 if much worse	-0.0058	0.0358		0.0315	0.0207	
Stress included						
t2012	-0.0009	0.0121		0.0004	0.0022	
PSS	0.0071	0.0029	**	0.0013	0.0006	**
Unemployment included						
t2012	0.0009	0.0121		0.0006	0.0023	
1 if unemployed	0.0738	0.0387	*	0.0037	0.0056	
Income included						
t2012	0.0021	0.0120		0.0001	0.0023	
real income	-0.0008	0.0022		-0.0010	0.0005	*
Working hours included						
t2012	0.0041	0.0119		0.0001	0.0021	
working hours per workday	-0.0014	0.0012		-0.0004	0.0003	*

Results are presented as marginal effects. Sample weights are applied. Covariates controlled for are age, age squared, number of children, marital status, residence, education, prescription medication, and short-term crisis coefficient (t2009). ᵋMissing coefficient due to perfect predictability of underweight; hence optimal weight and underweight are combined in this estimation as a benchmark. *$p < 0.1$, **$p < 0.05$, ***$p < 0.01$

Table 6 Pooled logit model estimations - Mediation analysis: females

Dependent variable	Hypertension			Cardiovascular Disease		
	dy/dx	Robust SE		dy/dx	Robust SE	
Without mediators						
t2012	0.0258	0.0132	*	0.0007	0.0026	
BMI included						
t2012	0.0224	0.0127	*	0.0004	0.0020	
1 if underweight	-0.0235	0.0961		ε	ε	
1 if overweight	0.0606	0.0133	***	0.0002	0.0022	
1 if obese	0.1710	0.0196	***	0.0032	0.0026	
Alcohol included		0.0132				
t2012	0.0238	0.0224	*	0.0002	0.0021	
1 if daily drinker	-0.0830	0.0158	***	σ	σ	
1 if frequent drinker	-0.0365	0.0150	*	-0.0009 σ	0.0027 σ	
1 if seldom drinker	0.0068	0.0166		0.0010	0.0022	
1 if rare drinker	0.0185			0.0025	0.0025	
Smoking included						
t2012	0.0247	0.0133	*	0.0004	0.0020	
1 if daily smoker	-0.0358	0.0127	***	-0.0020	0.0022	
1 if weekly smoker	-0.0367	0.0440		-0.0053 δ	0.0028 δ	*
1 if seldom smoker	-0.0385	0.0351		δ	δ	
Perceived status in society included						
t2012	0.0260	0.0134	*	0.0005	0.0019	
1 if much better	-0.0354	0.0443		-0.0014	0.0054	
1 if considerably better	0.0013	0.0179		-0.0051	0.0023	**
1 if somewhat better	-0.0153	0.0131		-0.0025	0.0019	
1 if somewhat worse	-0.0112	0.0160		-0.0028	0.0020	
1 if considerably worse	-0.0123	0.0228		-0.0002	0.0031	
1 if much worse	-0.0048	0.0475		-0.0037	0.0025	
Stress included						
t2012	0.0258	0.0135	*	-0.0002	0.0020	
PSS	-0.0034	0.0029		0.0007	0.0004	
Unemployment included						
t2012	0.0256	0.0133	*	0.0004	0.0020	
1 if unemployed	0.0190	0.0284		0.0110	0.0081	
Income included						
t2012	0.0247	0.0134	*	0.0009	0.0020	
real income	-0.0014	0.0033		-0.0007	0.0006	
Working hours included						
t2012	0.0254	0.0135	*	0.0003	0.0021	
working hours per workday	-0.0033	0.0016	**	-0.0004	0.0003	

Results are presented as marginal effects. Sample weights are applied. Covariates controlled for are age, age squared, number of children, marital status, residence, education, prescription medication, and short-term crisis coefficient (t2009). $^{\varepsilon}$Missing coefficient due to perfect predictability of underweight; hence optimal weight and underweight are combined in this estimation as a benchmark. $^{\sigma}$Missing coefficient due to perfect predictability of daily drinker; hence daily drinker and frequent drinker are combined in this estimation. $^{\delta}$Missing coefficient due to perfect predictability of seldom smoker; hence seldom smoker and weekly smoker are combined in this estimation. $*p < 0.1$, $**p < 0.05$, $***p < 0.01$

Fig. 6 Regression results from fixed-effect models. Notes: Markers refer to point estimates from regressions. Horizontal lines refer to 90% confidence intervals

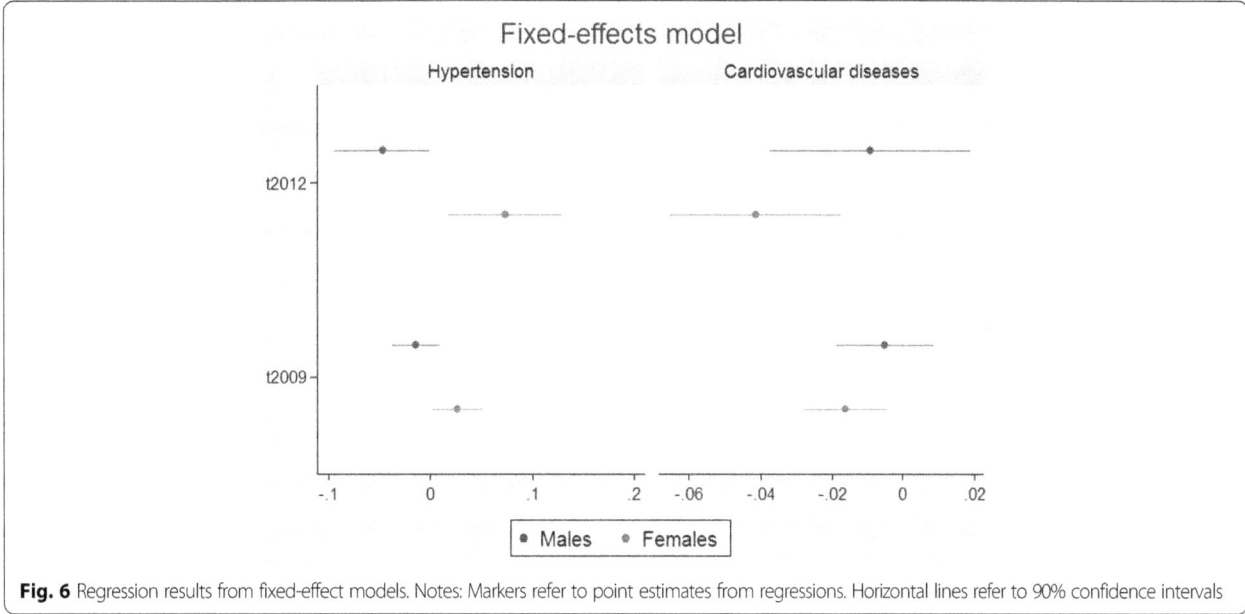

When comparing results from our main analysis to the pooled logit models in the sensitivity analysis we find that the linear probability fixed-effects model shows a recovery effect that is larger in magnitude and higher in statistical significance for hypertension in both genders and for cardiovascular diseases in females (Figs. 6 and 7, and Tables 3, 4, 5 and 6).

Sensitivity analysis – prescription medication
The results found when using prescription medication as the dependent variables paint a very similar picture as our main results, both when using fixed-effects models and pooled logit models in the estimations (see Tables 7 and 8). The sign of the coefficient for the recovery indicator is negative, and statistical significance is quite similar to our main results except in the case of hypertension in females where we do not find a statistically significant relationship when using prescription medication as a dependent variable (see Tables 3, 4, and 7). Predictably, a positive, highly statistical relationship is found between age and the use of prescription medication. Rather striking though, is the high statistical significance for the recovery indicator, especially when compared to our main results using diagnosis of the diseases as a dependent variable. The most obvious reason

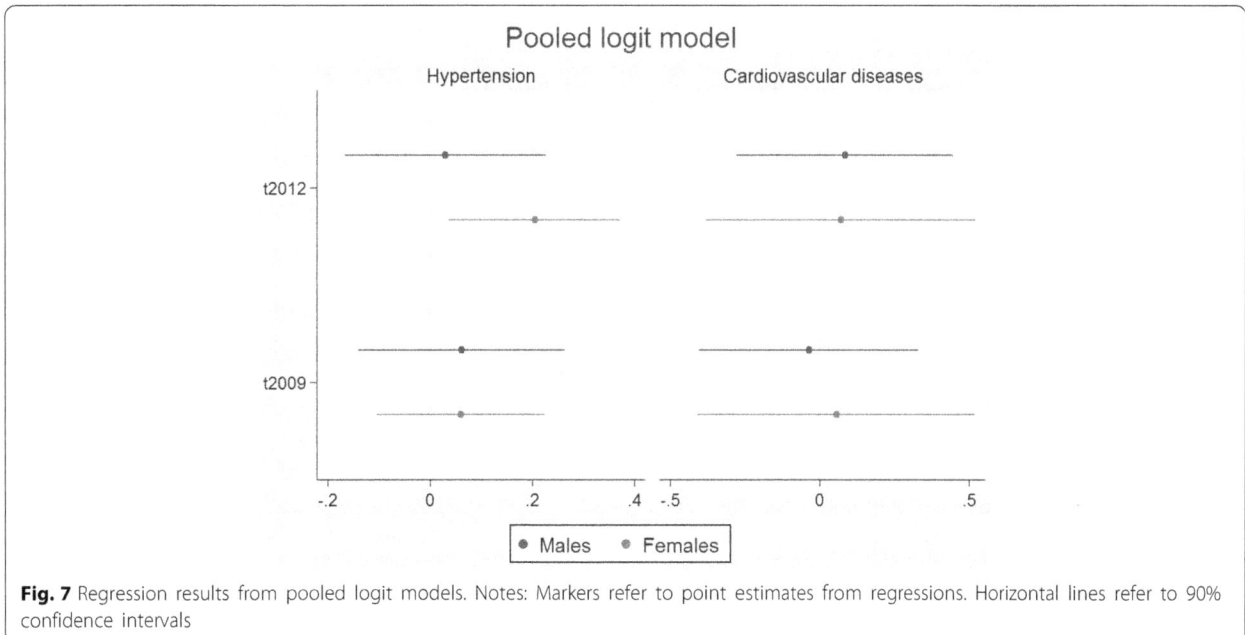

Fig. 7 Regression results from pooled logit models. Notes: Markers refer to point estimates from regressions. Horizontal lines refer to 90% confidence intervals

Table 7 Prescription medication usage in the last 2 weeks – fixed-effects model estimations

Dependent variable	Hypertension-medication			Cardiovascular & cholesterol-medication		
	dy/dx	Robust SE		dy/dx	Robust SE	
Males						
t2012	-0.0506	0.0226	**	-0.0303	0.0238	
t2009	-0.0157	0.0110		-0.0225	0.0100	**
Age squared	0.0003	0.0001	***	0.0002	0.0001	***
No. of children	-0.0030	0.0215		-0.0116	0.0200	
1 if rural	-0.0084	0.0189		-0.0378	0.0277	
1 if cohabiting	0.0061	0.0138		0.0054	0.0194	
1 if married	0.0217	0.0257		0.0312	0.0283	
1 if divorced	-0.0877	0.0733		0.0300	0.0387	
1 if widowed	-0.0743	0.0696		0.0224	0.0540	
n	4163			4260		
Females						
t2012	-0.0035	0.0227		-0.0564	0.0193	***
t2009	0.0076	0.0105		-0.0257	0.0088	***
Age squared	0.0001	0.0001	***	0.0002	0.0000	***
No. of children	-0.0239	0.0101	**	-0.0115	0.0049	**
1 if rural	0.0164	0.0195		0.0097	0.0140	
1 if cohabiting	-0.0004	0.0110		-0.0118	0.0113	
1 if married	0.0071	0.0182		-0.0075	0.0164	
1 if divorced	-0.0154	0.0311		0.0375	0.0264	
1 if widowed	0.0181	0.0431		0.0633	0.0566	
N	4790			4872		

Sample weights are applied. $*p < 0.1$, $**p < 0.05$, $***p < 0.01$

for this difference is that participants were asked about their usage of prescription drugs in the last 2 weeks, but when asked about a diagnosis of a disease no time perimeter was set in the questionnaires from 2007 to 2009 and it was 12 months in the questionnaire from 2012.

In light of the attrition between the original sample and the final sample used in our analysis an attrition analysis was performed. This was also done in an attempt to understand better the reversal of the relationship between the shorter-term crisis and hypertension found by Asgeirsdottir et al. [7] using panel estimations and the differing results from the methods used here. By comparing means between groups we found that there are more non-attritors who report having hypertension in general than attritors, but fewer who report having developed hypertension during the economic collapse, between 2007 and 2009. Our main internal validity concern is that participants who reported having developed hypertension or cardiovascular diseases in the years between 2007 and 2009 had attrited and were thus not a part of the sample in 2012. This was indeed found to be the case for cardiovascular diseases, but this hypothesis was however rejected in our attrition analysis in the case of hypertension (result

available in the supplementary online material). However, the sign of the coefficient is comparable in the attrition analysis between genders, thus not explaining the differing results found in our analyses.

Discussion

A priori the recovery effects under examination here are not known, where one could well imagine that health effects influenced by changes in the economy could diminish or even disappear with the stabilization of economic conditions. Conversely, some diseases take time to emerge, e.g. because of persistent exposure to stressful circumstances caused by ambient economic conditions. Cardiovascular diseases have both elements of cumulative build up, as well as sensitivity to immediate circumstances.

The results found using fixed-effects models and pooled logit models were consistent across some dimensions while conflicting across others. When effects were found for females, they consistently showed hypertension to be greater during the recovery period than the boom. However, while fixed-effects estimations revealed statistically significant results for both genders (in opposite

Table 8 Prescription medication usage in the last 2 weeks – pooled logit model estimations

Dependent variable	Hypertension-medication			Cardiovascular & cholesterol-medication		
	dy/dx	Robust SE		dy/dx	Robust SE	
Males						
t2012	0.0265	0.0093	***	0.0143	0.0070	**
t2009	0.0153	0.0097		0.0025	0.0055	
Age	0.0238	0.0016	***	0.0130	0.0011	***
Age squared	-0.0002	0.0000	***	-0.0001	0.0000	***
No. of children	-0.0066	0.0028	**	-0.0037	0.0016	**
1 if rural	-0.0004	0.0070		-0.0021	0.0043	
1 if cohabiting	0.0245	0.0226		0.0206	0.0157	
1 if married	0.0017	0.0151		0.0002	0.0097	
1 if divorced	-0.0421	0.0127	***	-0.0111	0.0114	
1 if widowed	-0.0009	0.0205		0.0416	0.0259	
educ2	-0.0030	0.0087		-0.0092	0.0051	*
educ3	0.0291	0.0122	**	0.0028	0.0062	
educ4	0.0004	0.0124		-0.0142	0.0073	*
educ5	0.0038	0.0134		0.0090	0.0105	
N	4151			4250		
Pseudo R-squared	0.206			0.206		
Females						
t2012	0.0203	0.0105	*	0.0101	0.0034	***
t2009	0.0166	0.0107		0.0036	0.0027	
Age	0.0178	0.0021	***	0.0064	0.0007	***
Age squared	-0.0001	0.0000	***	0.0000	0.0000	***
No. of children	0.0025	0.0032		0.0002	0.0008	
1 if rural	0.0186	0.0091	**	-0.0007	0.0020	
1 if cohabiting	-0.0099	0.0209		-0.0007	0.0066	
1 if married	-0.0035	0.0169		0.0018	0.0045	
1 if divorced	-0.0098	0.0207		0.0094	0.0081	
1 if widowed	0.0092	0.0223		0.0050	0.0063	
educ2	-0.0214	0.0205		-0.0003	0.0054	
educ3	-0.0150	0.0099		-0.0026	0.0027	
educ4	-0.0327	0.0114	***	-0.0045	0.0034	
educ5	-0.0429	0.0142	***	-0.0074	0.0051	
n	4774			4856		
Pseudo R-squared	0.184			0.214		

Sample weights are applied. *$p < 0.1$, **$p < 0.05$, ***$p < 0.01$

directions), statistically significant results were found only for females using pooled logit models. Furthermore, pooled cross-sectional estimations reported in the supplementary online material showed statistically significant results for men only. Our sensitivity analysis using prescription medication as a dependent variable supported our main results to a large extent, with the exception of hypertension in females where the recovery indicator was not statistically significant. A priori we did not expect

such similarities to emerge since the definition of the outcome variables are quite different, as is the time frame for each one (participants were asked about their use of prescription medication in the last two weeks, but when asked about the diagnosis of a medical condition the time frame indicated in the questionnaires from 2007 to 2009 was simply "in the past" and in the 2012 questionnaire it was changed to "the last 12 months"). As people's memory can become less reliable as time goes by, the accuracy in answers is arguably better with a shorter time-frame for participants to consider, but on the other hand not all who are diagnosed with a disease decide to use medication to combat the disease. Therefore it is not obvious which variable better captures what we want to measure – the long-term exposure of the economic collapse on health. Thus it's important to view the results from the primary estimations and sensitivity analysis together as a whole.

Previously published results by Asgeirsdottir et al. [7] showed statistically significant hypertension effects of the crisis in the short term in males only. Our results using pooled data in a similar fashion as they did showed a different timing of responses across genders; with males showing a more immediate response and dwindling with time (not statistically significant), and females showing a delayed response during the economic recovery as opposed to the height of the crisis in 2009.

Although our results using fixed-effects models point to a negative relationship between long-term exposure to the crisis (recovery indicator) and cardiovascular diseases (statistically significant for females), those results were found to be affected by attrition. Perhaps not surprisingly, those results were not found to be stable across estimation strategies, with no statistically significant relationship found using pooled logit models. Those results are though reported for completeness as was done in the study on short-term effects of the crisis [7].

Not all our results are robust to changes in the estimation model used. However, the coefficient that remained stable and statistically significant was the recovery indicator when estimating hypertension in females. Furthermore, bias due to attrition was not found to be present in those estimations. Our main conclusion is thus that during the economic recovery in 2012, when the dust was settling after the economic collapse, Icelandic women had an increased probability of having hypertension compared to the boom year 2007.

In light of the commonalities of our research and that of Asgeirsdottir et al. [7], the causes of the differences in results are worth further attention and even further exploration in future research. As mentioned earlier, the nature of diseases can vary. This could explain why the elevated hypertension during the recovery period in men is no longer found when a balanced panel is used, but has instead appeared in women. However, this would not explain why the gender effects are reversed when new individuals in both 2007 and 2012 are studied, as found in the cross-sectional estimations reported in the supplementary online material. If death of males who previously reported having hypertension is the main cause of the altered results between years, or the different results found between estimation methods, that in itself would be noteworthy, but results for the attrition analysis did not confirm a systematic attrition of males in particular. Information on the

fate of individual participants is however not accessible at this time, barring us from that line of research.

This later-time appearance of a female response in the panel data is also interesting as the male-only effect in the previous study had been somewhat puzzling, especially in light of research showing a stronger short-term stress response to the crisis in females than in men using the same data as we examine (waves from 2007 to 2009), where the male stress response was largely measured without statistical significance [5]. Similarly a female-only result was reported for the change in attendance at cardiac emergency departments in Reykjavík, Iceland immediately following the economic collapse in October 2008, which was not observed at other emergency departments [8]. Even further, misuse of alcohol had been reported to go down to a greater extent for males than for females [2]. Those are all results that would suggest a greater effect on female hypertension and CVD than on males, which made the previous results puzzling. The current findings may indicate a lingering female response that may have taken longer to come through. That would be in line with some previous findings, although it has to be kept in mind that the found effects could also be the immediate result of a growing economy in 2012, rather than a delayed effect of the crisis.

This study has both strengths and limitations. The main strengths lie in the comparability to the study by Asgeirsdottir et al. [7], providing additional information on the fates of the same individuals under study using both a pooled logit model as they did as well as using a balanced panel to examine individual fixed effects. Additionally, in the supplementary online material we report results for the pooled cross-sectional estimations, and thus results for always-in-participants and new participants in 2012 can be compared and the possibility of a selection bias in the always-in sample is dealt with. Furthermore, in the supplementary online material we include a mediation analysis using fixed effects which allows for the possibility of moderated mediation. In such a model one could hypothesize various interactions and pathways; marriage may provide some risk sharing, the presence of children in the household could give people less flexibility in adjusting to the crisis, for example by relocating for a different job. Although the current approach is kept in line with the previously published literature, we have included an example of one such pathway, where we add an interaction term of the recovery indicator and the possible mediating factor. Further exploration of this type is a possible avenue for further research.

Moreover, a notable strength is the health outcomes chosen to explore, cardiovascular morbidity, that are available at an individual basis, but most previous studies have used aggregate mortality data, both disease-specific mortality [44, 83] and overall mortality [38, 42, 44, 84]. Death is the severest outcome, and only focusing on that can mask some real health effects that do nevertheless affect people's lives. The study adds to the literature, although results cannot be directly compared with those studies utilizing mortality outcomes.

The analysis by Gudlaugsson et al. [66] of the latest data in *Health and well-being of Icelanders* shows that the health of young Icelandic women, as reported by themselves, has deteriorated across the spectrum in the period between 2007 and 2012. This applies to both mental and physical conditions. The opposite was found for young males, who generally reported better health in 2012 than 2007. These results complement those found in our panel estimations, but also raise questions on why changes in health are materializing differently for males and females. The analysis by Gudlaugsson et al. [66] uses the full dataset available, i.e. all 2012 participants regardless of whether they are new to the sample or not (as well as those who did not fulfil our specifications) and is not in accordance with our results using new entrants in 2012 (results in the supplementary online material), where the economic-recovery indicator shows a stronger association to hypertension in males than females. Although we find a consistently positive link between long-term exposure to the crisis into the recovery period and hypertension in females, both methods used here reveal an unexplained difference in the size of the recovery coefficient between genders. Although fluctuations in the prevalence of hypertension of Icelanders (see Fig. 3) could theoretically be an explanation for our findings, our limited analysis of patterns in related data on hypertension suggests otherwise. First and foremost, a steady decline in the prevalence of hypertension among cardiovascular patients after 2008 suggests that the economic collapse had a beneficial impact on that specific patient group; Icelanders suffering from hypertension were not admitted to the hospital because of cardiovascular diseases to the same extent as before. Given the lack of available data on overall prevalence of hypertension in Icelanders, the aggregate data on cardiovascular patients at Landspitali University Hospital probably gives the strongest clue on the true incidence of hypertension in Iceland. Furthermore, predicted hypertension prevalence, drug use, and circulatory-disease mortality suggest that our findings for females represent a deviation from pre-crisis trends and thus signify a true longer-term crisis impact. Further research is well warranted on that issue.

Conclusions

We find that during the economic recovery in 2012, Icelandic women had an increased probability of having hypertension compared to the boom year 2007. For males,

the results were more ambiguous. This study adds to the strand of literature concerning the relationship between economic cycles and health. Results from other studies regarding this relationship are mixed between settings, and thus our results conform to some while being conflicting to others. We provide results based on individual-level morbidity data, whereas the literature mostly contains studies using mortality data due to data restrictions. The small size of the Icelandic economy might diminish the generalizability of our results, but having said that, the country is a western country, in which the health-care system and health status rival most western societies and standards of living are also comparable. This leads us to conclude that the generalizability and comparability of our results are fairly strong.

Abbreviations
BMI: Body mass index; CVD: Cardiovascular disease; ISK: Icelandic kronas; PSS: Perceived stress scale

Funding
The project was funded by the Icelandic Research Fund (IRF grant number 130611-052) and The University of Iceland Eimskip Fund. The data collection was financed and carried out by the Directorate of Health Iceland (and formerly the Public Health Institute of Iceland). The authors would like to thank the Directorate for access to the data.

Authors' contribution
The work was carried out and led by KHB, Ph.D. student of Economics at the University of Iceland. This includes statistical work as well as the writing of the paper. The work was done under close collaboration and supervision of her Ph.D. thesis supervisor TLA who is a professor at the Department of Economics – University of Iceland. SHJ professor at the University of Iceland, who is also a data analyst at the Directorate of Health, has partly overseen the collection of the data used in the study. He was thus an instrumental advisor and collaborator with expertise on practicalities of the data. All authors read and approved the final manuscript.

Competing interests
The authors declare that they have no conflict of interest.

Author details
[1]Faculty of Economics, University of Iceland, Oddi v/Sturlugotu, 101 Reykjavik, Iceland. [2]Faculty of Social and Human Sciences, University of Iceland, Oddi v/Sturlugotu, 101 Reykjavik, Iceland.

References
1.   Asgeirsdottir TL, Berndsen HH, Gudmundsdottir BP, Gunnarsdottir BA, Halldorsdottir HJ. The effect of obesity, alcohol misuse and smoking on

employment and hours worked: evidence from the Icelandic economic collapse. Rev Econ Househ. 2016;14(2):313–35.

2. Asgeirsdottir TL, Corman H, Noonan K, Olafsdottir T, Reichman NE. Was the economic crisis of 2008 good for Icelanders? impact on health behaviors. Econ Hum Biol. 2014;13:1–19.

3. Asgeirsdottir TL, Corman H, Noonan K, Reichman NE. Lifecycle effects of a recession on health behaviors: boom, bust, and recovery in Iceland. Econ Hum Biol. 2016;20:90–107.

4. Olafsdottir T, Hrafnkelsson B, Asgeirsdottir TL. The Icelandic economic collapse, smoking, and the role of labor-market changes. Eur J Health Econ. 2014. English.

5. Hauksdottir A, McClure C, Jonsson SH, Olafsson O, Valdimarsdottir UA. Increased stress among women following an economic collapse - a prospective cohort study. Am J Epidemiol. 2013;177(9):979–88.

6. McClure CB, Valdimarsdóttir UA, Hauksdóttir A, Kawachi I. Economic crisis and smoking behaviour: prospective cohort study in Iceland. BMJ Open. 2012;2(5). doi:10.1136/bmjopen-2012-001386.

7. Asgeirsdottir TL, Olafsdottir T, Ragnarsdottir DO. Business cycles, hypertension and cardiovascular disease: evidence from the Icelandic economic collapse. Blood Press. 2014;23(4):213–21.

8. Gudjonsdottir GR, Kristjansson M, Olafsson O, Arnar DO, Getz L, Sigurdsson JA, et al. Immediate surge in female visits to the cardiac emergency department following the economic collapse in Iceland: an observational study. Emerg Med J. 2012;29(9):694–8.

9. Asgeirsdottir TL, Zoega G. On the economics of sleeping. Mind Soc. 2011; 10(2):149.

10. Olafsdottir T, Asgeirsdottir TL. Gender differences in drinking behavior during an economic collapse: evidence from Iceland. Rev Econ Househ. 2015;13(4):975–1001.

11. Asgeirsdottir TL, Ragnarsdottir DO. Health-income inequality: the effects of the Icelandic economic collapse. Int J Equity Health. 2014;13(1):50. doi:10. 1186/1475-9276-13-50. PubMed PMID.

12. Jonsdottir S, Asgeirsdottir TL. The effect of job loss on body weight during an economic collapse. Eur J Health Econ. 2014;15(6):567–76. English.

13. Asgeirsdóttir TL, Olafsson SP, Zoega G. Sleep and the management of alertness. Mind Soc. 2016;15(2):169–89.

14. The Prime Minister's Office. Address to the Nation by H.E. Geir H. Haarde, Prime Minister of Iceland, October 6th 2008. 2008 [updated October 9th 2013]. Available from: http://eng.forsaetisraduneyti.is/news-and-articles/nr/ 3035.

15. World Bank. World development indicators-Google public data explorer 2015 [cited 2015 July 14th]. Available from: http://www.google.com/publicdata/ explore?ds = d5bncppjof8f9_&met_y = ny_gdp_mktp_kd_zg&%20idim = country:USA:IND:GBR&hl = en&dl = en#!ctype = l&strail = false&bcs = d&nselm = h&met_y = ny_gdp_mktp_kd_zg&scale_y = lin&ind_y = false&rdim = region&idim = country:USA:IND:GBR:ISL:ESP:PRT&ifdim = region&tstart = 1152835200000&tend = 1373760000000&hl = en_US&dl = en&ind = false.

16. Duxbury C. Iceland's Central Bank Sees Economic Recovery but Flags Risks 2014 [cited 2015 July 14th]. Available from: http://www.wsj.com/articles/ icelands-central-bank-sees-economic-recovery-but-flags-risks-1405695810.

17. Mingels G. Out of the Abyss: Looking for Lessons in Iceland's Recovery 2014 [updated January 10th 2014; cited 2015 July 14th]. Available from: http:// www.spiegel.de/international/europe/financial-recovery-of-iceland-a-case-worth-studying-a-942387.html.

18. Greenstein T. Iceland's Stabilized Economy Is A Surprising Success Story: Forbes; 2013 [updated July 14th 2015]. Available from: http://www.forbes. com/sites/traceygreenstein/2013/02/20/icelands-stabilized-economy-is-a-surprising-success-story/.

19. International Monetary Fund. Iceland: Sixth Post-Program Monitoring Discussions-Staff Report; Press Release; and Statement by the Executive Director for Iceland 2015 [cited 2015 July 14th]. Available from: http://www. imf.org/external/pubs/ft/scr/2015/cr1572.pdf.

20. Zawadzki S. Iceland prepares to come in from the financial cold: Reuters; 2015 [cited 2015 July 14th]. Available from: http://www.reuters.com/article/ 2015/04/02/us-iceland-economy-insight-idUSKBN0MT0WE20150402.

21. O'Brien M. The miraculous story of Iceland: The Washington Post; 2015 [October 17th 2016]. Available from: https://www.washingtonpost.com/ news/wonk/wp/2015/06/17/the-miraculous-story-of-iceland/.

22. The Special Investigation Commission. Report of the Special Investigation Commission (SIC); Chapter 21: Causes of the collapse of the Icelandic Banks - Responsibility, Mistakes and Negligence. 2010.

23. The Special Investigation Commission. Report of the Special Investigation Commission (SIC); Chapter 12: Verðbréfamarkaðir. 2010.

24. Economics T. Iceland Stock Market n.d. [cited October 17th 2016]. Available from: http://www.tradingeconomics.com/iceland/stock-market.

25. BBC News. How did Iceland clean up its banks? : BBC News; 2016 [cited October 18th 2016]. Available from: http://www.bbc.com/news/business-35485876.

26. Statistics Iceland. Employment, unemployment and labour force - Original Data - Montly 2003-2016 n.d. [cited October 17th 2016]. Available from: http://px.hagstofa.is/pxen/pxweb/en/Samfelag/Samfelag__vinnumarkadur__ vinnumarkadur/VIN00001.px/table/tableViewLayout1/?rxid = 07c0d8b2-a5b9- 4bc0-a75c-a40e871fd831.

27. Statistics Iceland. Labour market and wages n.d. [cited October 17th 2016]. Available from: http://px.hagstofa.is/pxen/pxweb/en/Efnahagur/Efnahagur__ thjodhagsreikningar__efnahagslegar_skammtimatolur/THJ00117.px/table/ tableViewLayout1/?rxid = 07c0d8b2-a5b9-4bc0-a75c-a40e871fd831.

28. Bergovec M, Mihatov S, Prpic H, Rogan S, Batarelo V, Sjerobabski V. Acute myocardial-infarction among civilians in Zagreb city area. Lancet. 1992; 339(8788):303. PubMed PMID: WOS:A1992HB52900029. English.

29. Bergovec M, Mihatov S, Prpic H, Heitzler VN, Rogan S, Batarelo V, et al. Influence of the War induced stress in Croatia on the incidence and mortality of acute ischemic-heart-disease. Wiener Med Wochenschr. 1992; 142(19):430–2. PubMed PMID: WOS:A1992KD61800002. German.

30. Aoki T, Fukumoto Y, Yasuda S, Sakata Y, Ito K, Takahashi J, et al. The great east Japan earthquake disaster and cardiovascular diseases. Eur Heart J. 2012;33(22):2796–803. PubMed PMID: WOS:000311303700010. English.

31. Aoki T, Fukumoto Y, Yasuda S, Sakata Y, Ito K, Takahashi J, et al. Increased incidence of heart failure in the east Japan earthquake. J Card Fail. 2012; 18(10):S123–S4. PubMed PMID: WOS:000310180000014. English.

32. Leor J, Poole WK, Kloner RA. Sudden cardiac death triggered by an earthquake. N Engl J Med. 1996;334(7):413–9. PubMed PMID: WOS: A1996TU69600001. English.

33. Baumhakel M, Kindermann M, Kindermann I, Bohm M. Soccer world championship: a challenge for the cardiologist. Eur Heart J. 2007;28(2):150– 3. PubMed PMID: WOS:000244259600006. English.

34. Zimmerman FH, Fass AE, Katz DR, Cole SP. Safety of spectator sports: blood pressure and heart rate responses in baseball and football fans. J Clin Hypertens. 2010;12(10):816–7.

35. Wilbert-Lampen U, Leistner D, Greven S, Pohl T, Sper S, Volker C, et al. Cardiovascular events during world Cup soccer. N Engl J Med. 2008;358(5): 475–83. PubMed PMID: WOS:000252722900005. English.

36. Carroll D, Ebrahim S, Tilling K, MacLeod J, Smith GD. Admissions for myocardial infarction and world Cup football: database survey. Br Med J. 2002;325(7378):1439–42. PubMed PMID: WOS:000180188600007. English.

37. Kloner RA, McDonald S, Leeka J, Poole WK. Comparison of total and cardiovascular death rates in the same city during a losing versus winning super bowl championship. Am J Cardiol. 2009;103(12):1647–50. PubMed PMID: WOS:000267407000004. English.

38. Gerdtham UG, Ruhm C. Deaths rise in good economic times: evidence from the OECD. Econ Hum Biol. 2006;4(3):298–316.

39. Ruhm C. Recessions, healthy no more? J Health Econ. 2015;42:17–28.

40. Ruhm C. A healthy economy can break your heart. Demography. 2007;44(4): 829–48. PubMed PMID: ISI:000251734100010. English.

41. Ruhm C. Good times make you sick. J Health Econ. 2003;22(4):637–58. PubMed PMID: ISI:000184078500007. English.

42. Neumayer E. Recessions lower (some) mortality rates: evidence from Germany. Soc Sci Med. 2004;58(6):1037–47.

43. Tapia Granados JA, Ionides EL. Mortality and macroeconomic fluctuations in contemporary Sweden. Eur JPopulation. 2011;27(2):157–84. PubMed PMID: ISI:000290574800002. English.

44. Ruhm C. Are recessions good for your health? Q J Econ. 2000;115(2):617–50.

45. Stuckler D, Basu S, Suhrcke M, Coutts A, McKee M. The public health effect of economic crises and alternative policy responses in Europe: an empirical analysis. Lancet. 2009;374(9686):315–23. PubMed PMID: ISI:000268508200029. English.

46. Haider AW, Larson MG, Franklin SS, Levy D. Systolic blood pressure, diastolic blood pressure, and pulse pressure as predictors of risk for congestive heart failure in the Framingham Heart Study. Ann Intern Med. 2003;138(1):10–6. PubMed PMID: WOS:000180996200002. English.

47. Lawes CMM, Vander Hoorn S, Rodgers A, Hypertens IS. Global burden of blood-pressure-related disease, 2001. Lancet. 2008;371(9623):1513–8. PubMed PMID: WOS:000255668300027. English.

48. Lee DS, Massaro JM, Wang TJ, Kannel WB, Benjamin EJ, Kenchaiah S, et al. Antecedent blood pressure, body mass index, and the risk of incident heart failure in later life. Hypertension. 2007;50(5):869–76. PubMed PMID: WOS: 000250518200012. English.

49. Lloyd-Jones DM, Larson MG, Leip EP, Beiser A, D'Agostino RB, Kannel WB, et al. Lifetime risk for developing congestive heart failure - the Framingham heart study. Circulation. 2002;24:3068–72. PubMed PMID: WOS:000179785000027. English.

50. Mills KT, Bundy JD, Kelly TN, Reed JE, Kearney PM, Reynolds K, et al. Global disparities of hypertension prevalence and control. A systematic analysis of population-based studies from 90 countries. Circulation. 2016;134(6):441.

51. Forouzanfar MH, Alexander L, Anderson HR, Bachman VF, Biryukov S, Brauer M, et al. Global, regional, and national comparative risk assessment of 79 behavioural, environmental and occupational, and metabolic risks or clusters of risks in 188 countries, 1990–2013: a systematic analysis for the global burden of disease study 2013. Lancet. 2013;386(10010):2287–323.

52. Mukamal KJ, Conigrave KM, Mittleman MA, Camargo CA, Stampfer MJ, Willett WC, et al. Roles of drinking pattern and type of alcohol consumed in coronary heart disease in Men. N Engl J Med. 2003;348(2):109–18.

53. Ruhm C. Healthy living in hard times. J Health Econ. 2005;24(2):341–63.

54. Matthews KA, Salomon K, Brady SS, Allen MT. Cardiovascular reactivity to stress predicts future blood pressure in adolescence. Psychosom Med. 2003; 65(3):410–5. Epub 2003/05/24. eng.

55. Huang C-J, Webb HE, Zourdos MC, Acevedo EO. Cardiovascular reactivity, stress, and physical activity. Front Physiol. 2013;4:314.

56. McEwen BS, Stellar E. Stress and the individual: mechanisms leading to disease. Arch Intern Med. 1993;153(18):2093–101.

57. Lundin A, Lundberg I, Hallsten L, Ottosson J, Hemmingsson T. Unemployment and mortality—a longitudinal prospective study on selection and causation in 49321 Swedish middle-aged men. J Epidemiol Community Health. 2010;64(01):22–8.

58. Eliason M, Storrie D. Does job loss shorten life? J Hum Resour. 2009;44(2): 277–302. PubMed PMID: ISI:000265444000001. English.

59. Moser KA, Fox AJ, Goldblatt PO, Jones DR. Stress and heart-disease: evidence of associations between unemployment and heart disease from the OPCS longitudinal study. Postgrad Med J. 1986;62(730):797–9. PubMed PMID: ISI:A1986D516800021. English.

60. Gallo WT, Teng HM, Falba TA, Kasl SV, Krumholz HM, Bradley EH. The impact of late career job loss on myocardial infarction and stroke: a 10 year follow up using the health and retirement survey. Occup Environ Med. 2006;63(10):683–7.

61. Gallo WT, Bradley EH, Falba TA, Dubin JA, Cramer LD, Bogardus ST, et al. Involuntary job loss as a risk factor for subsequent myocardial infarction and stroke: findings from the health and retirement survey. Am J Ind Med. 2004; 45(5):408–16. PubMed PMID: ISI:000221245200002. English.

62. Strully KW. Job loss and health in the U.S. labor market. Demography. 2009; 46(2):221–46. PubMed PMID: ISI:000268057900001. English.

63. Grossman M. Concept of health capital and demand for health. J Polit Econ. 1972;80(2):223–5. PubMed PMID: ISI:A1972M451700001. English.

64. Grossman M. Demand for health - theoretical and empirical investigation. Nber Occas Pap Natl Bur Econ Res. 1972;119:1–115. PubMed PMID: WOS: A1972S050500001. English.

65. Xu X, Kaestner R. The business cycle and health behaviors. 2010.

66. Gudlaugsson JO, Magnusson KT, Jonsson SH. Heilsa og líðan Íslendinga 2012: Framkvæmdaskýrsla (Health and Wellbeing of Icelanders 2012. Project Report). Reykjavík: Directorate of Health; 2014.

67. Statistics Iceland. Consumption and sales value of drugs by main therapeutic groups 1989-2015 n.d. [cited 2017 February 6th]. Available from: http://px. hagstofa.is/pxen/pxweb/en/Samfelag/Samfelag__heilbrigdismal__ heilbrigdisthjonusta/HEI08101.px/table/tableViewLayout1/?rxid = b55fddaf-5d24-4e01-885f-299513510b32.

68. OECD. OECD Health Statistics 2015 2015 [August 11th 2015]. Available from: http://stats.oecd.org/index.aspx?DataSetCode = HEALTH_STAT.

69. Wilkins K, Campbell NRC, Joffres MR, McAlister FA, Nichol M, Quach S, et al. Blood pressure in Canadian adults. Health Reports. 2010. 21(1). PubMed PMID: WOS:000295504900003. English.

70. Kearney PM, Whelton M, Reynolds K, Muntner P, Whelton PK, He J. Global burden of hypertension: analysis of worldwide data. Lancet. 2005;365(9455):217–23.

71. Yoon SS, Gu Q, Nwankwo T, Wright JD, Hong Y, Burt V. Trends in blood pressure among adults with hypertension: United States, 2003 to 2012. Hypertension. 2015;65(1):54–61.

72. Yoon S, Ostchega Y, Louis T. Recent trends in the prevalence of high blood pressure and its treatment and control, 1999-2008. Hypertension. 2010;56(5): E65–E. PubMed PMID: WOS:000283240400068. English.

73. Thamm M. [Blood pressure in Germany–current status and trends]. Gesundheitswesen. 1999 Dec;61 Spec No:S90-3. Epub 2000/03/22. Blutdruck in Deutschland–Zustandsbeschreibung und Trends. ger.

74. McAlister FA, Wilkins K, Joffres M, Leenen FHH, Fodor G, Gee M, et al. Changes in the rates of awareness, treatment and control of hypertension in Canada over the past two decades. Can Med Assoc J. 2011;183(9):1007–13.

75. Warttig SL, Forshaw MJ, South J, White AK. New, normative, English-sample data for the short form perceived stress scale (PSS-4). J Health Psychol. 2013;18(12):1617–28.

76. MacKinnon DP, Krull JL, Lockwood CM. Equivalence of the mediation. Confounding Suppression Effect Prev Sci. 2000;1(4):173.

77. Hayes AF, Preacher KJ. Statistical mediation analysis with a multicategorical independent variable. Br J Math Stat Psychol. 2014;67(3):451–70.

78. Baron RM, Kenny DA. The moderator mediator variable distinction in social psychological-research - conceptual, strategic, and statistical considerations. J Pers Soc Psychol. 1986;51(6):1173–82. PubMed PMID: WOS:A1986F285400010. English.

79. Edwards JR, Lambert LS. Methods for integrating moderation and mediation: a general analytical framework using moderated path analysis. Psychol Methods. 2007;12(1):1–22. PubMed PMID: WOS:000244988200001. English.

80. Preacher KJ, Rucker DD, Hayes AF. Addressing moderated mediation hypotheses: theory, methods, and prescriptions. Multivar Behav Res. 2007; 42(1):185–227. PubMed PMID: WOS:000247879400007. English.

81. Sobel M. Effect analysis and causation in linear structural equation models. Psychometrika. 1990;55(3):495–515. English.

82. Mackinnon DP, Dwyer JH. Estimating mediated effects in prevention studies. Eval Rev. 1993;17(2):144–58.

83. Ruhm C. Macroeconomic Conditions, Health and Mortality. National Bureau of Economic Research Working Paper Series. 2004. No. 11007. doi:10.3386/ w11007.

84. Dehejia R, Lleras-Muney A. Booms, busts, and babies' health. Q J Econ. 2004; 119(3):1091–130. PubMed PMID: WOS:000223100200009. English.

5

Discrete-choice modelling of patient preferences for modes of drug administration

Ebenezer Kwabena Tetteh[*], Steve Morris and Nigel Titcheneker-Hooker

Abstract

The administration of (biologically-derived) drugs for various disease conditions involves consumption of resources that constitutes a direct monetary cost to healthcare payers and providers. An often ignored cost relates to a mismatch between patients' preferences and the mode of drug administration. The "intangible" benefits of giving patients what they want in terms of the mode of drug delivery is seldom considered. This study aims to evaluate, in monetary terms, end-user preferences for the non-monetary attributes of different modes of drug administration using a discrete-choice experiment. It provides empirical support to the notion that there are significant benefits from developing patient-friendly approaches to drug delivery. The gross benefits per patient per unit administration is in the same order of magnitude as the savings in resource costs of administering drugs. The study argues that, as long as the underlying manufacturing science is capable, a patient-centred approach to producing drug delivery systems should be encouraged and pursued.

Keywords: Discrete-choice experiments, Drug administration, Manufacturing, United Kingdom

Introduction

A recent systematic review [1] notes that administration of multiple drug doses over time requires different types of medical resources and hence can have a non-trivial impact on the monetary costs of healthcare delivery. This argument, however, does not consider the non-monetary hedonic characteristics (attributes) of administering drugs that are linked to the preferences of patients for different modes of drug administration. That is to say, a full accounting of the societal costs and benefits of resources expended on drug administration should take into account both the direct monetary and indirect non-monetary costs and benefits. This is because a given mode of drug administration that incurs the lowest monetary cost to healthcare payers or providers may incur hidden indirect costs in terms of a mismatch with what is preferred by end-users, be it patients or otherwise healthy people [2].

It is crucial therefore to understand and assess the characteristics (attributes) of drug administration – such that better drugs can be developed and manufactured

tailored to patients' preferences. The importance of this is evident from a report published by the Knowledge Transfer Network (HealthTech and Medicines) on "[t]he future of high value manufacturing [in the pharmaceutical, biopharmaceutical and medical device sectors] in the UK" [3]. The report identified, among a number of factors, the importance of: (1) early consideration of manufacturing needs, (2) flexible production facilities; (3) reducing cost to the UK National Health Services [NHS] and (4) the delivery of better services and improved health outcomes to patients. The last, in particular, focussed on the need for more stable, effective medicines; novel ways of administering them; and smart [packaging] technologies to monitor usage by patients. A full understanding of end-user preferences for modes of drug administration is necessary if objective (4) above is to be achieved.

In this study, we aim to evaluate the attributes of drug administration, focusing on the preferences of patients, or otherwise healthy people from the UK general public. We do this using a discrete choice experiments (DCE) that – in contrast to interviews, focus groups and other in-person surveys – supports quantitative estimation of

---

* Correspondence: e.tetteh@ucl.ac.uk; kwabetteh@yahoo.com
University College London, Gower Street, London WC1E 6BT, UK

the strength of end-user preferences for different attributes and how they are traded off against one another. In addition, a DCE supports monetary valuation of different attribute combinations that produce estimates of the indirect benefits to end-users. By monetizing preferences, a comparison with the direct monetary costs of administering biologic drugs can be made. The direct monetary costs of administration can be predicted using the algorithm developed by Tetteh and Morris [4]. And we will argue that these predicted cost estimates plus preference valuations measured in this paper should be considered in (bio)manufacturing decision-making. This is the kind of information manufacturers need in order to make patient-friendly drugs that have low administration costs. The use of such evidence in pre-market R&D and manufacturing decisions should yield drug products with added value.

Cost-effectiveness assessments, from a healthcare payer perspective, will capture the added value in terms of savings in drug administration costs. This is not the case for indirect end-user benefits. The comfort of an improved mode of drug administration is seldom considered in evidence-based medicine and often seen as "luxury". The DCE conducted in this study however shows the monetary value of intangible end-user benefits (what some may consider luxury that can be ignored) is significant. This finding is most relevant to (bio)pharmaceutical manufacturers as they are the translators of promising (biologic) drug candidates into medicines that offer positive direct health benefits relative to placebo or existing treatments. The pertinent issue here is whether healthcare payers recognize and are willing to pay for the indirect benefits to end-users, besides the direct health benefits. If they do, manufacturers will be faced with the right incentives to produce drugs that make significant contribution to patient care.

Background

Our starting point was the observation that drug administration is one part of the whole packaged good or service we call health or medical care. Preferences for different modes of drug administration reflect a derived demand for the direct health benefits offered by a given drug product. The mode of drug administration simply constitutes a vehicle via which these direct health benefits are delivered to a patient. The willingness to pay for a marketed drug product will include valuations of the direct health benefits it offers plus valuations of the means by which these direct health benefits are delivered. A DCE in which drug products are identical in every aspect except their mode of administration, provides the means of evaluating the attributes of drug administration separately. The attributes and attribute-levels chosen in such a DCE should be realistic and relevant to manufacturing decisions and/or consumer (end-user) choices.

Under the premise of utility-maximizing behaviour, an end-user (indexed s) will choose a given mode of administering a drug if the utility derived from that choice is the maximum among J alternative ways of administering that same drug. This represents J differentiated product versions of the same drug. Following Manski [5], the utility (U_{sj}^*) from choosing alternative $j(=1, 2, ..., J)$ from among a set of J discrete products has: one, a systematic, explainable or observable component, V_{sj} that is a function of the attributes of drug administration; and two a random unexplainable error term, ϵ_{sj}. We can write the following:

$$U_{sj}^* = V_{sj}\left(\boldsymbol{\beta}_{jk}\mathbf{X}_{jk}\right) + \epsilon_{sj}$$
$$\boldsymbol{\beta}_{jk}\mathbf{X}_{jk} = \boldsymbol{\beta}_k'\mathbf{X}_k' + \beta_p C_p + \sum_{j=1}^{J-1}ASC_j$$

(1)

where X_{jk} is a vector of attribute-levels decomposed into X_k', a vector of generic non-monetary attribute-levels and C_p, the cost associated with alternative j. $\boldsymbol{\beta}_{jk}$ is a vector of preference coefficients, decomposed into β_k', a vector of coefficients for the non-monetary attributes and β_p, coefficient for the cost attribute. The random error term (ϵ_{sj}) could refer to effects of unobserved attributes; imperfect information on alternative products available; measurement error; misspecification of the utility function; heterogeneity in preferences or simply random behaviour [6]. ASC_j is an alternative-specific-constant to capture peculiar effects of each alternative product that are not reflected in the attributes. ($\sum_{j=1}^{J-1}ASC_j$ may be considered as the mean of ϵ_{sj}.)

Given a sample of end-users (S), a number of choice sets or situations (N) faced by each end-user and prior knowledge of the $\boldsymbol{\beta}_{jk}$ vector, the probability (P) that product $j(=1)$ will be chosen above the other $J - 1$ products can be estimated using the basic multinomial logit (MNL) model [7] as:

$$P_{1ns}(y_1 = 1) = P_{1ns}\left(U_1^* > U_j^*\right) = \frac{\exp(\mu[V_{1ns}])}{\sum_{j=1}^J \exp(\mu[V_{jns}])}D(\epsilon_{sj})$$
$$= \exp(-\epsilon_{sj})\exp(-\exp(\mu\epsilon_{sj})); F(\epsilon_{sj}) = \exp(-\exp(\mu\epsilon_{sj}))$$

(2)

where y denotes the choices made such that $y_1 = 1$ if product $j(=1)$ is selected and zero otherwise. The term μ is a positive scale parameter that is inversely related to the error variance (σ_{ϵ^2}) of the panel of choices made.

Equation (2) requires $D(\epsilon_{sj})$, a Gumbel (log-Weibull) probability density function for independent and identically distributed (IID) error terms, where $F(\epsilon_{sj})$ is the corresponding cumulative density function. Since the error terms are specific to each choice dataset, μ is usually normalized to one for the basic MNL model – indicating homoskedastic (constant) error variance. With preference coefficients fixed or invariant over end-users, and IID error terms, we have the so-called independence from [ir]relevant alternatives (IIA) assumption – which suggests the ratio of choice probabilities is independent of the inclusion or omission of other products.

Methods

Attributes, attribute-levels and experimental designs

In conducting our DCE, we first set out to identify a common set of relevant attributes and attribute-levels for different modes of drug administration. We do this via a selective review of literature investigating different modes of administering drugs [8–14]. Table 1 below shows our selected set of attributes, definitions of these attributes and their levels.

Considering the mode of administration is simply a vehicle for delivering the direct health benefits offered by a drug to patients, we opted to specify the alternative products as drugs that are identical in every aspect apart from the manner in which they are administered to patients. We used a forced-choice format of presenting survey respondents with two unlabelled drugs A and B. We did not include an "opt-out" alternative as we found it difficult to imagine that people will choose not to have a clinically-beneficial drug simply because the way in which the drug is administered is not what they prefer.

The next step was to develop the experimental designs that will form the basis of our survey questionnaires. The designs were created from fractional-factorial designs for estimating only *main effects* of the attribute-levels. This was done in SAS v. 9.3, using a set of macros and programming codes written by Kuhfeld [15, 16], as follows. We first used the macro "MktRuns" to gain some insights as to the appropriate number of runs, i.e., the sizes of candidate set-designs we could use. The "MktRuns" macro suggested (among others) the following sizes: 48 runs (=24 choice sets), 72 runs (=36 choice sets) and 144 runs (=72 choice sets). We then used the macro "MkTex" to create corresponding candidate set-designs in 48, 72 and 144 runs. Using the macro "ChoicEff", we identified and evaluated the statistical efficiency of the best experimental design containing 24 choice sets and drawn from these candidate set-designs. We found a 24 choice-set design with a relative D-efficiency of 65%. This was developed from the candidate set-design with 48 runs.

To test the integrity of the experimental designs above (since we had no prior information on the attribute coefficients), we merged them with simulated pre-pilot discrete-choice data using the macro "MktMerge". Given the artificial dataset created, we estimated a basic MNL model using the macro "phChoice" and SAS PHREG procedure. Compared with the other competing 24 choice-set designs

Table 1 Attributes, definitions and attribute-levels

Attributes	Definitions	Levels
Method of drug administration	This attribute refers to the route by which therapeutically-active drug products are physically administered into a patient. The attribute-levels include all other "needle-free" methods of drug administration to capture the preferences of patients who desire oral drug delivery and/ or have a fear of needles.	1. Intravenous delivery 2. Subcutaneous delivery 3. Intramuscular delivery 4. Needle-free delivery
Dosing frequency	This attribute refers to the frequency of administering a drug for a single full course of treatment. Dosing frequency associated with repeated treatments should not be considered.	1. Once every six months 2. Once every month 3. Once every week 4. Once every day
Setting	This attribute refers to place (clinical and non-clinical settings) where a given drug is administered. Clinical settings include, for example, hospitals, outpatient clinics, care homes, offices of general practitioners/physicians etc. Non-clinical settings include home, schools and other public places.	1. Clinical 2. Non-clinical + self-administration* 3. Non-clinical + supervision*
Disruption to daily activities	This attribute refers to how a given method of drug administration or dosing frequency disrupts the daily activities of patients. Disruptions could be due to, for example, repeated venepuncture and, in the extreme, immobility (hospitalization for the sole purpose of drug administration).	1. None 2. Moderate but manageable 3. Moderate but I can't cope 4. Severe
Risk of adverse events	This attribute refers to features of drug administration that might cause discomfort or injury to patients or health-staff administering drugs. This could be local or generalized adverse events such as indurations; damage to nerves and blood vessels; abscess formation around the sites of injection etc. This is separate from side-effects of the drug molecule itself.	1. None 2. Moderate 3. Severe
Cost	This attribute refers to the additional time and travel costs borne out-of-pocket by the patient each time they have to take or their medicines or it has to be given to them by health workers.	1. £0 2. £10 3. £50 4. £100

Notes: * This refers to the situation where people, if properly trained, could self-administer the drug in a non-clinical setting; or otherwise, their medications will have to be delivered to them under the supervision of qualified healthcare professional, for example, a community or district nurse. Given this set of attributes and attribute-levels, we have a full factorial of 2304 (= $4^4 3^2$) possible profiles or treatment combinations

developed from candidate set-designs with 72 and 144 runs, the design developed from the candidate with 48 runs, produced the lowest estimates of standard errors over *all* attribute-coefficients for the same simulated choice data. It also had the highest number of statistically significant attribute-coefficients.[1] We therefore chose this design for our survey questionnaire.

However, there is a trade-off here: an experimental design with the highest possible D-efficiency may impose greater cognitive burden (task complexity) on survey respondents. One has to balance a desire for near-optimal designs with the possibility of collecting irrational or inconsistent choices [17]. We therefore, using the macro "MktBlock", partitioned our chosen experimental design into two versions – such that each block version contained a sequence of 12 randomly allocated choice tasks.

Survey administration

From the blocked experimental designs above, we developed two draft versions of the survey questionnaire. Each questionnaire was split into three sections. The first section provided a preamble with information about the purpose of the study and the hypothetical constructed context in which respondents had to make their choices. It also provided descriptions of the attributes and attribute-levels as well as an example of a completed choice set as a guide for the survey respondents (see Fig. 1 below). The second section contained the actual sequence of 12 choice questions or situations; and the third section collected anonymized information on individual respondents' characteristics. We did not collect any data on respondents' stated non-attendance to the attributes as this was not an objective of this study. The anonymized format of the questionnaires meant we did not require ethical approval prior to administering the survey.

Before sending the questionnaires out, we carried out a small-scale informal pilot of the draft versions of the questionnaires with no more than five people from the UK general public (given the time and resources available for this study). We asked recipients of the questionnaires to check the wording of the questionnaire; to ensure that the instructions were clear and to identify what might be perceived as implausible combination of attributes and attribute-levels. The respondents found all combinations of attributes and attribute-levels plausible, although some combinations may not be technologically feasible (given the current state of manufacturing or formulation science). We found that it took, on average, 15–20 min to complete each block version of the questionnaire. Following the pilot phase, we made small wording changes to the questionnaire to improve clarity.

We determined that a minimum sample size of 200 survey respondents will be adequate for meaning analyses. This was not derived from statistical sampling theory requiring accurate prior estimates of preference

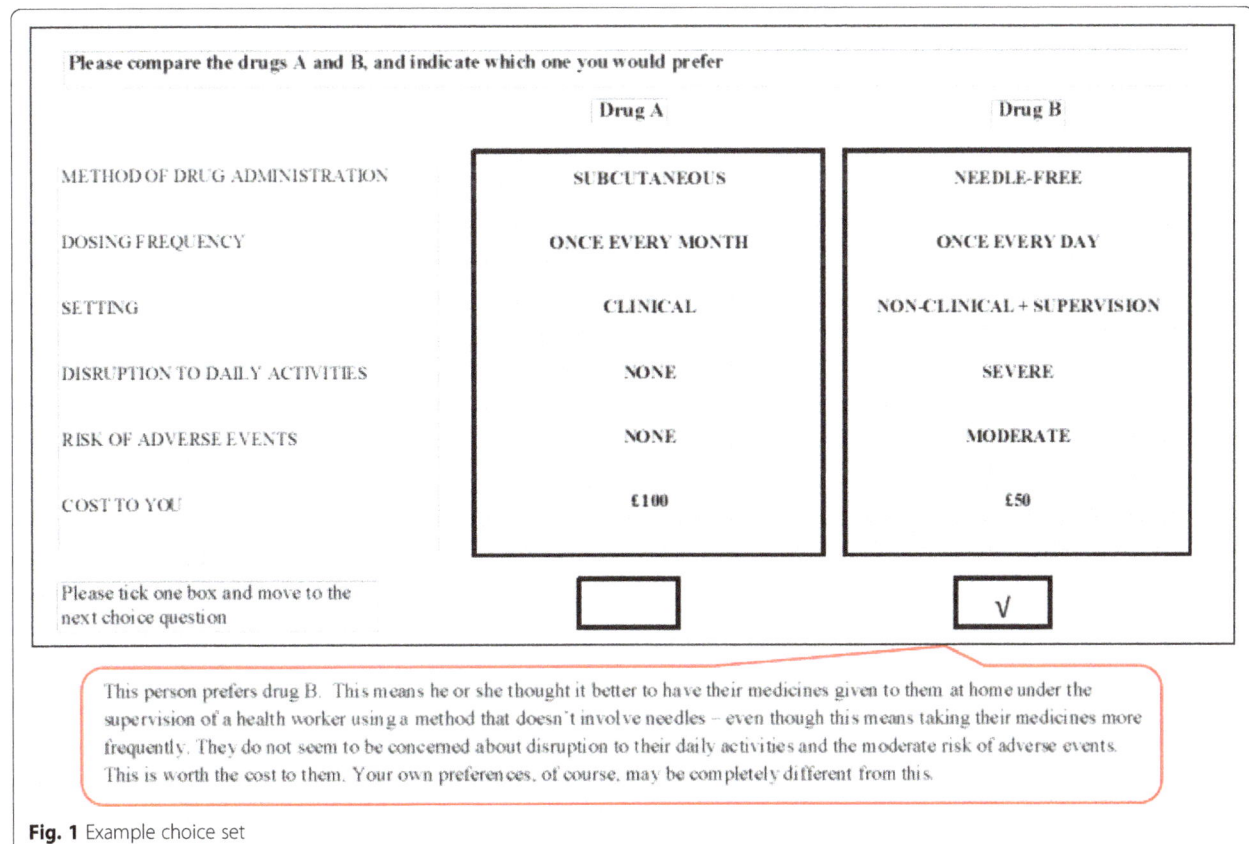

Please compare the drugs A and B, and indicate which one you would prefer	Drug A	Drug B
METHOD OF DRUG ADMINISTRATION	SUBCUTANEOUS	NEEDLE-FREE
DOSING FREQUENCY	ONCE EVERY MONTH	ONCE EVERY DAY
SETTING	CLINICAL	NON-CLINICAL + SUPERVISION
DISRUPTION TO DAILY ACTIVITIES	NONE	SEVERE
RISK OF ADVERSE EVENTS	NONE	MODERATE
COST TO YOU	£100	£50
Please tick one box and move to the next choice question		√

This person prefers drug B. This means he or she thought it better to have their medicines given to them at home under the supervision of a health worker using a method that doesn't involve needles – even though this means taking their medicines more frequently. They do not seem to be concerned about disruption to their daily activities and the moderate risk of adverse events. This is worth the cost to them. Your own preferences, of course, may be completely different from this.

Fig. 1 Example choice set

coefficients or choice probabilities/proportions. It is a pragmatic choice determined by the research budget and it is consistent with the range of sample sizes reported in Bridges et al. [17]. With the help of a commercial vendor (Survey Monkey), the questionnaires were administered online to a sample of people from the UK general population. It took roughly 2 weeks for the vendor to complete the web-based surveys.

Econometric modelling

To explore plausible explanations (unobserved heterogeneity, variation in preferences, respondent fatigue etc.) for the observed sequence of choices in the data collected, we estimated a number of econometric models. As our starting point, we estimated a basic MNL model. The IID/IIA assumption underlying this model (with normalization of the scale parameter to one), however, is equivalent to saying that all survey respondents have the same preferences and/or that unobserved variation around these preferences are similar. For this reason, some researchers will argue that all estimates derived from the basic MNL model are biased. We therefore considered alternative econometric models that relax the IID/IIA restriction.

We considered a heteroskedastic multinomial (HMNL) model, where the scale parameter is no longer normalized to one but considered a variable that must be estimated. The error terms are therefore no longer IID distributed, and a typical approach is to express the scale parameter as a function of a vector of respondents' characteristics ($\mathbf{Z}$). The probability of an individual choosing alternative product j from among a set of competing products, in a given choice situation, is then given by:

$$P_{jns}\left(y_j = 1\right) = \frac{\exp\left(\exp(\alpha\mathbf{Z}_s)\beta_{jk}\mathbf{X}_{jk}\right)}{\sum_{j=1}^{J}\exp\left(\exp(\alpha\mathbf{Z}_s)\beta_{jk}\mathbf{X}_{jk}\right)} \quad (3)$$

where α is a vector of coefficients reflecting the influence of respondents' characteristics on the error variance. If $\hat{\alpha}$ is not statistically different from zero, we revert back to or close to the basic MNL model. If $\hat{\alpha}$ is statistically significant different from zero, then it is possible to *exogenously* determine subpopulations with somewhat identical preferences [18].

A variant of the HMNL model is the entropy multinomial (EMNL) model in which the scale parameter is a function of entropy (E): a measure of the information content or uncertainty represented in the probability distribution of a discrete random variable, in this case the choice variable y. In DCE literature, entropy summarizes the impact of task complexity or respondent fatigue due to the number of choice alternatives; the number and correlation between attributes and attribute-levels; and similarity between the alternatives. The relationship between the scale parameter and entropy of each choice situation can be expressed as:

$$\mu_{ns} = \exp\left(\theta_1 E_{ns} + \theta_2 E_{ns}^2\right)$$
$$E_{ns} = -\sum_{j=1}^{J}\widehat{P_{jns}}\log\left(\widehat{P_{jns}}\right)$$

$$(4)$$

where $\widehat{P_{jns}}$ is the estimated choice probability from the basic MNL model; θ_1, θ_2 are parameters associated with entropy. The linear term $\widehat{\theta_1}$ measures deviation from maximum entropy, i.e., completely random choices whilst the quadratic term $\widehat{\theta_2}$ identifies non-linearity in the relationship above. The case of $\widehat{\theta_1} > 0$ indicates entropy is either offset by exertion of more effort and/or (independent of effort) respondents' under-estimation of the differences between choice alternatives. Researchers often treat the case of $\widehat{\theta_1} < 0$ and $\widehat{\theta_2} > 0$ as indicative of respondent fatigue (declining effort) as a survey respondent works through a sequence of choice sets [19, 20].

Next we considered the mixed multinomial (MMNL) model in which $\boldsymbol{\beta}$ varies randomly across individual respondents. Typically, these random coefficients are drawn from a mixture of continuous parametric distributions denoted by $f(\beta|\delta)$, where δ refers to parameters of that mixture distribution. The choice probability for alternative product j (out of all J products) is then given by:

$$P_{jns}\left(y_j = 1\right) = \int_{\beta_{sjk}}\left[\frac{\exp\left(\beta_{sjk}\mathbf{X}_{jk}\right)}{\sum_{j=1}^{J}\exp\left(\beta_{sjk}\mathbf{X}_{jk}\right)}\right].f(\beta|\delta)\partial\beta_{sjk}$$

$$(5)$$

where the values of β_{sjk} are drawn from the continuous mixture distribution $f(\beta|\delta)$ [21]. Here we assumed the individual-specific non-price preference coefficients that had no statistically significant effects in the basic MNL model are normally distributed and correlated with a price coefficient that is log-normal distributed and constrained to be negative. This combination of random attribute-coefficients and extreme-value (Gumbel) distributed error terms, however, means the MMNL model cannot be solved analytically but approximated via simulations with a finite number of draws.

Finally, we considered a latent-class multinomial (LCMNL) model that assumes attribute-coefficients are drawn from a mixture of non-parametric discrete distributions, representing C latent classes of homogenous subpopulations. It is not known a priori which latent class an individual belongs to; and the probability of latent-class membership (π) can be estimated as:

Table 2 Explanatory variables

Variables	Definitions (Effects coding)
INTRAVENOUS	=1 if a drug is administered intravenously (1, 0, 0, −1)
SUBCUTANEOUS	=1 if a drug is administered subcutaneously (0, 1, 0, −1)
INTRAMUSCULAR	=1 if a drug is administered ntramuscularly (0, 0, 1, −1). The reference category (−1) is administration via needle-free routes
DOSFREQ	Continuous variable referring to the number of unit administrations over a one year period for a single full course of treatment
NONCLINICAL_SELF	=1 if a drug is self-administered in non-clinical settings (1, 0, −1)
NONCLINICAL_SUPV	=1 if a drug is administered in non-clinical settings under the supervision of a qualified healthcare professional (0, 1, −1). The reference category (−1) is drug administration in clinical settings
DDA_MODERATE1	=1 if a given mode of administration is associated with moderate but manageable disruption to respondents' daily activities (1, 0, 0, −1)
DDA_MODERATE2	=1 if a given mode of drug administration is associated with moderate disruptions to daily activities that a respondent cannot cope with (0, 1, 0, −1)
DDA_SEVERE	=1 if a given mode of drug administration is associated with severe disruption to the respondent's daily activities (0, 0, 1, −1). The reference category (−1) is a mode of administration that carries no risk of disruption to patients' daily activities
RAE_MODERATE	=1 if the risk of adverse events associated with a given mode of drug administration s moderate (1, 0, −1)
RAE_SEVERE	=1 if the risk of adverse events associated with a given mode of drug administration is severe (0, 1, −1). The reference category (−1) is drug delivery that is associated with no risk of adverse events
COST	Continuous variable indicating the time and travel costs borne by patients per unit administration
A	Alternative-specific constant = 1 for drug option A (1, −1). The reference point, drug option B = −1
FEMALE	=1 if survey respondent is female (1, −1). The reference category (−1) are males

Table 2 Explanatory variables *(Continued)*

RESPONDENTAGE	Continuous variable indicating the age of a survey respondent
VOCATIONAL	=1 if the highest level of education attained by a respondent is vocational training (1, 0, −1)
GCSEs_O + A	=1 if the highest level of education attained by a respondent is GCSEs O' and A' levels (0, 1, −1). The reference category (−1) are respondents with "higher education"
EMPLOYED	=1 if respondent is employed (1, −1). The reference category (−1) are those who are currently unemployed
INCOME_1	=1 if respondent's annual household income is under £15,000 (1, 0, 0, 0, −1)
INCOME_2	=1 if respondent's annual household income is between £15,000 and £29,999 (0, 1, 0, 0, −1)
INCOME_3	=1 if respondent's annual household income is between £30,000 and £49,999 (0, 0, 1, 0, −1)
INCOME_4	=1 if respondent's annual household income is between £50,000 and £75,000 (0, 0, 0, 1, −1). The reference category (−1) are respondents with annual household income in excess of £75,000
PRIOR_ILLNESS	=1 if a survey respondent had received medical treatment under the advice or guidance of a qualified health worker over the past year (1, −1). The reference category (−1) are those who remained healthy over the past year

$$\pi_{cs}(\gamma) = \frac{\exp(v_c + \gamma_c \mathbf{Z_s})}{1 + \sum_{c=1}^{C-1} \exp(v_c + \gamma_c \mathbf{Z_s})} \quad (6)$$

where $\sum_{c=1}^{C} \pi_c = 1$, the vector γ $(=\gamma_1, \gamma_2, \ldots, \gamma_C)$ refers to the effect of individuals' characteristics on class membership, and v_c is a vector of class-specific constants [22]. Unconditional on class membership, the probability (P^*) of observing the sequence of N choices that an individual respondent makes is given by:

$$P^*(y_{Ns} = 1) = \sum_{c=1}^{C^*} \pi_{cs} \prod_{n=1}^{N} \prod_{j=1}^{J} \left(\frac{\exp(\beta_{cjk} \mathbf{X_{jk}})}{\sum_{j=1}^{J} \exp(\beta_{cjk} \mathbf{X_{jk}})} \right)^{y_s}$$

$$(7)$$

where the optimal number of latent classes C^* is determined by: (1) estimating a series of LCMNL models with different numbers of latent classes; (2) choosing the preferred model using the lowest consistent Akaike

Information Criterion [cAIC] and/or Bayes Information Criterion [BIC]; and (3) making judgements on the trade-off between improved log-likelihoods and increase in standard errors (loss in precision) of the attribute-coefficients as the number of latent-classes gets large.

We estimated the models in STATA v. 11 using the attribute-based (**X**) and respondent-characteristics (**Z**) variables in Table 2 below. The **Z** variables are those in the shaded region of Table 2. The values of our explanatory variables are effects coded rather than 0–1 dummies to ensure the alternative-specific constant and other constant terms carry no information about the reference or omitted categories. See Bech and Gyrd-Hansen [23].

Measuring patient benefits

The outputs of the models above allow us to compute, first, the marginal willingness-to-pay (MWTP) for a given change in an attribute (level) or a bundle of attributes. MWTP is the marginal rate of substitution between the non-monetary attributes (singly or in a bundle) and the price/cost attribute – assuming there is only one product available that will be chosen with a 100% certainty. For our purposes, we only computed $\widehat{\text{MWTP}}$ for a *single* non-monetary attribute (= $-\hat{\beta}_k/\hat{\beta}_p$). Classical confidence intervals were generated using 100 bootstrap replicates of $\widehat{\text{MWTP}}$. Admittedly, a higher number of replicates is needed for more precise estimation but we prefer this procedure as it is: (1) computationally less demanding; (2) uses actual data from respondents without making parametric assumptions about the distribution of $\widehat{\text{MWTP}}$ [24]; and (3) compatible with all STATA estimators for the HMNL, EMNL, MMNL and LCMNL models.

Second, we estimated the incremental welfare gain or loss from switching (changing) from one product to another using the expected compensating variation (ECV). This is a more valid measure of welfare benefits when there is uncertainty about which product will be chosen. For discrete-choice probabilities estimated using an MNL-type model, ECV is formally computed as follows:

$$\text{ECV} = -1\lambda \left[\ln \sum_{j=1}^{J} \exp\left(\widehat{V_j^0}\right) - \ln \sum_{j=1}^{J} \exp\left(\widehat{V_j^1}\right) \right]$$

(8)

where λ is the marginal utility of income proxied by the negative coefficient of the price/cost attribute; and the superscripts 0 and 1 denote the conditions before and after the change (switch). The log-sum expressions or "inclusive values" in the brackets effectively weight the systematic utilities by the probability that an alternative product will be chosen in each state. Analogous to a change in consumer surplus, ECV measures the amount of money that will have

to be extracted from an individual for them to remain indifferent between the initial (0) and final (1) states [25–27].

The ECV estimates computed in this study thus provides a monetary value of what might be considered intangible benefits of giving patients what they want in terms of the mode of drug delivery. From previous work [4], however, we know there are potential administration-cost savings to healthcare payers and providers from reformulating or reverse-engineering a drug product. To ascertain whether these intangible benefits are of any significant importance, we compared our ECV estimates with predicted administration cost savings of switching from one mode of drug delivery to another.

Results
Descriptive statistics

On completion of the DCE survey, we checked the data collected for incomplete sequence(s) of choices so as to avoid estimation biases due to discontinuous preferences ("noise") created by information overload, boredom, unfamiliarity with or lack of interest in the survey. We found that each survey respondent completed all 12 choice tasks. Our estimation sample thus provided 10,608 usable choice responses from 442 respondents. We had no information on the number of people the vendor approached in order to achieve the minimum number of respondents. It is not possible therefore to compute response rates for the survey although the choice data was collected from more than the minimum number of respondents specified. Table 3 provides a summary of the sample demographic characteristics. We make no argument that this sample is representative of the UK population.

Factors influencing choices

Table 4 shows the results from our econometric modelling. Given that we employed a forced-choice format for our survey with only two alternatives, we could not perform a Hausman-McFadden [28] statistical test for the IID/IIA assumption underlying the basic MNL model. However, the different results obtained from HMNL, EMNL, MMNL and LCMNL models suggest that the IID/IIA assumption would have been violated. The HMNL and EMNL models indicate non-constant error terms, whilst the MMNL and LCMNL models indicate variation in observed preferences across the survey respondents. Based on the log-likelihoods and Akaike Information Criterion (AIC), the LCMNL model with two latent classes[2] offers the best model fit to our data. That is to say, preference variation in our dataset can be conveniently represented by two homogenous subgroups of respondents.

That said, the other models provide useful insights on the choice behaviour of respondents. For example, a Lagrangian Multiplier test for heteroskedastic errors in the HMNL model showed statistically significant unobserved

Table 3 Demographic characteristics of sample

Characteristics (of 442 respondents)	N (% of sample)
Gender	
Male*	181 (40.95)
Female	261 (59.05)
Respondents' age	
17–34 years	151 (34.16)
35–49 years	155 (35.07)
≥ 50 years	136 (30.77)
Employment status	
Employed	307 (69.46)
Unemployed*	135 (30.54)
Household-income category	
< £15,000 (per year)	109 (24.66)
£15,000 – £29,999 (per year)	134 (30.32)
£30,000 – £49,999 (per year)	118 (26.70)
£50,000 – £75,000 (per year)	52 (11.76)
> £75,000 (per year)*	29 (6.56)
Highest education achieved	
GCSEs O & A levels	189 (42.76)
Higher education*	212 (47.96)
Vocational training	41 (9.28)
Prior illness (in the past year)	
Yes	178 (40.27)
No*	264 (59.73)

Notes: N = number of respondents; * indicates the reference category for the effects coding used (see also Table 2)

variation that is explained by gender, age, education and employment status. Other respondents' characteristics: prior illness within the past year and household-income were only statistically significant contributors to unobserved heterogeneity at the 10% level. (Note that Table 4 only reports selected findings on the set of contributors to unobserved heterogeneity in the HMNL model.) Similarly, a Lagrangian Multiplier test for heteroskedastic errors in the EMNL model showed statistically significant unobserved variation.[3] However, the statistically insignificant entropy parameters $(\widehat{\theta_1}, \widehat{\theta_2})$ of the EMNL model, with $\widehat{\theta_1} > 0$, suggested that respondent fatigue (perhaps offset by learning effects) could be ignored as plausible explanations for the sequence of choices observed. We believe this justifies our decision to block the experimental designs underlying the survey questionnaires. That aside, the improvement in log-likelihoods observed with the MMNL model, over and above that of the MNL model, confirm there are some significant variations in and correlations between the coefficients drawn from the continuous mixture distribution.

This heterogeneity and correlations in preferences, however, can be captured equivalently by the LCMNL model.

Focusing on the results of the LCMNL model, we observed the probability that any individual belongs to the first subgroup (latent-class 1) is determined by age, gender, and education; and not household income or prior illness suffered in the previous year. Conditional on membership of latent-class 1, the average or representative survey respondent is indifferent to needle-free modes of drug administration when compared with intravenous or subcutaneous routes conditional on the other attributes. Respondents are indifferent in the sense that coefficients for the INTRAVENOUS and SUBCUTANEOUS variables were not statistically different from zero. We interpret this to mean respondents are informed enough to know that, in some disease states, needle-free routes may not be the best or a feasible method of drug administration. On the other hand, respondents, on average, show a negative preference for intramuscular modes of drug delivery when compared with needle-free routes, perhaps because of the pain involved. Similarly, we observed a negative preference for drug administration modes that involve higher dosing frequency albeit the magnitude of the effect was small and close to zero. We observed also a positive preference for self-administration within a non-clinical setting and a negative statistically insignificant preference for drug administration in non-clinical settings under supervision. A probable explanation for this result is that if administering a drug requires supervision by a qualified healthcare professional, then one might be better off having the drug administered in a clinical setting.

Our results show a positive preference for "moderate but manageable" disruptions to daily activities and a negative preference for "severe" or "moderate but unmanageable" disruptions to daily activities. This suggests that respondents did take into account the hypothetical nature of the choice tasks: although possible (in the future), a mode of drug administration that is associated with zero disruption to daily activities may not be currently available or technologically feasible. Similarly, we observed a positive preference for modes of drug administration associated with a "moderate" risk of adverse events and a negative preference for modes of drug administration associated with "severe" risk of adverse events. Again, we observed, on average, some kind of mental accounting of the fact that a mode of drug delivery that has a zero risk of adverse events may not be available or technologically feasible.

Conditional on membership of latent-class 2, we observe similar choice patterns with the following exceptions. First, coefficients for the variables for moderate

Table 4 Econometric results

Dependent variable: CHOICE PROBABILITY						
Variables/Coefficients:	MNL model $\hat{\beta}$ (SE)	HMNL model $\hat{\beta}$ (SE)	EMNL model $\hat{\beta}$ (SE)	MMNL model $\hat{\beta}_s$ (SE)	LCMNL model $\hat{\beta}_1$ (SE)	$\hat{\beta}_2$ (SE)
INTRAVENOUS	−0.011 (0.091)	0.005 (0.057)	0.017 (0.042)	−0.026 (0.110)	−0.119 (0.439)	0.021 (0.123)
SUBCUTANEOUS	0.021 (0.043)	0.016 (0.027)	0.002 (0.019)	−0.016 (0.049)	−0.073 (0.130)	0.070 (0.060)
INTRAMUSCULAR	−0.136 (0.049)**	−0.090 (0.031)**	−0.111 (0.037)**	−0.123 (0.053)*	−0.560 (0.210)**	−0.219 (0.064)***
DOSFREQ	−0.001 (0.000)***	−0.0005 (0.000)***	−0.001 (0.000)**	−0.001 (0.000)***	−0.003 (0.001)***	−0.001 (0.000)**
NONCLINICAL_SELF	0.167 (0.037)***	0.108 (0.025)***	0.112 (0.038)**	0.210 (0.039)***	0.424 (0.128)***	0.146 (0.045)**
NONCLINICAL_SUPV	−0.122 (0.028)***	−0.078 (0.019)***	−0.067 (0.025)**	−0.120 (0.030)***	−0.124 (0.093)	−0.098 (0.037)**
DDA_MODERATE1	0.391 (0.033)***	0.239 (0.033)***	0.214 (0.074)**	0.437 (0.038)***	1.210 (0.150)***	0.264 (0.050)***
DDA_MODERATE2	−0.267 (0.042)***	−0.171 (0.032)***	−0.167 (0.059)**	−0.300 (0.046)***	−1.058 (0.141)***	−0.075 (0.061)
DDA_SEVERE	−0.525 (0.039)***	−0.336 (0.044)***	−0.308 (0.103)**	−0.588 (0.044)***	−1.376 (0.184)***	−0.324 (0.057)***
RAE_MODERATE	0.169 (0.034)***	0.108 (0.024)***	0.111 (0.041)**	0.212 (0.038)***	0.522 (0.141)***	0.067 (0.043)
RAE_SEVERE	−0.743 (0.039)***	−0.461 (0.056)***	−0.406 (0.138)**	−0.869 (0.044)***	−2.342 (0.215)***	−0.204 (0.059)***
COST	−0.008 (0.001)***	−0.005 (0.001)***	−0.004 (0.001)**	−0.0118 (0.040)***	−0.012 (0.002)***	−0.008 (0.001)***
A	−0.054 (0.054)	−0.033 (0.034)	0.002 (0.025)	−0.073 (0.066)	0.370 (0.274)	−0.122 (0.073)!
Entropy$\left(\theta_1^{\hat{}}, \theta_2\right)$	—	—	(1.026, 0.717)	—	—	
$\hat{a}_0$(FEMALE)	—	0.170 (0.035)***	—	—	—	
$\hat{a}_1$(VOCATIONAL)	—	−0.230 (0.085)**	—	—	—	
$\hat{a}_2$(GCSEs_O + A)	—	−0.199 (0.054)***	—	—	—	
$\hat{\pi}_c$	—	—	—	—	0.49	0.51
$\hat{\gamma}_c$(VOCATIONAL)	—	—	—	—	−0.892 (0.324)**	—
$\hat{\gamma}_c$(GCSEs_O + A)	—	—	—	—	0.577 (0.203)**	—
$\hat{\gamma}_c$(FEMALE)	—	—	—	—	0.285 (0.122)*	—
$\hat{\gamma}_c$ (RESPONDENTAGE)					0.024 (0.009)**	
Log-likelihood (AIC)	−2855.357 (5736.713)	−2812.19 (5670.381)	−2837.971 (5670.381)	−2782.51 (5611.019)	−2652.879 (5379.757)	

Notes: SE = standard error. For the HMNL and LCMNL models, we report *selected* effects of respondent-characteristics on the scale-parameter and latent-class membership. MMNL model was estimated using 500 Halton draws of correlated normally-distributed coefficients for the variables A, INTRAVENOUS and SUBCUTANEOUS and a log-normal distributed cost coefficient. *** $p < 0.001$ ** $p < 0.01$ * $p < 0.05$! $p < 0.10$. AIC = Akaike Information Criterion

risk of disruptions-to-daily-activities and moderate risk of adverse events were not statistically significant. That respondents belonging to latent-class 2 show indifference to these attribute-levels provides further support to our argument that respondents may have, in their decision choices, considered that drug delivery modes with zero disruptions to their daily activities and/or zero risk of adverse events are perhaps unavailable even though they are desirable. Second, the magnitudes of the coefficients for the INTRAVENOUS and SUBCUTANEOUS variables indicate a positive preference for these modes of drug administration relative to needle-free routes of administration. But since these effects are not statistically different from zero, we maintain the argument that respondents are generally indifferent to the choice between needle-free and intravenous/subcutaneous routes of drug administration.

For both latent-classes, we observe a small but statistically significant coefficient for the cost attribute. This suggests that our survey respondents have price inelastic "demands" for the attributes of drug administration we investigated in response to any (out-of-pocket) costs of accessing healthcare. This probably reflects two things. One, the fact that the UK NHS provides tax-funded insurance protection against the financial risks of ill health; and two, that the costs in question are by and large 'unavoidable': without spending resources on some form of a vehicle for administering a drug, patients will be unable to realize the direct health benefits offered by that drug.

Patient benefits and cost savings

Table 5 shows MWTP estimates for each of the non-cost attributes studied and the associated confidence intervals around these estimates. A positive $\widehat{MWTP}$ indicates a preference for an attribute taking into account the associated cost, whilst a negative $\widehat{MWTP}$ indicates a dispreference. As observed in Table 4, there are subtle differences in the MWTP estimates obtained from the different econometric models. We focus on estimates from the LCMNL model as this provided the best fit with the choice data collected. This shows a statistically significant and substantial willingness-to-pay for drug delivery modes that are associated with "moderate" disruption to daily activities and "moderate" risk of adverse events. There is also a statistically significant and substantial willingness-to-pay to avoid drug delivery modes that are associated with "moderate but unmanageable" or "severe" disruptions to daily activities. Similarly, there is a statistically significant and substantial willingness-to-pay to avoid drug delivery modes that are associated with "severe" risk of adverse events. Further, there is a statistically significant and substantial willingness-to-pay to avoid drug administration via the intramuscular route.

To evaluate the welfare change, i.e., the intangible benefits from manufacturing drugs in a patient-friendly manner, we considered the following. A given biologic drug C can be manufactured in two ways (C1 and C2). Assume, as we did in the survey, that both versions of the drug have the same molecule, efficacy and safety profile. In option C1, the drug can be manufactured for intravenous administration in clinical settings, and this mode of drug delivery is associated with "severe" risk of adverse events and "severe" disruptions to patients' daily activities. Option C2 is where a drug is manufactured for subcutaneous self-administration in non-clinical settings and this mode of drug delivery is associated with "moderate" risk of adverse events and "moderate" disruptions to patients' daily activities. In this case, we can compute the expected compensating variation ($\widehat{ECV}$) using eq. (8). Since household-income categories had no statistically significant effect on class membership in our preferred LCMNL model, we do not differentiate our $\widehat{ECV}$ by household-income category.

Based on the MNL model, switching from option C1 to C2 yields a welfare gain ($\widehat{ECV}$ per patient per unit administration) of -£296 (95% CI: -£302 to -£289). Based on the MMNL model, $\widehat{ECV}$ is: -£364 (95% CI: -£370 to -£358). Based on the LCMNL model with two latent-classes, and unconditional on latent-class membership, we obtained $\widehat{ECV}$ of -£435 (95% CI: -£524 to -£346). Note that the ECV is a measure of welfare gain, not welfare loss. The negative sign reflects the fact that ECV is the amount of money that has to be *taken from* the state of having option C2 so that the average respondent will be indifferent to option C1 (see equation 8). Note also that with our choice data failure to control for preference

Table 5 Marginal willingness to-pay estimates

Variables:	MNL model MWTP (95%CI)	HMNL model MWTP (95% CI)	EMNL model MWTP (95%CI)	MMNL model MWTP (95%CI)	LCMNL model MWTP (95%CI)
INTRAVENOUS	−2.12 (−4.09, −0.16)*	1.17 (−0.74, 3.08)	3.43 (1.73, 5.14)*	2.31 (−2.86, 7.49)*	5.85 (−50.38, 62.07)
SUBCUTANEOUS	2.35 (1.37, 3.32)*	2.60 (1.58, 3.63)*	0.23 (−0.52, 1.03)	−8.33 (−10.31, −6.34)*	2.42 (−7.76, 12.59)
INTRAMUSCULAR	−17.43 (−18.65, −16.22)*	−19.19 (−20.41, −17.97)*	−26.08 (−27.15, −25.01)*	−9.39 (−11, −7.77)*	−40.63 (−72.47, −8.80)*
DOSFREQ	−0.08 (−0.09, −0.08)*	−0.09 (−0.094, −0.085)*	−0.12 (−0.13, −0.12)*	−0.10 (−0.10, −0.09)*	−0.23 (−0.30, −0.17)*
NONCLINICAL_SELF	21.45 (20.51, 22.39)*	22.41 (21.48, 23.35)*	26.35 (25.55, 27.16)*	31.01 (29.87, 32.14)*	28.57 (21.40, 35.74)*
NONCLINICAL_SUPV	−15.45 (−16.06, −14.83)*	−15.74 (−16.36, −15.11)*	−15.46 (−15.95, −14.96)*	−19.83 (−20.64, −19.02)*	−15.53 (−26.04, −5.03)*
DDA_MODERATE1	50.09 (48.91, 51.27)*	49.40 (48.15, 50.65)*	50.14 (49.02, 51.27)*	58.88 (57.65, 60.11)*	84.71 (67.59, 101.82)*
DDA_MODERATE2	−34 (−35.15, −32.85)*	−35.24 (−36.51, −33.97)*	−38.86 (−39.89, −37.83)*	−43.13 (−44.35, −41.92)*	−58.84 (−72.28, −45.40)*
DDA_SEVERE	−66.36 (−67.74, −64.99)*	−68.64 (−70.14, −67.14)*	−71.55 (−72.80, −70.30)*	−73.64 (−75.15, −72.14)*	−94.50 (−117.91, −71.10)*
RAE_MODERATE	22.06 (21.20, 22.92)*	22.64 (21.74, 23.53)*	26.37 (25.59, 27.14)*	30.32 (29.23, 31.41)*	23.49 (17.29, 29.70)*
RAE_SEVERE	−94.65 (−96.64, −92.65)*	−94.77 (−96.85, −92.70)*	−94.75 (−96.58, −92.93)*	−116.08 (−117.65, −114.51)*	−130.32 (−165.12, −95.53)*

Notes: The 95% CIs above are "standard or classical confidence intervals" calculated using 100 bootstrapped replicates of MWTP. This is because accurate, less-erratic and reliable "bootstrap confidence intervals" require replications in the order of 1000, which would have been computationally demanding and time consuming [32]. The confidence intervals reported are therefore not exact. * indicates confidence interval does not include zero heterogeneity in the MNL model leads to an underestimation of welfare change. The same argument may not be applicable to other choice data. But how does our ECV estimates (of intangible benefits to patients) compare with savings in drug administration costs to a healthcare payer?

To answer this question, we used a regression-based algorithm to predict the cost of UK NHS resources that will be consumed in administering drugs C1 and C2. Details of this algorithm will be found elsewhere [4]. We maintained all previous assumptions made in computing estimates of ECV, and added the following. One, both drugs C1 and C2 are indicated for management of a chronic illness; two, product C2 is sold bundled with some of the equipment and consumables used in drug administration; and three, a single full treatment course of C1 over a year requires 10 unit administrations whilst a single full treatment course of C2 requires 5 unit administrations over a year. Direct monetary costs of administering drugs C1 and C2 were then estimated as:

$$\ln \widehat{ADMINCOST}_{C1} = 7.1499 - 3.2026(0) - 5.2737(0) + .428(10)$$
$$+ .404(0) - .2896(1) - .00106(10^2) - .3173(10)(1)$$

$$\widehat{ADMINCOST}_{C1} = \exp(7.8613) \cdot \hat{\Phi}(= 1.0792) = £2800.41$$

$$\ln \widehat{ADMINCOST}_{C2} = 7.1499 - 3.2026(1) - 5.2737(0) + .428(5)$$
$$+ .404(1) - .2896(1) - .00106(5^2) - .3173(5)(1)$$

$$\widehat{ADMINCOST}_{C2} = \exp(4.6099) \cdot \hat{\Phi}(= 1.3799) = £138.64$$

where $\hat{\phi} = 1.0792$ and 1.3799 are the subgroup-specific smearing factors for intravenous and subcutaneous products respectively.

The estimates above yield a cost saving of roughly £2662 per patient per year; or £532 per patient per unit administration of switching from C1 to C2. This is comparable to the absolute value of $\widehat{ECV}$: £435 derived from the LCMNL model.

Discussion

The non-zero MWTP and ECV estimates reported above provide a monetary measure of the "clinical usability" of a drug – where clinical usability has to do with the mode of drug administration as separate from considerations of efficacy, safety and/or value-for-money. Some might consider MWTP and ECV as old-fashioned, redundant metrics of welfare change – arguing that it is better to evaluate predicted choice probabilities for a selected group of products (bundles of attributes). However, such discrete demand analyses will not allow us to compare the monetary value of the intangible benefits from making patient-friendly medicines with the monetary savings in drug administration costs.

From our analyses, we found that the monetary value of the intangible benefits (from satisfied patients' preferences) is in the same order of magnitude as savings on the direct monetary costs of resources healthcare providers spend on drug administration. Our results also indicate a strong positive preference for modes of drug administration that are associated with some but not significant risks of adverse events and/or disruptions to patients daily activities. They also show a positive preference for self-administration of drugs in non-clinical settings – and a negative preference for drug administration in clinical settings or non-clinical settings under the supervision of a qualified healthcare professional. Advances in biopharmaceutical manufacturing such as pre-filled syringes, auto-injectors and pen injectors and other innovations that reduce the risk of adverse events and/or disruptions to daily activities clearly hit with these observations.

This argument, however, assumes that the state of biopharmaceutical manufacturing and formulation science is mature enough to support the desired innovations in making patient-friendly medicines and/or that the profit signals are strong enough to get manufacturers to consider end-user preferences. There might be, of course, practical manufacturing challenges that militate against reverse engineering product option C1 to C2. Nevertheless, our estimates indicate there are substantial benefits from developing patient-friendly drug delivery systems if the underlying formulation and manufacturing science makes it possible to do so. If these societal benefits are considered important by policy makers, then there is a case for public interventions to encourage manufacturing research in an attempt to achieve the desired goal of producing clinically usable medicines and drug delivery devices. With the right pricing and reimbursement environment, an additional incentive for manufacturers to consider the preferences of end-users may come from attempts to differentiate products in order to maintain or increase market shares.

For any given cohort of patients (end-users), a drug product that closely matches the preferences of the average representative end-user or consumer should enjoy higher demand volumes (keeping prices unchanged). Product differentiation along the lines of satisfying end-user preferences for the mode of drug administration may indeed create brand loyalty without manufacturers engaging in academic detailing or direct-to-consumer advertising. We would also expect additional demand inducement where manufacturing a drug product in a patient-friendly manner, amplifies the (incremental) direct health benefits derived from that drug. This is particularly important considering healthcare payers and providers' requirements for estimates of cost-effectiveness from manufacturers to demonstrate product value. Our ECV estimates measure indirect or intangible benefits assuming direct health benefits remain the same. So if healthcare payers and providers are willing to pay for the value of the drug delivery mode, and the discounted present value of private producer surplus of developing patient-friendly drug delivery systems (relative to other investment opportunities) is positive, then manufacturers should consider the switch from C1 to C2.

As with all research, a number of limitations apply to the arguments above.

First, the list of attributes evaluated in this study was taken from a selective literature review. Ideally, one would want to supplement this literature review with interviews and/or focus group discussions involving end-users. Given the time and resources available for this study, we were not able to apply these qualitative methods – which are of most value where there is a lack or dearth of existing (grey) literature. We therefore make no claim here that the selected set of attributes and attribute-levels are exhaustive of all characteristics of all possible modes of drug administration. We believe, however, that the selected attributes and attribute-levels in Table 1 are realistic, relevant and suited for investigating the gross welfare benefits (consumer surplus) from manufacturing patient-friendly medicines. Second, the levels "none", "moderate" and "severe" for the attribute risk-of-adverse-events, for example, will be understood differently by different respondents with different backgrounds. The attribute-levels were chosen to represent a natural categorical ordering of risk or severity; but the strength of respondents' preferences could be influenced by differences in attribute perception. Unfortunately, we did not include variables constructed to measure attribute perceptions in our analysis. Differences in attribute perception will appear as preference heterogeneity in the MMNL and LCMNL models we estimated. Or, with preferences restricted to be the same, appear as unobserved heterogeneity in the HMNL and EMNL models. We cannot therefore make any statements about the precise impacts of differences in attribute perception on choices. What we know is: age, gender and education affect variation in individual preferences; and the same set of respondent characteristics plus employment status influence unobserved heterogeneity.

Third, it might be argued that our ECV estimates depend on the cost levels chosen. However, Hanley et al. [29] have shown that using different levels for the cost attribute may not result in statistically significant differences in estimates of welfare change albeit there is a possibility that such differences might be significant when the ECV estimates are employed in cost-benefit analyses, for example. See also Slothuus et al. [30]. In our study, we believe that the chosen cost range with an upper limit of £100 adequately captures out-of-pocket access costs that NHS patients are most likely to pay. Considering also the near zero coefficients, we will argue that cost levels

beyond £100, and any non-linearity in the cost-attribute effects, are unlikely to change the arguments above. Fourth, some might argue that $\widehat{ECV}$ derived from the LCMNL model suffers from ecological fallacy – as they are based on the average weighted coefficients over two latent-classes. For that matter (erroneous) conclusions that apply at the aggregate level may not apply at the latent-class level. However, we do not know a priori which latent-class a given respondent belongs to. Since we cannot assume fixed class membership, the reported $\widehat{ECV}$, which is unconditional on class membership, is a valid measure of welfare change.

Finally, we have only evaluated the preferences of mostly healthy people from the UK general public at a given point in time. If preferences change over time, our estimates may no longer be valid albeit we will not expect any dramatic differences from what we have reported. A possible avenue for future research is to repeat the analysis here using a panel data of discrete choices collected over time. That aside, it is well known that end-user preferences for healthcare interventions in healthy states are not the same as when they are in sick states – and that people make decisions behind a "veil of experience", i.e., they prefer products and services that they have previously experienced [31]. Hence, our sample which was dominated by healthy people may bias our estimates. We did indeed recognize the issue and it is for this reason we linked the variable PRIOR_ILLNESS to the scale parameter in the HMNL model – to partially account for health-state-dependent preferences and the experience-good features of healthcare. What is more the variable for prior illness was not a statistically significant predictor of preference heterogeneity in the LCMNL model. We did not ask survey respondents the type of illness (acute or chronic) they had experienced. The variable for prior illness therefore is crude and it says nothing about the number of visits to a health facility in the past year or the severity of illness and whether this affects respondents' cognitive abilities. It is then possible that specific patient-populations (for example, those suffering from Alzheimer's, diabetes or some form of cancer) may have preferences that differ from that of the sample we studied. We leave this issue of health-state-dependent preferences for future research.

Conclusions

In this study, we attempted to estimate the monetary value of end-user preferences for a generic set of attributes of different modes of drug administration. We found a non-trivial marginal willingness-to-pay for drug delivery systems associated with zero or moderate risk of adverse events and/or disruption to patients' daily activities. We also found a high marginal willingness-to-pay for self-administration of drugs in non-clinical settings. In addition, we estimated that the monetary value of making patient-friendly medicines could be as large as the savings on direct monetary costs of drug administration to healthcare payers and providers. We argue that as long as there is recognition of the value of the drug delivery mode (besides the value of drug molecules in improving health outcomes); and the underlying manufacturing science is capable, a patient-centred approach to producing beneficial drugs and drug delivery systems should be encouraged and pursued.

Endnotes

[1]Note that our simulated discrete-choice data were not derived from known utility functions or a known β vector. Our interests are in the robustness of the attribute-coefficients ($\hat{\beta}$) and not how $\hat{\beta}$ closely approximates prior or "true" values of β. The lower standard errors and high number of statistically significant coefficients, obtained from the same MNL model estimated with the same simulated dataset, confirms the efficiency gain from our chosen experimental design.

[2]In determining C^*, we estimated a number of LCMNL models with 2–10 latent-classes. To increase the speed of computation, we estimated these models without the Z variables in the class-membership function, i.e., equation (6). We found the closest competitor to the LCMNL with two-classes (cAIC = 5522.461, BIC = 5495.461) was an LCMNL with four classes (cAIC = 5528.196, BIC = 5473.196). We chose the two-class LCMNL model on the basis of precision loss in the estimated coefficients: the fourth latent-class of the LCMNL model with four-classes had no statistically significant coefficients.

[3]Because the measure of entropy is derived from choice probabilities predicted from the MNL model, it is in effect an "endogenous" explanatory variable that might bias the coefficients of the EMNL model. In Table 4, we observe that, even if these coefficients are biased, they are consistent with that of the MNL and HMNL models. What is more, the primary purpose of the EMNL model is to assess respondents' (fatigued) reactions to the choice tasks, i.e., we are interested mostly in equation (4) and not equation (3).

Acknowledgements
This study formed part of the corresponding author's doctoral thesis and benefited from a grant disbursed under the UCL Grand Challenges on Human Wellbeing. Additional funding from the UK Engineering & Physical Sciences Research Council (EPSRC) for the EPSRC Centre for Innovative Manufacturing in Emergent Macromolecular Therapies is gratefully acknowledged. Financial support from the consortium of industrial and governmental users is also acknowledged. The funders or sponsors had no role in the study design; analysis and interpretation of the study results, or the decision to submit for publication. The statements, views and conclusions expressed in this paper are those of the authors and not necessarily those of the authors' affiliated institutions (in the past or present). The authors take full responsibility for all errors.

Authors' contributions
All authors read and approved the final manuscript and its draft versions.

Competing interests
The authors declare that they have no competing interests.

References
1. Tetteh E, Morris S. Systematic review of drug administration costs and implications for biopharmaceutical manufacturing. Appl Health Econ Health Policy. 2013;11:1–12.
2. Chess R. Economics of drug delivery. Pharm Res. 1998;15(2):172–4.
3. Knowledge Transfer Network. The future of high value manufacturing in the UK: Pharmaceutical, biopharmaceutical & medical device sectors. Available from URL: https://connect.innovateuk.org/documents/3112383/10498355/Health+KTN+−+The+future+of+of+High+Value+Manufacturing+in+the+UK+Pharmaceutical%20Biopharmaceutical+&+Medical+Device+Sectors+−+2013/738f33cc-a53f-417c-910f-339f4727489f [Accessed: 29 Oct 2014].
4. Tetteh E, Morris S. Evaluating the administration costs of biologic drugs: development of a cost algorithm. Heal Econ Rev. 2014;4(1):26.
5. Manski CF. The structure of random utility models. Theor Decis. 1977;8(3):229–54.
6. Palma A, Gordon MM, Papageorgiou YY. Rational choice under an imperfect ability to choose. Am Econ Rev. 1994;84(3):419–40.
7. McFadden D. Conditional logit analysis of qualitative choice behavior. In: Zarembka P, editor. Frontiers in econometrics. New York: Academic Press; 1974. p. 105–42.
8. Benjamin L. Physicians' preferences for prescribing oral and intravenous anticancer drugs: a discrete choice experiment. Eur J Cancer. 2012;48(6):912.
9. Augustovski F, Beratarrechea A, Irazola V, Rubinstein F, Tesolin P, Gonzalez J, et al. Patient preferences for biologic agents in rheumatoid arthritis: a discrete-choice experiment. Value Health. 2013;16(2):385–93.
10. Huynh TK, Oÿstergaard A, Egsmose C, Madsen OR. Preferences of patients and health professionals for route and frequency of administration of biologic agents in the treatment of rheumatoid arthritis. Patient Preference Adherence. 2014;8:93.
11. Parker SE. Pharmacoeconomics of intravenous drug administration. PharmacoEconomics. 1992;1(2):103–15.
12. Dychter SS. Subcutaneous drug delivery: a route to increased safety, patient satisfaction, and reduced costs. Infus Nurs. 2012;35(3):154.
13. McDowell SE, Mt-Isa S, Ashby D, Ferner RE. Where errors occur in the preparation and administration of intravenous medicines: a systematic review and Bayesian analysis. Qual Saf Health Care. 2010;19(4):341–5.
14. Keers RN, Williams SD, Cooke J, Ashcroft DM. Prevalence and nature of medication administration errors in health care settings: a systematic review of direct observational evidence. Ann Pharmacother. 2013;47(2):237–56.
15. Kuhfeld WF, Tobias RD. Large factorial designs for product engineering and marketing research applications. Technometrics. 2005;47(2):132–41.
16. Kuhfeld WF. Marketing research methods in SAS experimental design, choice, conjoint, and graphical techniques. 2009.
17. Bridges JFP, Hauber AB, Marshall D, et al. Conjoint analysis applications in health - a checklist: a report of the ISPOR good research practices for conjoint analysis task force. Value Health. 2011;14(4):403–13.
18. Louviere JJ, Islam T, Wasi N, Street D, Burgess L. Designing discrete choice experiments: do optimal designs come at a price? J Consum Res. 2008;35(2):360–75.
19. Swait J. Choice environment, market complexity, and consumer behavior: a theoretical and empirical approach for incorporating decision complexity into models of consumer choice. Organ Behav Hum Decis Process. 2001;86(2):141–67.

20. de Bekker-Grob EW, Rose JM, Bliemer MC. A closer look at decision and analyst error by including nonlinearities in discrete choice models: implications on willingness-to-pay estimates derived from discrete choice data in healthcare. PharmacoEconomics. 2013;31(12):1169–83.
21. Hole AR. Estimating mixed logit models using maximum simulated likelihood. Stata J. 2007;7(3):388–401.
22. Pacifico D. Fitting nonparametric mixed logit models via expectation-maximization algorithm. Stata J. 2012;12(2):284–98.
23. Bech M, Gyrd-Hansen D. Effects coding in discrete choice experiments. Health Econ. 2005;14(10):1079–83.
24. Hole AR. A comparison of approaches to estimating confidence intervals for willingness to pay measures. Health Econ. 2007;16(8):827–40.
25. Lancsar E, Savage E. Deriving welfare measures from discrete choice experiments: inconsistency between current methods and random utility and welfare theory. Health Econ. 2004;13(9):901–7.
26. Ryan M. Deriving welfare measures in discrete choice experiments: a comment to Lancsar and savage (1). Health Econ. 2004;13(9):909–12.
27. Santos Silva JMC. Deriving welfare measures in discrete choice experiments: a comment to Lancsar and savage (2). Health Econ. 2004;13(9):913–8.
28. Hausman J, McFadden D. Specification tests for the multinomial logit model. Econometrica. 1984:1219–40.
29. Hanley N, Adamowicz W, Wright RE. Price vector effects in choice experiments: an empirical test. Resour Energy Econ. 2005;27(3):227–34.
30. Slothuus Skjoldborg U, Gyrd-Hansen D. Conjoint analysis. The cost variable: an Achilles' heel? Health Econ. 2003;12(6):479–91.
31. Salkeld G, Ryan M, Short L. The veil of experience: do consumers prefer what they know best? Health Econ. 2000;9(3):267–70.
32. Efron B. Better bootstrap confidence intervals. J Am Stat Assoc. 1987;82(397): 171–85.

6

Valuing productivity loss due to absenteeism: firm-level evidence from a Canadian linked employer-employee survey

Wei Zhang[1,2] [iD], Huiying Sun[1], Simon Woodcock[3] and Aslam H. Anis[1,2]*

Abstract

In health economic evaluation studies, to value productivity loss due to absenteeism, existing methods use wages as a proxy value for marginal productivity. This study is the first to test the equality between wage and marginal productivity losses due to absenteeism separately for team workers and non-team workers. Our estimates are based on linked employer-employee data from Canada. Results indicate that team workers are more productive and earn higher wages than non-team workers. However, the productivity gap between these two groups is considerably larger than the wage gap. In small firms, employee absenteeism results in lower productivity and wages, and the marginal productivity loss due to team worker absenteeism is significantly higher than the wage loss. No similar wage-productivity gap exists for large firms. Our findings suggest that productivity loss or gain is most likely to be underestimated when valued according to wages for team workers. The findings help to value the burden of illness-related absenteeism. This is important for economic evaluations that seek to measure the productivity gain or loss of a health care technology or intervention, which in turn can impact policy makers' funding decisions.

Keywords: Productivity loss, Absenteeism, Marginal productivity, Wage, Teamwork, Valuation

JEL codes: J31, D24, I12, I15

Introduction

It is still under debate whether we should take account of productivity gains or losses from a health care intervention in economic evaluation studies [1, 2]. Cost-effectiveness studies, for example, are routinely used to determine the eligibility of health technologies such as pharmaceuticals for coverage under national or provincial health plans. The inclusion of productivity losses in such analyses would have a significant influence on determinations of cost-effectiveness, leading to different resource allocation decisions. Krol et al. find that accounting for productivity costs can either increase or

decrease the incremental cost-effectiveness ratio (ICER) between treatment arms [3, 4]. Thus, cost-effectiveness studies that account for productivity losses are useful in identifying interventions with a potentially broad impact, and do not necessarily lower the ICERs of an intervention.

Despite robust arguments in favour of including productivity loss in evaluation studies [3–6], current methods to value productivity loss are limited. Existing methods usually quantify productivity loss using wages as a proxy for marginal productivity [1, 7, 8]. However, wages may not equal marginal productivity for many reasons, making it a poor proxy and reducing the accuracy of estimated productivity loss. In imperfect labour markets, wages may not equal marginal productivity due to inequities, such as race or gender discrimination, whereby an identifiable group routinely receives lower wages. More commonly, risk-averse workers might willingly

* Correspondence: aslam.anis@ubc.ca
[1]Centre for Health Evaluation and Outcome Sciences, St. Paul's Hospital, 588-1081 Burrard Street, Vancouver, BC V6Z1Y6, Canada
[2]School of Population and Public Health, University of British Columbia, 2206 East Mall, Vancouver, BC V6T1Z3, Canada
Full list of author information is available at the end of the article

accept a wage below their marginal productivity in exchange for job security, e.g. allowances for sick days [9, 10].

A wedge between a worker's wage and marginal productivity may also arise if a job involves team production or if the firm output is time-sensitive [9, 11]. Pauly et al. presented a general model demonstrating that when there is a team production and substantial team-specific human capital, the value of lost output to the firm from an absence will exceed the daily wage of the absent worker and could be as large as the total output of the team [9]. Similarly, the cost of an absence will exceed the wage when a firm incurs a penalty if it misses an output target due to the absence. In both situations, the productivity loss could be reduced if replacements are found who are either inexpensive or are close substitutes for the absent worker.

Although there are many reasons that wage may not equal marginal productivity, there is still lack of empirical evidence on their equality with regard to absenteeism and team participation. This is the first study to empirically test the wage and marginal productivity losses due to absenteeism and measure the multiplicative effect of absenteeism for team workers. This study examines the theoretical implications on the relationship between wages and productivity when a job is involved in team production. Its findings will help determine whether wages can be used as a precise proxy of marginal productivity in estimating productivity loss due to illness-related absenteeism. In addition, we use a unique employer-employee data, the Workplace and Employee Survey (WES). The advantage of these data is that they contain information on a firm's output, capital, materials, other expenditures, payroll, and industry as well as its workers' age, sex, education, occupation, team participation status and absenteeism. The availability of such data allows us to test the equality of wage and marginal productivity for groups of workers with different characteristics. The WES is one of only a few linked employer-employee databases worldwide and the only one for Canada. Furthermore, we conduct robustness checks using alternative specifications and dropping some of the assumptions. We find that our estimates of wage and marginal productivity losses due to absenteeism appear relatively robust and reasonable. We also divide the full sample into small firm and large firms and examine whether our estimates vary by firm size.

The remainder of this paper is organized as follows. Section 2 contains the conceptual framework and a short review of related studies. In section 3, we present our empirical specification. Section 4 describes our data and defines the main variables. In section 5, we present

our findings and parameter estimates. Section 6 summarizes our findings and their implications for economic evaluators.

Background
Conceptual framework

A large literature has documented substantial wage differentials on the basis of firm size [12, 13], industry [14–16], group or non-group work [17, 18], union and non-union contracts [19, 20], business cycle [21, 22], competitiveness of the industry [23, 24], and government regulation [25, 26]. These wage gaps are conventionally estimated from a wage regression using individual-level data. Without an independent measure of worker productivity, however, it is difficult to determine whether these estimated wage differentials reflect productivity differentials or other factors such as wage discrimination [27, 28]. Hellerstein et al. have developed a framework to simultaneously estimate firm-level wage equations and production functions on population-based datasets that link employees' input to their employers' output [27, 28]. Their approach yields estimated marginal productivity differentials and wage differentials for workers with different characteristics, and a framework to test their equality.

Hellerstein and Neumark use Israeli labour market data to test whether the wage gap between men and women exceeds the gap between them (if any) in marginal productivity [27]. Hellerstein et al. use US population data to estimate wage and marginal productivity differentials for worker groups with different age, sex, and race characteristics [28]. Many recent studies have applied the Hellerstein et al. framework. For example, Haegeland and Klette analyze wage and productivity gaps among Norwegian workers grouped by sex, education and work experience [29]; van Ours and Stoeldraijer identify 13 studies on age, wage and productivity using linked employer-employee data [30].

Our theoretical framework is based on Pauly et al. [9]. They develop a general model to examine the magnitude and incidence of costs associated with absenteeism under alternative assumptions about firm size, the production function, the nature of the firm's product, and the competitiveness of the labor market. We test two key theoretical predictions of their model using the Hellerstein et al. [27] and Hellerstein and Neumark [28] framework.

The first prediction is that the productivity loss associated with a worker's absence will be larger than the wage in firms with team production. If a team worker is absent, the output of the entire team may be affected. Hence the impact on firm output exceeds the wage that would have been paid to the absent team worker. We test the hypothesis that the absence of team workers has a larger effect on firm-level production than wages (i.e., a significant difference between productivity effects and wage effects). In contrast, we hypothesize that the absence of non-team workers has a similar effect on production and wages.

The second prediction is that the difference between the wage and the productivity loss due to absence will be larger in small firms than large firms. While large firms can hire extra employees to ensure that a given output level can be maintained if a team worker is absent, small firms may not be able to afford this expense. We test whether the difference between productivity effects and wage effects is larger in small firms than large firms.

Previous literature on the impact of absenteeism and team on wages and production

A related literature seeks to uncover factors that determine or affect worker absence by modeling absence [17, 31–35] or focuses on the association between health conditions and absenteeism [36–39]. Few studies have estimated the impact of absenteeism on wages or production, and none have examined whether their impact varies by team work status and firm size.

Allen estimates the trade-off between wages and expected absence via a hedonic wage equation using individual worker level data in 1970s, and the effect of absenteeism on output per man-hour via a plant-level production function for manufacturing [40]. He finds a small difference between the wage effect and the productivity effect. However, he uses different data for the effects and does not estimate the two equations simultaneously. Thus, the absence-rate coefficients from the two equations might not be comparable.

Several studies have estimated the impact of absenteeism on productivity using plant-level data. In the production function of Allen [40], the elasticity of the absence rate is −0.015, meaning an increase in the absence rate from 0.1 to 0.2 reduces the output per man-hour by 1%. In addition, Mefford examines the effect of unions on productivity in 31 plants of a large multinational firm from 1975 to 82 [41]. He also includes the absence rate into the production function and finds that the elasticity of the absence rate is −0.033, implying if the absence rate increases from 0.1 to 0.2, productivity will decrease by 2.3%. The direction of the estimated effect in our study is consistent with these previous studies yet the magnitude of the effect size is greater.

Coles et al. introduced the idea of the shadow cost of absenteeism: the relatively high wage paid by firms requiring a low level of absenteeism, to compensate workers for attending work reliably [17]. They use just-in-time as an indicator of an assembly line production process. Using individual worker level data, they find an association between higher wages and lower absence rates; however, the relationship is almost twice as steep in just-in-time firms contrasted to non-just-in-time firms.

Measure of compensation

Wage rate versus the impact of absenteeism on aggregate wages

In the absenteeism literature, the measure of opportunity cost of absenteeism is usually proxied by the worker's wage rate (wage per unit time) taken from firm data. In this paper, however, the wage cost of absenteeism comes from an estimate of the impact of worker absenteeism on aggregate wages for workers at a firm. It may differ from a direct measure of the wage rate because the equilibrium wage incorporates any effects of absenteeism as a compensating differential. For example, the observed wage per day may vary much less between a firm where (for some exogenous reasons) absenteeism is common and one where it is rare than does the estimate from our wage regression. Most importantly, with only an aggregate measure of output available, we prefer to use the aggregate wages at the firm level in order to obtain the most comparable estimates. As Hellerstein et al. pointed out, by jointly estimating the firm-level production function and wage equation, we can conduct straightforward statistical tests of the equality of wages and marginal productivity [27]. Furthermore, the biases from some unobservables are more likely to affect the estimated absenteeism impacts on productivity and wages similarly when both are estimated at the firm level. Their impact on the tests of the equality of marginal productivity and wages is therefore diminished.

Payroll and non-wage benefits

In our main analysis, we use payroll as a measure of compensation. Payroll or wage is only part of the total employee compensation. Non-wage benefits are also available to employees, e.g., health related benefits (e.g. dental care, life insurance), pay related benefits (e.g. severance allowances), or pension related benefits. As a robustness test, we also use the total compensation (payroll plus non-wage benefits) as the outcome in our wage equation.

Measure of absenteeism

Because we are primarily interested in estimating the productivity loss due to illness for applications in health care economic evaluation studies, an ideal measure of absenteeism would reflect illness-related absences only. However, data limitations dictate that we rely on a broader measure of absenteeism. The WES data used in this study only measure absences due to paid sick leave, but not unpaid sick leave. Following the definition of Dionne and Dostie [32], our measure of absenteeism includes the number of days of paid sick leave; other paid leave encompassing education leave, disability leave, bereavement, marriage, jury duty, and union business; and unpaid leave. It does not include paid vacations, paid paternity/maternity leave, or absence due to strikes or lock-outs. Although our measure of absenteeism is broader than a pure measure of illness-related absenteeism, our findings are still useful to determine whether wages are a reasonable proxy of the productivity loss due to illness-related absenteeism under the assumption that illness-related absenteeism and other forms of paid and unpaid leave have a similar impact on wages and output.

Methods

Our empirical analysis is based on two firm-level equations which we specify and estimate jointly: a production function and a wage equation. The production function is used to capture productivity effects related to absenteeism and team work at the firm level, and the wage equation is to capture the corresponding wage effects. By simultaneously estimating the two equations, we can compare the productivity effects with wage effects to determine the equality of marginal productivity and wages. The traditional approach of estimating the wage equation alone to measure the impact of absenteeism does not fully capture productivity differentials associated with different levels of absenteeism.

We think it is useful to baseline our results with an estimate of economy-wide aggregate effects. Thus we begin by estimating a baseline model that restricts the effect of absenteeism to be the same for team workers and non-team workers and in small and large firms. We subsequently relax these restrictions by assuming that absenteeism affects team workers and non-team workers differently, and then by estimating our model separately for small and large firms.

Production function

Our baseline specification of the production function is an extension of the standard Cobb-Douglas [27, 28, 42, 43]. See Additional file 1: Appendix B for its complete deviation. Because the Cobb-Douglas form is restrictive, we assess the robustness of our estimates to more general alternatives described in Section 3.4.

For each workplace, we start with a simple Cobb-Douglas production function:

$$\ln Q_j = \alpha \ln L_j^A + \beta \ln K_j + \eta F_j + \mu_j \qquad (1)$$

where Q_j is output, measured as value added by firm j, L_j^A is an aggregate labour input defined below, K_j is the capital stock, F_j is a matrix of various firm characteristics, α, β are the elasticity of output with respect to labour and capital, respectively, η is a vector of parameters for firm characteristics and μ_j is the error term.

We divide the labour input into different worker types, that is, workers with different characteristics such as age, sex, education, occupation and team participation. If the total number of characteristics is I and workers are divided into V_i categories by each characteristic i, then the total number of worker types will be $\prod_{i=1}^{I} V_i$. Our aggregate labour input L_j^A can be simplified after making several assumptions: First, we assume perfect substitutability among all types of workers and different marginal productivity for each worker type [27, 28]. Second, we assume that the proportion or distribution of one type of worker defined by one characteristic is constant across all other characteristic groups, which is referred to as the *equi-proportionate restriction* [27, 28].[1] Third, we assume the relative marginal productivity of two types of workers within one characteristic group is equal to those within another characteristic group, which is referred to as the *equal relative productivity restriction* [27, 28].[2] Fourth, attendance rates have the same marginal impact on productivity for different worker types.

The aggregate labour input can then be written as (equation 8 from Additional file 1: Appendix B):

$$L_j^A = (1-a_j)^\theta \lambda_{0,I} L_j \left(1 + (\gamma_G-1)P_{Gj}\right) \qquad (2)$$
$$\prod_{i=1}^{I-1} \left(1 + \sum_{v=1}^{V_i-1} (\gamma_{iv}-1)P_{ivj}\right)$$

where a_j is the absence rate in firm j, L_j is the number of all workers in the firm j, P_{Gj} is the proportion of team workers among all workers in the firm j, $i = 1, 2, ..., I$-1 indicates worker characteristics other than team participation, $v_i = 1, 2, ..., V_i$-1 represents worker categories divided according to the worker characteristic i, $P_{ivj} = \frac{L_{ivj}}{L_j}$ is the proportion of the worker type iv among all workers in the firm j, θ is the parameter of (1-absence rate), i.e., the attendance impact on the marginal productivity for any worker type, $\lambda_{0,I}$ is the marginal productivity for the reference group when work force is divided by I characteristics and absence rate = 0, γ_G is the relative marginal productivity of team workers compared to non-team workers, and $\gamma_{iv} = \frac{\lambda_{iv}}{\lambda_{io}}$ is the relative marginal productivity of one worker type iv to the worker type $i0$ for each characteristic i.

By substituting L_j^A into the simple production function, equation 1, we obtain our baseline specification (equations 9 and 10 from Additional file 1: Appendix B), i.e., a "restricted model" as follows:

$$\ln Q_j = \beta_0 + \beta \ln K_j + \alpha \ln L_j + \alpha\theta \ln(1-a_j)$$
$$+ \alpha \ln\big(1 + (\gamma_G-1)P_{Gj}\big) + \alpha E_j + \eta Fj + \mu j \tag{3}$$

Where

$$E_j = \sum_{i=1}^{I-1} \ln\left(1 + \sum_{v=1}^{V_i-1}(\gamma_{iv}-1)P_{ivj}\right) \tag{4}$$

E_j refers to workforce characteristics other than team participation, and β_0 is a constant term that incorporates $a \ln\lambda_{0,I}$.

In addition, we relax the fourth assumption for teamwork participation, that is, the attendance impact on the marginal productivity for team workers (θ_G) is different from that for non-team workers (θ_N). A relatively "complete model" (equations 12 and 13 from Additional file 1: Appendix B) is therefore presented as:

$$L_j^A = \lambda_{0,I}(1-a_j)^{\theta_N} L_j \left(1 + \left(\gamma_G(1-a_j)^{\theta_G-\theta_N}-1\right)P_{Gj}\right) \tag{5}$$
$$\prod_{i=1}^{I-1}\left(1 + \sum_{v=1}^{V_i-1}(\gamma_{iv}-1)P_{ivj}\right)$$

and,

$$\ln Q_j = \beta_0 + \beta \ln K_j + \alpha \ln L_j$$
$$+ \alpha\theta_N \ln(1-a_j) + \alpha \ln\left(1 + \left(\gamma_G(1-a_j)^{\theta_G-\theta_N}-1\right)P_{Gj}\right)$$
$$+ \alpha E_j + \eta F_j + \mu_j$$
$$\tag{6}$$

Wage equation

Applying the same approach as above, wage effects can be estimated through the relationship between payroll and average absence rate and share of workers participating in a team at the firm level. We write the aggregate wage w_j as the sum of wage for each worker type. Applying the same assumptions in the production function, the aggregate wage can be simplified as:

$$w_j = w_{0,I}(1-a_j)^\zeta L_j(1 + (\phi_G-1)P_{Gj}) \tag{7}$$
$$\prod_{i=1}^{I-1}\left(1 + \sum_{v=1}^{V_i-1}(\phi_{iv}-1)P_{ivj}\right)$$

where w_j is the annual payroll of firm j, $w_{0,I}$ is the wage for the reference group when work force is divided by I

characteristics, ζ is the parameter of attendance rate, i.e., the attendance impact on wages for any worker type, ϕ_G is the relative wage of team workers to non-team workers, $\phi_{iv} = \frac{w_{iv}}{w_{i0}}$ is the relative wage of one worker type iv to the worker type $i0$ for each characteristic i other than team participation.

After log transforming equation 7, the "restricted model" for wage equation is written as:

$$\ln w_j = \beta_{w0} + \beta_w \ln K_j + \alpha_w \ln L_j + \zeta \ln(1-a_j)$$
$$+ \ln\big(1 + (\phi_G-1)P_{Gj}\big) + E_{wj} + \eta_w F_j + \mu_{w,j} \tag{8}$$

where,

$$E_{wj} = \sum_{i=1}^{I-1}\ln\left(1 + \sum_{v=1^{V_i-1}}(\phi_{iv}-1)P_{ivj}\right) \tag{9}$$

β_{w0} is a constant term incorporating $w_{0,I}$, α_w, β_w are the elasticity of wage with respect to labour and capital, respectively, η_w is a vector of parameters for firm characteristics and $\mu_{w,j}$ is the error term.

Correspondingly, we assume the attendance impact on wages differ by team participation and thus the relatively "complete model" becomes:

$$w_j = w_{0,I}(1-a_j)^{\zeta_N} L_j\left(1 + \left(\phi_G(1-a_j)^{\zeta_G-\zeta_N}-1\right)P_{Gj}\right) \tag{10}$$
$$\prod_{i=1}^{I-1}\left(1 + \sum_{v=1}^{V_i-1}(\phi_{iv}-1)P_{ivj}\right)$$

and

$$\ln w_j = \beta_{w0} + \beta_w \ln K_j + \alpha_w \ln L_j$$
$$+ \zeta_N \ln(1-a_j)$$
$$+ \ln\left(1 + \left(\phi_G(1-a_j)^{\zeta_G-\zeta_N}-1\right)P_{Gj}\right)$$
$$+ E_{wj} + \eta_w F_j + \mu_{w,j} \tag{11}$$

where ζ_N is the impact of attendance rate for non-team workers and ζ_G is the impact of attendance rate for team workers.

Estimation

We estimate the production function and wage equation simultaneously via nonlinear least squares (NLS) [27, 28]., under the assumption that errors are correlated across equations (nonlinear seemingly unrelated regression).[3] All observations are weighted using linked weights provided by Statistics Canada. All standard errors are computed as Statistics Canada's recommended procedure [44] using 100 sets of provided bootstrap sample weights.

Our null hypothesis of primary interest is that the attendance coefficient in the production function equals the coefficient in the wage equation. In the restricted model, the equality of marginal productivity and wage is tested by comparing the attendance coefficients, θ and ζ. In the complete model, we compare the two coefficients for team workers, θ_G and ζ_G, and those for non-team workers, θ_N and ζ_N, respectively. We also test the equality of relative productivity of team workers to non-team workers and their relative wage by comparing $(\lambda_G - 1)$ and $(\phi_G - 1)$.

In order to examine whether parameter estimates vary by firm size, we conduct our analyses separately on two sub-samples: small firms with less than 20 employees and large firms (the remainder).

Robustness

We undertake further analyses to assess the robustness of our estimates. First, we relax restrictions on the functional form of our production function by estimating a specification using the much more flexible translog form. Second, we re-estimate our model using total compensation (payroll plus non-wage benefits) instead of payroll as the outcome of the wage equation.

Third, a key issue in the estimation of production functions is the potential correlation between input levels and unobserved firm-specific productivity shocks. Firms that have a large positive productivity shock may respond by using more inputs, giving rise to an endogeneity issue [45]. Following Hellerstein et al. [27], we address this issue by using value-added as the measure of output in the production function to avoid estimating a coefficient on materials. We also attempt to correct for the potential bias by estimating the model on first differences, which eliminates the effect of any time-invariant unobserved heterogeneity that jointly affects productivity and wages. We also apply Levinsohn and Petrin's approach [46] using intermediate inputs (expenses on materials which are subtracted out in our value-added production function) to address the simultaneity problem. Specifically, we estimate parameters of our value-added production function using NLS by adding a third-order or a fourth-order polynomial approximation in capital and material inputs [47].

Finally, we conduct sensitivity analyses to examine the impacts of some of the assumptions embodied in our baseline specification. We relax the equi-proportionate restriction between occupation, age, sex, education (> university bachelor versus bachelor and below) and team participation, respectively.[4] That restriction also implies that the firm-average absence rate is common to all worker types. To test the impact of this assumption, we allow the average absence rate to differ for team workers and non-team workers in each firm. That is, the firm-average absence rate in the complete model is replaced with the firm-average absence rate of team workers and the absence rate of non-team workers, correspondingly, as follows.

$$
\begin{aligned}
L^A_j &= \left(1-a_{Gj}\right)^{\theta_G} \lambda_{G,0,I-1} L_{Gj} \prod_{i=1}^{I-1}\left(1+\sum_{v=1}^{V_i-1}(\gamma_{iv}-1)P_{ivj}\right) \\
&+ \left(1-a_{Nj}\right)^{\theta_N} \lambda_{N,0,I-1} L_{Nj} \prod_{i=1}^{I-1}\left(1+\sum_{v=1}^{V_i-1}(\gamma_{iv}-1)P_{ivj}\right) \\
&= \lambda_{0,I}\left(1-a_{Nj}\right)^{\theta_N} L_j \left(1+\left(\gamma_G \frac{(1-a_{Gj})^{\theta_G}}{(1-a_{Nj})^{\theta_N}}-1\right)P_{Gj}\right) \\
&\prod_{i=1}^{I-1}\left(1+\sum_{v=1}^{V_i-1}(\gamma_{iv}-1)P_{ivj}\right)
\end{aligned}
$$

(12)

and

$$
\begin{aligned}
\ln Q_j &= \beta_0 + \beta \ln K_j \\
&+ \alpha \ln L_j + \alpha \theta_N \ln\left(1-a_{Nj}\right) \\
&+ \alpha \ln\left(1+\left(\gamma_G \frac{(1-a_{Gj})^{\theta_G}}{(1-a_{Nj})^{\theta_N}}-1\right)P_{Gj}\right) \\
&+ \alpha E_j + \eta F_j + \mu_j
\end{aligned}
$$

(14)

Data

The WES is a survey of Canadian employers and employees conducted by Statistics Canada over the period 1999–2006 [48].[5] These data have been used to estimate age-based wage and productivity differentials [49] and to compare wages and marginal productivity for workers with different levels of education and technology use [50, 51].

The sampling frame for the WES includes all Canadian workplaces[6] in the Statistics Canada Business Registry that had paid employees in March of the survey year. The sampling frame for employees comprises all employees working at or on paid leave from the targeted workplaces in March. In each year between 1999 and 2006, Statistics Canada surveyed a representative sample of approximately 6000 workplaces. The initial sample of workplaces was refreshed in odd-number years (2001, 2003, and 2005) to reflect attrition and firm births. In 1999–2005, Statistics Canada randomly sampled approximately 20,000 employees of sampled firms. The number of employees sampled from a firm was proportional to size, up to a maximum of 24. In workplaces with fewer than 4 employees, all employees were sampled. Sampled workers were surveyed for two years, and a new sample of workers was drawn in the next odd-numbered year.

Ethical approval for this study is not required because it was based exclusively on the WES conducted by Statistics Canada and we did not directly approach the study subjects. Our analysis is based on the pooled data 1999, 2001, 2003, and 2005 cross-sections.[7] We further restrict the sample to workplaces with at least one employee interviewed, operating for profit, and with positive output. Our sample includes 18,381 observations on 7766 unique workplaces. There are 7784 observations for small firms and 10,597 for large firms. Table 1 illustrates the transition from the gross workplace sample to our final sample in detail.

Outcome variables

Our outcome variable in the wage equation is the firm's total annual payroll. Our outcomes variables in the production function is the firm's output. Following Turcotte and Rennison [50, 51], we define output as value added, where value added is measured as annual gross operating revenues minus expenses on materials.[8] Expenses on materials equal annual gross operating expenditures minus total gross payroll and expenditures on non-wage benefits and training.

Independent variables of interest

Our measure of absenteeism is the absence rate of the firm's employees. This is defined as the number of days of total leave taken by employees, including paid sick leave, other paid leave (e.g., education leave, disability leave, bereavement, marriage, jury duty, union business) and unpaid leave [32] in the past 12 months or since the employee started his/her current job (if less than 12 months), divided by the total number of 'usual workdays'[9] over the same time period. The absence rate for a firm is the average absence rate for the employees surveyed at that firm. We define the firm's attendance rate as one minus the absence rate.

We identify workers as being a member of a team based on their reported participation in "a self-directed work group (semi-autonomous work group or mini-enterprise group) that has a high level of responsibility for a particular product or service area" [48].[10] In our analysis, team workers are those who report participating in such a group 'frequently' or 'always' and non-team workers are those who report participating in such a group 'occasionally' or 'never'.

The L_j in our baseline specification is measured by the number of total employees employed by each workplace.

Table 1 Transition from the gross sample to the final sample

	Observations	Workplaces
Gross sample	43832	9372
At least one employee without attrition[a]	36579	8875
For profit	31786	7931
Value added >0	30416	7812
Odd years	18381	7766
Small firms	7784	3870
Large firms	10597	4385

[a]In even survey years, employees who had a different employer or left his employer and did not have a new employer were considered as attrition

Estimation of our production function also requires a measure of the firm's capital stock. Unfortunately, there is no such measure in the WES. We therefore impute the firm's capital stock following the approach of Dostie [49] and Turcotte and Rennison [50, 51]. Our imputed capital measure equals the five-year average capital stock in the firm's industry, divided by the number of firms in each industry represented by the WES. The industry capital stock measure is the geometric (infinite) end-year net stock of non-residential capital reported in CANSIM Table 031–0002, obtained from Statistics Canada.[11]

Control variables in our empirical specification include other characteristics of the firm's workforce (firm-average proportion of employees grouped by age, sex, education, occupation, race, immigration status, and membership in union or collective bargaining agreement, separately, included in E_j), workplace characteristics (an indicator for selling into an international market, an indicator for foreign country ownership, region, and industry included in F_j), and calendar year dummies. More details on the definition of all variables we used in the study can be found in Additional file 1: Appendix A.

Table 2 provides descriptive statistics for variables used in our analysis. At the workplace level, the average absence rate is low (0.02), of which 65% is unpaid leave, 19% is paid sick leave and 16% is other paid leave. The share of workers in teamwork is 8%. The average age is 40 years old and the share of female workers is 54%. Only 38% of workplaces have at least 5 employees surveyed. The average number of employees per firm is 15 and most firms (85%) fall in the category of 1–19 employees. There are more large firms sampled in the WES survey than small firms (Table 1). However, the small firms are assigned higher sampling weights than large firms to represent their much greater number in the Canadian economy.

Results

Table 3 presents parameter estimates for our baseline model, which provides an estimate of the economy-wide aggregate effect of absenteeism. With the full set of controls, our estimate of the overall effect of attendance on marginal productivity (0.46) is almost identical to its estimated effect on wages (0.47). We cannot reject the hypothesis that the two coefficients are the same at conventional significance levels. These coefficients can be interpreted as elasticities: a 1% decline in the attendance rate reduces productivity by 0.95*0.46% = 0.44%[12] and wages by 0.47%.

In Table 4, we relax our baseline specification by allowing the coefficient on the attendance rate to differ for team workers and non-team workers. The impact of attendance is much larger for team workers: coefficients

Table 2 Descriptive statistics at workplace level

Variables	Weighted mean	Standard deviation
Value added (,000)	1393.333	38.705
Log value added	12.526	0.026
Total wage (,000)	524.346	10.281
Log wage	11.892	0.021
Employment	14.982	0.242
Capital stock (,000)	1254.673	59.224
Absence rate	0.019	0.001
Proportion of workers participating in a team	0.079	0.003
Other workforce characteristics		
Age	40.472	0.175
Proportion of workers by age		
Age <35	0.353	0.006
35 ≤ Age < 55	0.525	0.007
55 ≤ Age	0.123	0.005
Proportion of female workers	0.542	0.007
Proportion of workers by level of education		
< High school	0.130	0.005
High school graduate only	0.203	0.007
Under university bachelor (completed/some college or university)	0.539	0.007
University bachelor	0.092	0.003
> University bachelor	0.035	0.002
Proportion of workers by occupation		
Managers/professionals	0.269	0.005
Technical/trades/marking/sales/clerical/administrative	0.463	0.007
Production workers	0.200	0.006
Others	0.068	0.004
Proportion of ethnic minorities	0.187	0.006
Proportion of immigrants	0.179	0.006
Proportion of employees with bargaining agreement	0.046	0.002
Workplace characteristics	%	
Establishment size		
1–19 employees	84.7	
20–99 employees	13.5	
100–499 employees	1.6	
500 employees or more	0.2	
Number of employees surveyed[a]		
1	12.3	
2	16.8	
3	22.9	

Table 2 Descriptive statistics at workplace level *(Continued)*

4	9.9
>=5	38.0
International market	5.1
Foreign country owned	3.3
Industry	
Forestry, mining, oil, and gas extraction	1.5
Labour intensive tertiary manufacturing	3.3
Primary product manufacturing	1.2
Secondary product manufacturing	2.0
Capital intensive tertiary manufacturing	2.6
Construction	8.2
Transportation, warehousing, wholesale	12.1
Communication and other utilities	1.3
Retail trade and consumer services	33.7
Finance and insurance	5.3
Real estate, rental and leasing operations	4.2
Business services	13.2
Education and health services	9.7
Information and cultural industries	1.7
Region	
Atlantic	8.3
Quebec	21.0
Ontario	37.2
Alberta	11.7
British Columbia	14.9
Manitoba	3.0
Saskatchewan	3.8
Year[a]	
1999	25.2
2001	24.2
2003	24.2
2005	26.3

Employer weight is used for workplace characteristics; linked weight is used for workforce characteristics
[a]unweighted estimates

are 2.38 in the production function and 1.43 in the wage equation. In this specification, the total effect of attendance (or absenteeism) on wages and productivity depends on both these coefficients and the proportion of employees that work in a team. Fig. 1. plots the rate at which productivity and wages decline when the absence rate increases by 0.1, at various levels of the firm's absence rate and proportion of team workers. For example, at a firm where all employees work in teams, an increase in the absence rate from 0.1 to 0.2 reduces output by 23.4% and wages by 15.5%. At a firm where 20% of employees work in teams, output would only decline by

Table 3 Parameter estimates for the restricted model

	Production	P value	Wage	P value
Baseline controls[a]				
Log (total no. of employees)	0.94 (0.02)***	<0.001	1.04 (0.01)***	<0.001
Log (capital)	0.04 (0.01)***	<0.001	0.05 (0.01)***	<0.001
Attendance rate	0.42 (0.12)***	<0.001	0.41 (0.07)***	<0.001
Team	0.66 (0.19)***	<0.001	0.40 (0.08)***	<0.001
Difference in attendance rate coefficients	0.01 (0.10)	0.958		
Difference in team coefficients	0.26 (0.14)*	0.056		
All controls[b]				
Log (total no. of employees)	0.95 (0.02)***	<0.001	1.08 (0.01)***	<0.001
Log (capital)	0.00 (0.01)	0.931	−0.03 (0.01)***	0.002
Attendance rate	0.46 (0.13)***	<0.001	0.47 (0.07)***	<0.001
Team	0.26 (0.11)**	0.021	0.08 (0.05)	0.110
Difference in attendance rate coefficients	−0.01 (0.10)	0.953		
Difference in team coefficients	0.18 (0.09)**	0.037		

[a]Model adjusted for employment, capital stock, and years; [b]Adjusted for employment, capital stock, occupation, age, sex, education, race, immigrant, bargaining agreement, international market, foreign owned, region, industry and year; Standard error in the bracket; ***$p \leq 0.01$; **$0.01 < p \leq 0.05$; *$0.05 < p \leq 0.1$

8.6% and wages by 7.2%. Correspondingly, the difference between the attendance impact on marginal productivity and the impact on wage for team workers is also larger than that for non-team workers (0.95 versus −0.02) (Table 4). However, the gap is not statistically significant.

In Table 5, we further relax our baseline restrictions by estimating the model separately on sub-samples of small and large firms. The impact of non-team workers' attendance on output and wages is smaller for small firms than for large firms: coefficients are 0.47 versus 1.32 in the production function and 0.44 versus 1.08 in the wage equation. As hypothesized, the difference between the two effects are not significantly different from zero in small firms (0.03) or large firms (0.24). In contrast, the impact of team workers' attendance is much larger for small firms than for large firms. The productivity coefficients are 4.97 versus −0.76, and the wage coefficients are 2.25 versus −0.33, for small and large firms respectively. The difference between the attendance impact on output and that on wages is much larger in small firms (2.72) than in large firms (−0.43). The results suggest that in a large firm where all employees work in teams, absenteeism do not have any substantial impact on output or wages. On the other hand, absenteeism significantly reduces output and wages in small firms where all employees work in teams. The reduction in output is significantly higher than the reduction in wages at the 10% significance level. The results are consistent with our hypothesis that the absence of team workers has a larger effect on firm-level production than wages in small firms.

Our estimates of the relative productivity and the relative wage of team workers versus non-team workers

imply that team workers are more productive and earn more than non-team workers in the full sample (Tables 3 and 4). This difference is statistically significant at the 5% level in the specification including all controls. The difference between relative productivity and relative wage is larger in small firms but smaller in large firms (Table 5). This implies that on average, the higher wages paid to team workers are considerably less than their productivity differential relative to non-team workers.

In Additional file 1: Appendix C, we present parameter estimates for all covariates that are included in the models of Table 3 to Table 5, as well as the results of various robustness checks. These include estimates based on a translog production function (estimated on the full sample) and using total compensation (payroll plus non-wage benefits) as the outcome of the wage equation. The estimates from these alternative specifications are similar to what we have obtained above. When we consider different absence rates for team workers and non-team workers, the coefficients do not change much, which suggests our main analyses are robust. When the equi-proportionate restriction is dropped for occupation, age, sex and education with team participation, the estimated coefficients change only slightly.[13] Nevertheless, the qualitative nature of the results stay the same after relaxing these assumptions.

We have also re-estimated the model by excluding the capital stock and the attendance rate coefficients remain virtually identical. Therefore, we believe that our parameter estimates are robust to our (imperfect) measure of the capital stock.

We address the potential endogeneity of absenteeism and team work status in several ways. First, we have

Table 4 Parameter estimates for the complete model

	Production	P value	Wage	P value
Baseline controls[a]				
Log (total no. of employees)	0.94 (0.02)***	<0.001	1.04 (0.01)***	<0.001
Log (capital)	0.04 (0.01)***	<0.001	0.05 (0.01)***	<0.001
Attendance rate, non-team workers	0.37 (0.12)***	0.002	0.38 (0.07)***	<0.001
Attendance rate, team workers	2.78 (1.44)*	0.054	1.83 (0.84)**	0.029
Team	0.75 (0.17)***	<0.001	0.45 (0.08)***	<0.001
Difference in attendance coefficients, non-team workers	−0.01 (0.10)	0.876		
Difference in attendance coefficients, team workers	0.95 (0.95)	0.318		
Difference in team coefficients	0.30 (0.12)**	0.011		
All controls[b]				
Log (total no. of employees)	0.95 (0.02)***	<0.001	1.08 (0.01)***	<0.001
Log (capital)	0.00 (0.01)	0.935	−0.03 (0.01)***	0.002
Attendance rate, non-team workers	0.43 (0.13)***	<0.001	0.45 (0.07)***	<0.001
Attendance rate, team workers	2.38 (1.40)*	0.090	1.43 (0.75)*	0.058
Team	0.32 (0.12)**	0.012	0.10 (0.05)**	0.041
Difference in attendance coefficients, non-team workers	−0.02 (0.10)	0.816		
Difference in attendance coefficients, team workers	0.95 (1.00)	0.341		
Difference in team coefficients	0.21 (0.10)**	0.030		

[a]Model adjusted for employment, capital stock, and years
[b]Adjusted for employment, capital stock, occupation, age, sex, education, race, immigrant, bargaining agreement, international market, foreign owned, region, industry and year; Standard error in the bracket; ***$p \leq 0.01$; **$0.01 < p \leq 0.05$; *$0.05 < p \leq 0.1$

estimated the equations in first differences to remove any time invariant components of the model as a sensitivity analysis. The first differences estimates reported in Additional file 1: Appendix C are similar to the NLS estimates. Differencing does not eliminate the effect of correlated transitory shocks, however, and these are another potential source of bias. For example, a chemical spill accident may instigate sick leave and a reduction in output. Employee work attendance decisions also depend on the slope of the wage-absence tradeoff, which may introduced simultaneity problems [40]. In the presence of correlated transitory shocks or simultaneity, an

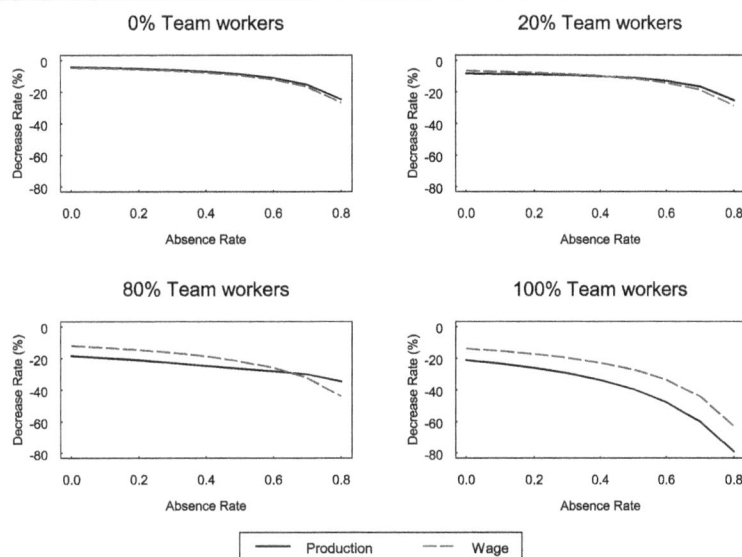

Fig. 1 Rate at which output and wages decline for a 0.1 increase in the absence rate, at various levels of the firm's absence rate and proportion of team workers

Table 5 Parameter estimates for the complete model by firm size

	Small firms				Large firms			
	Production	P value	Wage	P value	Production	P value	Wage	P value
Baseline controls[a]								
Log (total no. of employees)	0.87 (0.03)***	<0.001	1.04 (0.02)***	<0.001	1.07 (0.02)***	<0.001	1.01 (0.02)***	<0.001
Log (capital)	0.03 (0.01)***	0.005	0.04 (0.01)***	<0.001	0.09 (0.01)***	<0.001	0.08 (0.01)***	<0.001
Attendance rate, non-team workers	0.39 (0.14)***	0.005	0.36 (0.08)***	<0.001	1.95 (0.80)**	0.015	1.66 (0.58)***	0.004
Attendance rate, team workers	6.34 (2.25)***	0.005	3.01 (1.03)***	0.004	−0.57 (0.76)	0.449	−0.02 (0.70)	0.974
Team	0.75 (0.27)***	0.005	0.35 (0.10)***	<0.001	0.71 (0.15)***	<0.001	0.63 (0.12)***	<0.001
Difference in attendance coefficients, non-team workers	0.04 (0.11)	0.745			0.29 (0.36)	0.429		
Difference in attendance coefficients, team workers	3.33 (1.59)**	0.036			−0.55 (0.70)	0.431		
Difference in team coefficients	0.40 (0.21)*	0.056			0.08 (0.10)	0.433		
All controls[b]								
Log (total no. of employees)	0.88 (0.03)***	<0.001	1.07 (0.02)***	<0.001	1.10 (0.02)***	<0.001	1.03 (0.02)***	<0.001
Log (capital)	0.00 (0.02)	0.939	−0.03 (0.01)***	0.006	0.00 (0.01)	0.879	−0.01 (0.01)	0.263
Attendance rate, non-team workers	0.47 (0.14)***	0.001	0.44 (0.06)***	<0.001	1.32 (0.70)*	0.061	1.08 (0.47)**	0.021
Attendance rate, team workers	4.97 (1.87)***	0.008	2.25 (0.95)**	0.018	−0.76 (0.73)	0.300	−0.33 (0.64)	0.609
Team	0.33 (0.18)*	0.073	0.06 (0.06)	0.260	0.19 (0.10)*	0.054	0.09 (0.07)	0.213
Difference in attendance coefficients, non-team workers	0.03 (0.12)	0.811			0.24 (0.37)	0.511		
Difference in attendance coefficients, team workers	2.72 (1.49)*	0.068			−0.43 (0.72)	0.549		
Difference in team coefficients	0.27 (0.16)*	0.091			0.10 (0.07)	0.157		

Small firms are those with less than 20 employees; large firms are the remainder
[a]Model adjusted for employment, capital stock, and years
[b]Adjusted for employment, capital stock, occupation, age, sex, education, race, immigrant, bargaining agreement, international market, foreign owned, region, industry and year; Standard error in the bracket; ***$p \leq 0.01$; **$0.01 < p \leq 0.05$; *$0.05 < p \leq 0.1$

instrumental variable (IV) approach [30, 52, 53] can be used to consistently estimate parameters. We have estimated IV specifications of our model using the lagged attendance rate as an instrument. However this instrument turns out to be weak (F-statistic < 10), and we were unable to identify other valid instruments in the WES. We therefore adopt the Levinsohn and Petrin approach [46] and obtain estimates similar to our main findings. Overall, we find our estimates to be stable across different specifications, and this provides strong evidence in support of our main conclusions that wages underestimate the productivity loss due to absenteeism in the presence of team production, especially in small firms.

Discussion and conclusions

This study is the first to test the equality of the estimated absenteeism impacts on marginal productivity and wages using linked employer-employee data. Our findings support the theoretical predictions of Pauly et al. [9, 11] and provide compelling evidence that the productivity loss due to worker absence exceeds the wage for team workers, especially in small firms.

Our findings highlight that the productivity loss due to absenteeism among team workers substantially exceeds the wage in small firms. Interestingly, such a wage-productivity gap is absent in large firms. This may reflect differences in compensation policy between large and small firms, or differences in substitution possibilities. While team workers are more productive and earn higher wages than non-team workers, our findings further imply that their higher marginal productivity exceeds the wage premium they receive. Moreover, although we find that wages underestimate the productivity loss due to absenteeism for team workers, our estimates indicate that wages are reasonable estimate of the productivity loss due to absenteeism for non-team workers.

It is worth noticing that this study is an aggregate or ecologic study that has focused on the effect of team work at the firm level rather than at individual worker level due to a lack of individual-level output data. Thus, it might be subject to ecological bias. According to Greenland and Morgenstern [54], ecological bias can occur if confounders or other factors affecting output or wages are differentially distributed across firms (i.e., confounding by firms) or when the effects of absenteeism and team work on output and wages vary across firms (i.e., effect modification by firms). To minimize the bias, in our regression models, we have adjusted for firms' workforce characteristics that potentially affect output and wages, which were derived from individual-level worker data. Furthermore, we are more interested in the equality of the effects of absenteeism and team work in the two equations: production equation and wage equation. By jointly estimating the two equations at the firm level, the bias is more likely to affect the estimated effects on output and wages similarly [27] and thus the impact of bias on the tests of the equality of marginal productivity and wages might be diminished.

Collectively, our findings help to value the burden of illness-related absenteeism, by establishing situations where the wage can be used as a reasonable proxy for lost productivity, and situations where it will underestimate the loss. This is important for economic evaluations that seek to measure the productivity gain or loss of a health care technology/intervention, which in turn can impact policy makers' funding decisions. Other researchers have proposed a multiplier to adjust wages to estimate the productivity burden of illness or the productivity gain from a health care intervention [9, 11, 55]. Our study provides a justification for such a multiplier. In practice, the productivity loss can be estimated by calculating the measured number of absent workdays due to health problems, multiplied by the daily wage and the multiplier.

Finally, we have deliberately avoided being prescriptive with respect to the method that should be employed in measuring productivity losses in economic evaluations. We believe that the appropriate measurement approach (which we focus on above) has many dimensions and in this study our intention was to highlight the welfare economic implications of under/over estimating productivity impacts due to absenteeism. We hope that the debate on the inclusion or exclusion of productivity losses in economic evaluations will be informed by this work over and above the normative aspects of the controversy.

Endnotes

[1]For example, older workers are assumed to be equally represented among team workers and non-team workers; the distribution of absence rate is the same across different worker types.

[2]For instance, the relative marginal productivity of older workers versus younger workers among team workers is assumed to be the same as those among non-team workers.

[3]We have also estimated the equations in first differences to remove the firm-level fixed effects. The estimates were similar to the NLS estimates but very

imprecise due to the large number of implied firm effects relative to the sample size. The results are included in Appendix C.

[4]For example, when dropping the restriction between sex and team participation, we allow the proportion of team workers to differ in female and male employees. The new specification includes the proportion of female team workers, proportion of male team workers and proportion of female non-team workers as the independent variables.

[5]Only employers were surveyed in 2006.

[6]Employers in Yukon, Nunavut, and the Northwest Territories are excluded from the survey, as are those operating in crop production, animal production, fishing, hunting and trapping, private households, religious organizations and public administration.

[7]We do not use data from even-numbered years for two reasons. First, employee attrition is high in their second survey year and is likely nonrandom [56]. Second, many sampled workers change employers between survey years and only limited information is collected about their new employer.

[8]Using value added as an output measure helps address the potential endogeneity of materials by avoiding estimation of a coefficient on materials [27, 50, 51]. Another advantage of a value-added specification is that it improves comparability of data across industries and across workplaces within industries when their degree of vertical integration differs [27].

[9]The total number of usual workdays equals to the number of days per week that employees usually work multiplied by the number of weeks per year they usually work.

[10]More information on self-directed work group was provided in the question, i.e., "In such systems, part of your pay is normally related to group performance. Self-directed work groups: 1) Are responsible for production of a fixed product or service, and have a high degree of autonomy in how they organize themselves to produce that product or service. 2) Act almost as 'businesses within businesses'. 3) Often have incentives related to productivity, timeliness and quality. 4) While most have a designated leader, other members also contribute to the organization of the group's activities."

[11]Although firms in the WES are classified into industries according to 6-digit North American Industry Classification System (NAICS) (a total of 837 unique industries), the capital stock information provided by Statistics Canada is only available for 247 industries at varying levels of NAICS detail (2–6 digits, depending on industry). The 247 industries are not exclusive because both higher level and lower level of their NACIS are included for some industries. Eventually, a total of exclusive 201 NACISs are used: 2 in 2 digits, 70 in 3 digits,

107 in 4 digits, 20 in 5 digits and 2 in 6 digits. Hence, to impute a net stock estimate, we had to impute some firm's capital stock using the average value in a higher-level aggregate of the firm's industry.

[12]Note the output elasticity of labour is 0.95.

[13]Results are not presented but will be available upon request.

Funding
This study was supported by a Canadian Institutes of Health Research (CIHR) operating grant (#231571). Wei Zhang was funded by the CIHR Doctoral Research Award in the Area of Public Health Research and is supported by the Michael Smith Foundation for Health Research Postdoctoral Fellowship Award.

Authors' contributions
WZ designed the study, applied for the access to the data, performed the statistical analysis, interpreted the analysis results, and wrote the manuscript. HS participated in the development of the econometric models, the interpretation of the analysis results, and the finalization of the manuscript. SW and AHA participated in the design of the study and the interpretation of the data, and wrote the final manuscript. All authors read and approved the final manuscript.

Competing interests
The authors declare that they have no competing interests.

Ethics approval and consent to participate
This is a secondary use of the survey data held by Statistics Canada and is exempted from an ethical review. 1) The survey data have been collected through the provisions of the Statistics Act, respondents are informed that the survey is voluntary and that all information collected remains confidential and is solely used for statistical research purposes. 2) The individual data records are anonymous. 3) Access to the survey data is provided through legislation and regulation. Statistics Canada has a comprehensive regime of policies and procedures to protect the confidentiality of respondents, and to prosecute violations of legislation and disciplinary procedures for violations of regulations to protect respondent confidentiality (Statistics Canada, 2015. Mitigation of risk to respondents of Statistics Canada's surveys. URL http://www.statcan.gc.ca/eng/rdc/mitigation).

Author details
[1]Centre for Health Evaluation and Outcome Sciences, St. Paul's Hospital, 588-1081 Burrard Street, Vancouver, BC V6Z1Y6, Canada. [2]School of Population and Public Health, University of British Columbia, 2206 East Mall, Vancouver, BC V6T1Z3, Canada. [3]Department of Economics, Simon Fraser University, 8888 University Drive, Burnaby, BC V5A 1S6, Canada.

References
1. Drummond MF. Methods for the economic evaluation of health care programmes. 3rd ed. Oxford: Oxford University Press; 2005.
2. Gold MR, Siegel JE, Russell LB, Weinstein MC, editors. Cost-Effectiveness in Health and Medicine. 1st ed. New York: Oxford University Press; 1996.
3. Krol M, Papenburg J, Koopmanschap M, Brouwer W. Do productivity costs matter?: the impact of including productivity costs on the incremental costs of interventions targeted at depressive disorders. Pharmacoeconomics. 2011;29:601–19.
4. Krol M, Papenburg J, Tan SS, Brouwer W, Hakkaart L. A noticeable difference? Productivity costs related to paid and unpaid work in economic evaluations on expensive drugs. Eur J Health Econ. 2016;17:391–402.
5. Johannesson M, Jönsson B, Jönsson L, Kobelt G, Zethraeus N. Why should economic evaluations of medical innovations have a societal perspective? London: Office of Health Economics; 2009. Report No.: No. 51.
6. Jönsson B. Ten arguments for a societal perspective in the economic evaluation of medical innovations. Eur J Health Econ. 2009;10:357–9.
7. Berger ML, Murray JF, Xu J, Pauly M. Alternative valuations of work loss and productivity. J Occup Environ Med. 2001;43:18–24.
8. Johannesson M. The willingness to pay for health changes, the human-capital approach and the external costs. Health Policy. 1996;36:231–44.
9. Pauly MV, Nicholson S, Xu J, Polsky D, Danzon PM, Murray JF, et al. A general model of the impact of absenteeism on employers and employees. Health Econ. 2002;11:221–31.
10. Zhang W, Bansback N, Anis AH. Measuring and valuing productivity loss due to poor health: A critical review. Soc Sci Med. 2011;72:185–92.
11. Pauly MV, Nicholson S, Polsky D, Berger ML, Sharda C. Valuing reductions in on-the-job illness: "presenteeism" from managerial and economic perspectives. Health Econ. 2008;17:469–85.
12. Brown C, Medoff J. The Employer Size-Wage Effect. J Polit Econ. 1989;97:1027–59.
13. Fox JT. Firm-Size Wage Gaps, Job Responsibility, and Hierarchical Matching. J Labor Econ. 2009;27:83–126.
14. Goux D, Maurin E. Persistence of Interindustry Wage Differentials: A Reexamination Using Matched Worker-Firm Panel Data. J Labor Econ. 1999;17:492–533.
15. Groshen EL. Sources of Intra-Industry Wage Dispersion: How Much Do Employers Matter? Q J Econ. 1991;106:869–84.
16. Krueger AB, Summers LH. Efficiency Wages and the Inter-Industry Wage Structure. Econometrica. 1988;56:259–93.
17. Coles M, Lanfranchi J, Skalli A, Treble J. Pay, Technology, and the Cost of Worker Absence. Econ Inq. 2007;45:268–85.
18. Hamilton BH, Nickerson JA, Owan H. Team Incentives and Worker Heterogeneity: An Empirical Analysis of the Impact of Teams on Productivity and Participation. J Polit Econ. 2003;111:465–97.
19. Card D, Lemieux T, Riddell WC. Unions and wage inequality. J Labor Res. 2004;25:519–59.
20. Freeman RB, Medoff JL, Feeman RB. What Do Unions Do? New York: HarperCollins Canada / Basic Books; 1984.
21. Hoynes H. The Employment, Earnings, and Income of Less Skilled Workers Over the Business Cycle [Internet]. National Bureau of Economic Research; 1999 Jun. Report No.: 7188. Available from: http://www.nber.org/papers/w7188
22. Dustmann C, Glitz A, Vogel T. Employment, wages, and the economic cycle: Differences between immigrants and natives. Eur Econ Rev. 2010;54:1–17.
23. Borjas GJ, Ramey VA. Foreign Competition, Market Power, and Wage Inequality. Q J Econ. 1995;110:1075–110.
24. Guadalupe M. Product Market Competition, Returns to Skill, and Wage Inequality. J Labor Econ. 2007;25:439–74.
25. Fortin NM, Lemieux T. Institutional Changes and Rising Wage Inequality: Is there a Linkage? J Econ Perspect. 1997;11:75–96.
26. Koeniger W, Leonardi M, Nunziata L. Labor Market Institutions and Wage Inequality. Ind Labor Relat Rev. 2007;60:340–56.
27. Hellerstein JK, Neumark D, Troske KR. Wages, Productivity, and Worker Characteristics: Evidence from Plant-Level Production Functions and Wage Equations. J Labor Econ. 1999;17:409–46.
28. Hellerstein JK, Neumark D. Sex, Wages, and Productivity: An Empirical Analysis of Israeli Firm-Level Data. Int Econ Rev. 1999;40:95–123.
29. Hægeland T, Klette TJ. Do higher wages reflect higher productivity? Education, gender and experience premiums in a matched plant-worker data set. In: Haltiwanger JC, Lane JI, Spletzer JR, Theeuwes JJM, Troske KR, editors. The creation and analysis of employer-employee matched data. New York: Elsevier; 1999. p. 231–59.
30. van Ours JC, Stoeldraijer L. Age, wage and productivity [Internet]. IZA; 2010. Report No.: 4765. Available from: http://econpapers.repec.org/paper/izaizadps/dp4765.htm.
31. Brown S, Sessions JG. The Economics of Absence: Theory and Evidence. J Econ Surv. 1996;10:23–53.
32. Dionne G, Dostie B. New Evidence on the Determinants of Absenteeism Using Linked Employer-Employee Data. Ind Labor Relat Rev. 2007;61:108–20.

33. Heywood JS, Jirjahn U. Teams, Teamwork and Absence. Scand J Econ. 2004; 106:765–82.
34. Markussen S, Røed K, Røgeberg OJ, Gaure S. The anatomy of absenteeism. J Health Econ. 2011;30:277–92.
35. Ose SO. Working conditions, compensation and absenteeism. J Health Econ. 2005;24:161–88.
36. Darr W, Johns G. Work strain, health, and absenteeism: a meta-analysis. J Occup Health Psychol. 2008;13:293–318.
37. Dewa CS, Loong D, Bonato S, Hees H. Incidence rates of sickness absence related to mental disorders: a systematic literature review. BMC Public Health. 2014;14:205.
38. Keech M, Beardsworth P. The impact of influenza on working days lost: a review of the literature. Pharmacoeconomics. 2008;26:911–24.
39. Neovius K, Johansson K, Kark M, Neovius M. Obesity status and sick leave: a systematic review. Obes Rev. 2009;10:17–27.
40. Allen SG. How Much Does Absenteeism Cost? J Hum Resour. 1983;18: 379–93.
41. Mefford RN. The Effect of Unions on Productivity in a Multinational Manufacturing Firm. Ind Labor Relat Rev. 1986;40:105–14.
42. Cobb CW, Douglas PH. A theory of production. Am Econ Rev. 1928;18: 139–65.
43. Zhang W, Sun H, Woodcock S, Anis A. Illness related wage and productivity losses: Valuing "presenteeism.". Soc Sci Med. 2015;147:62–71.
44. Statistics Canada. Guide to the Analysis of the Workplace and Employee Survey [Internet], Report No.: Catalogue no. 71–221-GIE. Ottawa: Statistics Canada; 2004. Available from: http://www.statcan.gc.ca/pub/71-221-g/71-221-g2007001-eng.pdf.
45. Griliches Z, Mairesse J. Production Functions: The Search for Identification [Internet]. National Bureau of Economic Research; 1995. Report No.: 5067. Available from: http://www.nber.org/papers/w5067
46. Levinsohn J, Petrin A. Estimating Production Functions Using Inputs to Control for Unobservables. Rev Econ Stud. 2003;70:317–41.
47. Petrin A, Poi BP, Levinsohn J. Production Function Estimation in STATA using Inputs to Control for Unobservables. Stata J. 2004;4:113–23.
48. Statistics Canada. Workplace and Employee Survey (WES) [Internet]. [cited 2014 Feb 25]. Available from: http://www23.statcan.gc.ca/imdb/p2SV.pl?Function=getSurvey&SDDS=2615
49. Dostie B. Wage, productivity and aging [Internet]. IZA; 2006. Report No.: 2496. Availabe from: http://econpapers.repec.org/paper/izaizadps/dp2496.htm.
50. Turcotte J, Rennison LW. The Link between Technology Use, Human Capital, Productivity and Wages: Firm-level Evidence. Int Productivity Monit. 2004;9: 25–36.
51. Turcotte J, Rennison LW. Productivity and wages: Measuring the effect of human capital and technology use from linked employer- employee data [Internet]. Department of Finance; 2004 [cited 2013 May 25]. Available from: http://www.fin.gc.ca/pub/pdfs/wp2004-01e.pdf
52. Aubert P, Crépon B. La productivité des salariés âgés: une tentative d'estimation. Économie et Statistique. 2003;368:95–119.
53. Crépon B, Deniau N, Pérez-Duarte S. Wages, Productivity and Worker Characteristics: A French Perspective [Internet]. Centre de Recherche en Economie et Statistique; 2003. Report No.: 2003–04. Available from: https://ideas.repec.org/p/crs/wpaper/2003-04.html
54. Greenland S, Morgenstern H. Ecological Bias, Confounding, and Effect Modification. Int J Epidemiol. 1989;18:269–74.
55. Zhang W, Bansback N, Boonen A, Severens JL, Anis AH. Development of a composite questionnaire, the valuation of lost productivity, to value productivity losses: application in rheumatoid arthritis. Value Health. 2012;15: 46–54.
56. Pendakur K, Woodcock S. Glass ceilings or glass doors? Wage disparity within and between Firms. J Bus Econ Stat. 2010;28:181–9.

7

The relationship between target joints and direct resource use in severe haemophilia

Jamie O'Hara[1], Shaun Walsh[2], Charlotte Camp[2]* ⓘ, Giuseppe Mazza[3], Liz Carroll[4], Christina Hoxer[5] and Lars Wilkinson[5]

Abstract

Objectives: Target joints are a common complication of severe haemophilia. While factor replacement therapy constitutes the majority of costs in haemophilia, the relationship between target joints and non drug-related direct costs (NDDCs) has not been studied.

Methods: Data on haemophilia patients without inhibitors was drawn from the 'Cost of Haemophilia across Europe – a Socioeconomic Survey' (CHESS) study, a cost assessment in severe haemophilia A and B across five European countries (France, Germany, Italy, Spain, and the United Kingdom) in which 139 haemophilia specialists provided demographic and clinical information for 1285 adult patients. NDDCs were calculated using publicly available cost data, including 12-month ambulatory and secondary care activity: haematologist and other specialist consultant consultations, medical tests and examinations, bleed-related hospital admissions, and payments to professional care providers. A generalized linear model was developed to investigate the relationship between NDDCs and target joints (areas of chronic synovitis), adjusted for patient covariates.

Results: Five hundred and thirteen patients (42% of the sample) had no diagnosed target joints; a total of 1376 target joints (range 1–10) were recorded in the remaining 714 patients. Mean adjusted NDDCs for persons with no target joints were EUR 3134 (standard error (SE) EUR 158); for persons with one or more target joints, mean adjusted NDDCs were EUR 3913 (SE EUR 157; average mean effect EUR 779; $p < 0.001$).

Conclusions: Our analysis suggests that the presence of one or more target joints has a significant impact on NDDCs for patients with severe haemophilia, ceteris paribus. Prevention and management of target joints should be an important consideration of managing haemophilia patients.

Keywords: Haemophilia, Cost of illness, Target joints, Burden of disease, Arthropathy, Synovitis

Background

Haemophilia is an inherited, lifelong bleeding disorder characterised by prolonged traumatic or spontaneous bleeding due to a lack of clotting factor in the body. Haemophilia is a recessive X-linked disorder and primarily affects males; symptoms are present from infancy [1]. The two most common forms of the condition are Haemophilia A (Factor VIII deficiency) and Haemophilia B (Factor IX deficiency). Global incidence of haemophilia A is approximately 1 in every 5000 male births; haemophilia B is approximately six times rarer than haemophilia A [2].

Bleed events may be musculoskeletal or mucosal in nature but are most commonly observed in the joints of the body. In the absence of preventative 'prophylaxis' factor replacement therapy, most persons with severe haemophilia (<1% of normal factor level) will develop a first haemarthrosis between the ages of 1 and 5 years. Approximately four-fifths of bleed events occur in the knees, elbows, and ankles; arthroses in the hip, shoulder, carpus, or small hand or foot joints are less frequently observed [3].

Repeat intra-articular bleed events within a short timeframe (3–6 months) are associated with chronic synovial inflammation and in the longer term induce haemophilic arthropathy [4]. Such joints, known as target joints, exhibit continuous swelling and reduced range of motion;

* Correspondence: charlotte.camp@hcdeconomics.com
[2]HCD Economics, The Innovation Centre, Daresbury WA4 4FS, UK
Full list of author information is available at the end of the article

repeat acute and subacute haemarthoses lead to irreversible degradation of the joint, resulting in chronic pain and poor physical function and requiring orthopaedic intervention, ranging from removal of the synovium to replacement or fusion of the joint [5]. Bleed frequency, as well as age, body mass index, and inhibitor formation are known drivers of joint disease and functional limitation in persons with severe haemophilia [6–8]. The economic burden of frequent hospitalisations and palliative joint surgeries is reinforced by the psychosocial impact of chronic pain and disability, including limited employment opportunities, decreased social participation, and poor mental health [9, 10].

Prophylaxis regimens initiated at a young age (≤4 years of age) are shown to reduce bleed frequency and joint deterioration later into adulthood [5], and are therefore considered the benchmark in care for severe haemophilia [2]. However, introduction of universal prophylaxis has been protracted in many developed countries, due to a lack of evidence regarding clinical benefits of prophylaxis initiation later into adolescence and adulthood, as well as the substantial per-capita costs associated with replacement therapy [11–13]. Prophylaxis replacement therapy has recently undergone tentative economic evaluation by several European organisations. There is a need for greater clarity regarding the economic impact of care for persons with severe haemophilia in Europe, specifically regarding the cost of management of individuals with musculoskeletal complications, and in particular those patients receiving suboptimal therapy protocols.

The objective of this paper is to explore the relationship between target joints and direct medical costs for persons with severe haemophilia, and the extent to which health resource utilisation and direct medical costs (excluding replacement therapy) in severe haemophilia are driven by long-term clinical complications of the disease. While this topic has been explored to some detail within single-country studies [12, 14], this is the first to take a universal methodology across several European countries in assessing resource use and cost burden among persons with severe haemophilia.

Methods

Data source

Resource and cost data were gathered as part of the "Cost of Haemophilia across Europe – a Socioeconomic Survey (CHESS)", a prospective observational study in severe haemophilia A and B across five European countries (France, Germany, Italy, Spain, and the United Kingdom) undertaken in 2015 [15]. One hundred and thirty-nine haemophilia specialists provided demographic and clinical information for 1285 adults (≥18 years) via a web-based survey. A corresponding questionnaire covering indirect costs and health-related quality of life (HRQOL) measures was completed by patients.

Non drug-related direct costs (NDDCs) were an amalgam of 12-month ambulatory and secondary care costs gathered within the CHESS study, specifically incorporating: haematologist and other specialist consultant consultations, medical tests and examinations, surgeries relating to joint damage, bleed-related hospital admissions, and payments to professional care providers [15]. A unit cost database was developed for each country using publicly available information. A breakdown of individual cost elements of NDDCs is presented in Table 1.

Study exclusion criteria was limited to patients diagnosed with an inhibitor at the time of study capture ($n = 52$), due to a differing risk profile for bleeds and subsequent target joint development among these patients, and a higher utilisation of medical resources [16, 17].

Target joints

A 'target joint' as defined in the CHESS study encompasses any joint with known chronic synovitis; in contrast to previous clinical studies [18], study investigators were given discretion as to how this may be further defined with respect to bleed frequency and period of observation. In order to explore the differential impact of costs associated with lower and upper body joint deterioration, target joints were categorised into two groups based on their location. 'Upper body' target joints were those in the shoulders, elbows, wrists, neck, and spine; 'lower body' target joints consisted of hips, knees, and ankles. The target joint variable was assessed in three ways: as a binary 0/1 variable; as a binary 0/1 variable split into upper and lower body joints; and as a discrete variable.

Statistical analysis

Demographic and resource use data were compared between the sample of patients with no reported target joints and those with one or more reported target joints. Means were used to describe continuous variables; categorical variables are described as frequencies and proportions. Standard t-tests were conducted in order to test for between-group differences.

The marginal effect of the presence of one or more target joints on NDDCs was assessed using a generalized linear model (GLM). Medical cost data is often positively skewed with a large volume of zero values (i.e. no medical costs) and a long 'tail' from a select group of costly 'outlier' patients. The GLM is an extension of the linear regression framework (Eq. 1) suitable for nonparametric dependent variables [19, 20]. The GLM requires a link function relating the conditional mean to the covariates, and a distribution 'family' to specify the relationship between the variance and the mean [21]. The log-link function (Eq. 2) in combination with a gamma distribution

Table 1 National costs for CHESS resource units

Resource item	Baseline unit price (EUR)				
	France[a]	Germany[b]	Italy[c]	Spain[d]	UK[e]
Ambulatory care					
Haematologist visit (per visit)	25.99–45.99	20.88	27.32–23.17	65.69–113.54	124.71–228.57
Nurse visit (per visit)	81.74	34.28–38.42	15.11	20.92–37.46	19.36
Other specialist visit (per visit)	14.99–45.99	7.30–228.88	18.21–27.32	16.42–160	65.91–612.03
Blood test (per test)	1.89–53.96	0.50–112.50	2.11–17.22	4.78–98.37	4.29–7.67
Other test/examination (per test)	10.79–69.00	5.50–124.60	2.19–134.27	7.49–249.21	1.69–228.24
Hospitalisation					
Target joint surgery† (per surgery)	28.81–534.40	12.02–1719.43	33.48–1032.91	169.75–2156.33	1161.93–8397.52
Bleed event: ward stay (per day)	290.85	514.29	265	708.71	562.88
Bleed event: ICU stay (per day)	1174.60	1265	366	1559.24	1056.82
Professional caregiver (per hour)	8.30	27.43	7.39	13.66	24.56

Note. Ranges presented where more than one price is possible; ICU: intensive care unit; IU: International Units
†Arthrocentesis, arthrodesis, arthroplasty, arthroscopy, synovectomy
[a]Sources: Ameli, sante.gouv, ViDAL.fr, Catalogue Commun des actes médicaux
[b]Sources: Kbv.de, meinpharmaversand.de, Einheitlicher Bewertungsmaßstab, rote-liste service
[c]Sources: AIFA, agenziafarmaco.gov
[d]Sources: Oblikue e-salud, Agencia Española de Medicamentos y Productos Sanitarios
[e]Sources: National Schedule of Reference Costs, Electronic Medicines Compendium

(Eq. 3) is frequently used to estimate medical costs and was employed for this analysis [21]. A confirmatory analysis of the family and link functions was conducted using the modified Park test [20, 21].

$$NDDCs_{12mth} = \alpha + \beta_1(t\ argetjo\ ints) + \beta_2 x_1 + \cdots + \beta_n x_n \quad (1)$$

$Where\ i = 1, ..., n$

$$E[y|x] = f\left(x'\beta\right) = \exp\left(x'\beta\right) In(E[y|x]) = x'\beta \quad (2)$$

$$y \sim Var(y|x) \approx (E[y|x])^\lambda \quad (3)$$

A univariate estimate of the relationship between target joint status and NDDCs was first modelled (Model 1), followed by a multivariate estimate using country of residence, patient age, use of prophylaxis therapy regimen at the time of study capture, and number of haemophilia-related hospital admissions in the preceding 12 months as additional model covariates, added using a stepwise inclusion method (Model 2). Results are presented as average mean effects (AME). All statistical analysis was conducted using Stata 13 [22].

Results

Patient characteristics

The average age of study patients was 36 years old; the majority of patients in the study were receiving treatment prophylactically ($n = 708$; 57.7%) (Table 2). A total of 1376 target joints were recorded across the study population (mean 1.2 target joints; SD 1.37; range 0–10). Seven hundred and fourteen patients (58.2%) were reported diagnosed with one or more target joints. Target joints exclusively in the lower body were most commonly reported ($n = 371$ patients (52.3%)). More than four in ten patients with a reported target joint had undergone one or more surgeries on a target joint in the preceding 12 months, with joint aspiration (arthrocentesis) the most common procedure (200 patients, 28% of the target joint cohort).

Medical resource use

In all cases examined, patients with no target joints consumed less medical resources compared to patients with one or more target joints (Table 3). The largest between-group differences were reported for scheduled nurse consultations with 5.75 (SD 11.98) and 3.94 (SD 9.13) for the "has target joint" and "no target joint" groups respectively ($p < 0.001$). Physiotherapy visits were found to be lower in the no target joint group 0.89 (SD = 3.75) compared with patients with one or more target joints 3.14 (SD = 7.99) ($p < 0.001$). Patients with target joints attended a greater number of scheduled haemophilia consultations: 5.5 (SD = 4.36) and 4.7 (SD = 3.72) respectively ($p = 0.001$). The target joint group recorded 1.91 GP visits (SD = 3.78), with non-target joint patients reporting 1.35 visits (SD = 2.67; $p = 0.003$). Mean number of target joint surgeries in the affected group was 0.70. Rates of bleed-related hospital admissions were almost three times higher in the target joint cohort (mean 0.97 versus 0.36).

NDDCs

Mean NDDCs were EUR 3641 (SD 6157); per-patient NDDCs in the presence of one or more target joints –

Table 2 Patient characteristics ($N = 1227$)

Age (mean ± SD)	35.7 ± 14.6
Subtype (%)	
Haemophilia A	949 (77.3%)
Haemophilia B	278 (22.7%)
Country (%)	
UK	306 (24.9%)
Italy	271 (22.1%)
France	254 (20.7%)
Spain	206 (16.8%)
Germany	190 (15.5%)
Treatment strategy (%)	
On-demand	519 (42.3%)
Prophylaxis	708 (57.7%)
Target joints (mean ± SD)	1.1 ± 1.4
Number of target joints (patient n, %)	
Zero	518 (41.2%)
One	334 (46.4%)
Two	241 (34.0%)
Three or more	139 (19.6%)
Location of target joints (patient n, % of target joint cohort)	
Exclusively lower body	371 (52.3%)
Exclusively upper body	186 (26.2%)
Upper and lower body	152 (21.4%)
Surgeries to target joints in the previous 12 months (patient n, % of target joint cohort)	305 (42.7%)
Joint aspiration	200 (28.0%)
Endoscopic examination of joint	116 (16.2%)
Joint fusion	84 (11.8%)
Joint replacement	64 (9.0%)
Destruction/surgical removal of synovium	56 (7.8%)

Note. Values are means ± SD or numbers (%)

Table 3 12-month resource utilisation ($N = 1227$)

	No target joint ($n = 508$)	1+ target joints ($n = 714$)	P-Value
Outpatient haematologist consultations			
Scheduled	4.71	5.48	0.001
Unscheduled	1.15	1.84	0.001
Outpatient specialist nurse consultations			
Scheduled	3.95	5.75	0.003
Unscheduled	1.13	1.93	<0.001
Outpatient consultations – other specialties			
General practice	1.35	1.91	<0.001
General surgery	0.08	0.21	<0.001
Pain management	0.11	0.68	<0.001
Physiotherapy	0.89	3.14	<0.001
Tests and examinations			
Urinalysis	1.07	1.85	<0.001
X-ray	0.61	1.24	<0.001
Computed tomography	0.25	0.48	<0.001
Magnetic resonance imaging	0.25	0.52	<0.001
Radiography	0.36	1.05	<0.001
Ultrasonography	0.41	1.00	<0.001
Coagulation tests	1.82	3.11	<0.001
Target joint surgeries	n/a	0.70	n/a
Bleed event-related hospital admissions	0.36	0.97	<0.001

Multivariate analysis

The results of the multivariate analysis are presented in Table 4. A significant difference in costs was observed between the target joint and non-target joint cohorts: mean adjusted NDDCs for the non-target joint cohort were EUR 3134 (SE 158); for the target joint cohort, mean adjusted NDDCs were EUR 3913 (SE 157; AME EUR 779; $p < 0.001$). The mean average marginal effect (AME) of one or more upper body target joints was EUR 2646 (standard error (SE) 454); AME was EUR 2626 (SE 367) for individuals with one or more lower body target

regardless of number or location – was EUR 5046 (SD 7479) versus EUR 1684 for patients with no target joints. The number of target joints are positively correlated with NDDCs: individuals with one target joint reported mean NDDCs of EUR 3468 (SD 5595; $n = 332$) (Fig. 1); this increased to EUR 5585 (SD 7980; $n = 242$) for patients with two target joints; for those with three target joints mean NDDCs were EUR 7470 (SD 9396; $n = 70$).

Patients with at least one target joint in the upper body recorded mean NDDCs of EUR 5610 (SD 7861) (Fig. 2); patients with at least one lower body target joint reported mean NDDCs of EUR 5186 (SD 7594). The highest NDDCs were recorded among patients with both lower and upper body target joints (mean EUR 6696; SD 8461).

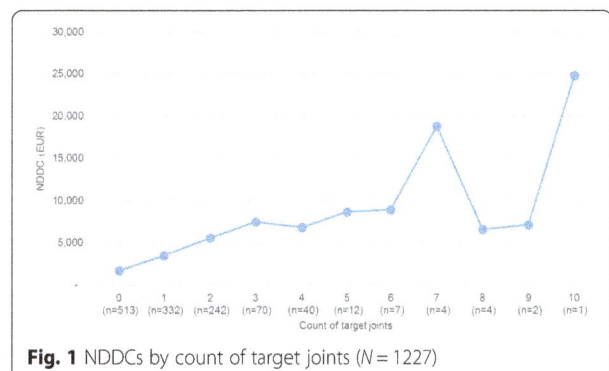

Fig. 1 NDDCs by count of target joints ($N = 1227$)

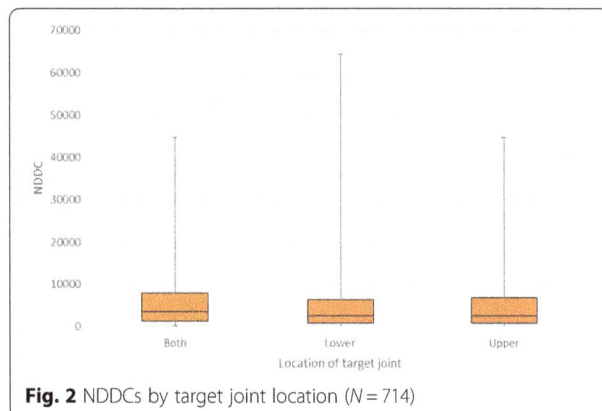

Fig. 2 NDDCs by target joint location (N = 714)

joints. When the analysis examined the impact of the location of the target joint, the AME for a lower body target joint was greater, at EUR 655 (SE 143). The AME for a patient with an upper body target joint was EUR 624 (SE 191).

Patient age was a negligible – albeit significant – driver of NDDCs: an additional year of life contributed just EUR 13.52 extra in costs (SD 3.48; $p < 0.001$). Somewhat unsurprisingly, an additional haemophilia-related hospitalisation was the most substantial contributor to NDDCs (AME 2681.52; SD 220.15; $p < 0.001$).

Discussion

This study has sought to quantify the economic burden associated with management and alleviation of joint-related complications in severe haemophilia. NDDCs represent a small proportion of total costs for persons with severe haemophilia (between 2% and 5% in most European studies) [14], and as a result their prioritisation for

Table 4 Multivariate Gamma regression analyses of NDDCs (N = 1227)

	Model 1	Model 2
Upper body target joint	2645.63 (454.07)	623.51 (191.13)**
Lower body target joint	2626.32 (367.36)	665.00 (143.57)**
Country[a]		
Germany		−711.36 (131.30)**
Italy		−562.68 (134.09)**
Spain		569.75 (254.91)*
UK		439.2861 (212.43)*
Age		13.52 (3.48)**
Haemophilia hospitalisation		2681.52 (220.15)**
On-demand treatment strategy		140.21 (59.65)*
	AIC = 18.13	AIC = 17.59
	BIC = −6939.61	BIC = −7600.63

Note. Values are average marginal effects (AMEs). Standard error shown in brackets. *Denotes 95% significance. **Denotes 99% significance
[a]Base factor: France

research has until now been limited. Nevertheless, it is critical to understand both physiological, psychosocial, and economic impacts of inadequate bleed control within haemophilia, and the longer-term repercussions of joint deterioration associated with suboptimal therapy and patient management. The results of this analysis suggest that cost drivers are not limited to surgical interventions, but in fact encompass more intensive ambulatory and outpatient care, including a higher volume of specialist visits, tests, and examinations among persons with severe haemophilia exhibiting chronic joint inflammation.

The CHESS study was a cross-sectional survey of clinicians and persons with severe haemophilia across five European countries, which captured a large volume of clinical and demographic information about consulting patients. However, we are limited in our ability to explore the causal relationship between management of haemophilia in early life and subsequent outcomes. Further work is required to understand the long-term impact of switching from on-demand to prophylaxis in late childhood and adulthood, when joint deterioration may already be present. Presence of target joints in the CHESS patient group is significantly higher among those receiving prophylaxis; whilst initially counterintuitive, it points to a large number of patients moving away from on-demand regimens due to poor bleed control and joint damage. As shown in previous work, this is particularly pertinent for those patients over the age of 30 years for whom prophylaxis in early childhood was not widely available. While the outcomes observed in this study population are not necessarily translatable to children born with haemophilia in the current era, suggestions of reducing access to prophylaxis give rise to a need to highlight the economic burden arising from conservative therapy among persons with severe haemophilia.

A target joint in this analysis is defined by the presence of chronic synovitis, the physiological manifestation of frequent intra-articular bleed events. In the more oft-observed scenario, sufficient time between bleed events (~3–4 weeks) allows for gradual alleviation of swelling and restoration of joint motion, via intensive infusions of replacement therapy and regular physiotherapy. Frequent recurrence of bleeding, however, precludes the reinstatement of a baseline level of motion, strength, and physical appearance; inadequate resolution of trauma arising from such events can in turn exacerbate bleed frequency. This cyclical process results in the longer term in a state of chronic synovitis and progressive arthropathy, due to excessive volumes of synovium and blood retained within the joint space and gradual deterioration of the joint tissue [4].

Other definitions in literature focus instead on the frequency of bleed events over a short-term (≤6 months) period in order to propose a diagnosis of a target joint.

The most recent International Society of Thrombosis and Hemostasis (ISTH) definition, for example, is one in which three or more spontaneous bleeds into a single joint occur within a consecutive 6-month period [23]. In the case of the ISTH guidelines, however, the joint ceases to be a target joint when there have been less than two bleeds into the joint within 12 consecutive months. While alternative definitions allow for more or less frequent bleeds and shorter or longer observation periods [24, 25], their commonality is the use of short-term bleed rates as a measure, and an observable follow-up period within which a target joint may no longer be defined as such.

In combination, these rules present a definition that is well-suited to clinical trials with finite follow-up periods and observable improvements in outcomes, but which lacks the consideration of the long-term complications associated with persistent bleed events. A recent paper published on behalf of the United Kingdom Haemophilia Centres Doctors Organisation (UKHCDO) highlights the long term changes effected to the soft tissue of the joint as a result of frequent bleed events, and thus a need for continuous, targeted monitoring of the afflicted joint beyond the period in which synovitis is observed [26]. Our choice of definition, therefore, encompasses an assumption of high bleed frequency via the identification of synovitis, as well as considering the long-term, irreversible changes to the joint tissue and structure that arise from repeat haemorrhage. We acknowledge, however, that there is substantial overlap between definitions.

Regardless of nuances in the definition of a target joint, the results presented in this study suggest that chronic synovitis in severe haemophilia is associated with greater intensity of patient management, resulting in higher levels of health resource use and direct medical costs. Approaches to minimising the long-term risk of joint damage and deterioration among these patients – beginning at a young age with proactive therapy protocols to minimise bleed frequency and severity – will serve to reduce future burdens on hospital systems and are a justification for continued access to preventative therapy protocols. Further studies should seek to incorporate the health-related quality of life impact of bleed events and joint disease, and hence to quantify the cost effectiveness of current therapy protocols among severe persons with haemophilia.

Conclusion

While non drug-related direct medical costs in severe haemophilia are small in relation to the costs of replacement therapy, our analysis demonstrates that the majority of individuals with this disease experience medical complications requiring substantial follow-up in the hospital setting. Further, the presence of one or more target joint can have a major impact on medical resource utilisation and subsequent costs for patients with severe haemophilia.

Abbreviations
AME: average mean effect; CHESS: 'The Cost of Haemophilia – a Socioeconomic Survey'; EUR: Euro; GLM: generalized linear model; HRQOL: health-related quality of life; ICU: intensive care unit; ISTH: International Society on Thrombosis and Haemostasis; IU: international units; PWH: people with haemophilia; SD: standard deviation; SE: standard error

Acknowledgements
Kind thanks to Ian Jacob (HCD Economics) for reviewing the manuscript drafts.

Funding
This study was funded by Novo Nordisk. Publication was not contingent upon study results.

Authors' contributions
JOH designed the study protocol. CC and SW analysed the data. JOH, SW, and CC wrote the manuscript. LC and GM provided non-clinical perspective for the analysis and manuscript. All authors reviewed the manuscript. All authors read and approved the final manuscript.

Competing interests
LW and CH are employees of Novo Nordisk.

Author details
[1]Faculty of Health and Social Care, University of Chester, Chester, UK. [2]HCD Economics, The Innovation Centre, Daresbury WA4 4FS, UK. [3]UCL Institute for Liver and Digestive Health, Royal Free Hospital, University College London, London, UK. [4]The Haemophilia Society, London, UK. [5]Novo Nordisk A/S, Vandtårnsvej 114, -2860 Søborg, DK, Denmark.

References
1. Liras A, Segovia C, Gabán AS. Advanced therapies for the treatment of hemophilia: future perspectives. Orphanet J. Rare Dis. 2012;7:97.
2. Srivastava A, Brewer AK, Mauser-Bunschoten EP, Key NS, Kitchen S, Llinas A, et al. WFH guidelines: guidelines for the management of hemophilia. Haemophilia. 2013;19:1–47.
3. Lobet S, Hermans C, Lambert C. Optimal management of hemophilic arthropathy and hematomas. J Blood Med Dove Press. 2014;5:207–18.
4. Mulder K, Llinás A. The target joint. Haemophilia. 2004;10(Suppl 4):152–6.
5. Manco-Johnson MJ, Soucie JM, Gill JC. Prophylaxis usage, bleeding rates and joint outcomes of hemophilia 1999 - 2010: a surveillance project. Blood. 2017;129:2368–75.
6. Monahan PE, Baker JR, Riske B, Soucie JM. Physical functioning in boys with hemophilia in the U.S. Am J Prev Med. 2011;41:S360–8.
7. Bladen M, Main E, Hubert N, Koutoumanou E, Liesner R, Khair K. Factors affecting the Haemophilia joint health score in children with severe haemophilia. Haemophilia. 2013;19:626–31.
8. Soucie JM, Wang C, Siddiqi A, Kulkarni R, Recht M, Konkle BA, et al. The longitudinal effect of body adiposity on joint mobility in young males with Haemophilia a. Haemophilia. 2011;17:196–203.
9. Iannone M, Pennick L, Tom A, Cui H, Gilbert M, Weihs K, et al. Prevalence of depression in adults with haemophilia. Haemophilia. 2012;18:868–74.
10. Cassis FRMY, Querol F, Forsyth A, Iorio A, HERO International Advisory Board. Psychosocial aspects of haemophilia: a systematic review of methodologies and findings. Haemophilia. 2012;18:e101–14.
11. World Federation of Hemophilia. Frequently asked questions about hemophilia [Internet]. 2012 [cited 2015 Jul 31]. Available from: http://www.wfh.org/en/page.aspx?pid=637#Life_expectancy.

12. Johnson KA, Zhou Z-Y. Costs of care in hemophilia and possible implications of health care reform. Hematology am. Soc. Hematol. Educ. Program. 2011;2011:413–8.

13. Henrard S, Hermans C, Devleesschauwer B, Speybroeck N. Oral presentations: abstracts. Eur J Public Health O. 2012;22:10–125.

14. Kodra Y, Cavazza M, Schieppati A, De Santis M, Armeni P, Arcieri R, et al. The social burden and quality of life of patients with haemophilia in Italy. Blood Transfus. SIMTI Servizi; 2014;12 Suppl 3:s567–s575.

15. O'Hara J, Hughes D, Camp C, Burke T, Carroll L. Diego D-AG. The cost of severe haemophilia in Europe: the CHESS study. Orphanet J Rare Dis. 2017;12(1):106.

16. Bohn RLRL, Aledort LM, Putnam K, Ewenstein B, Mogun H, Avorn JJ. The economic impact of factor VIII inhibitors in patients with haemophilia. Haemophilia. 2004;10:63–8.

17. Knight C. Health economics of treating haemophilia a with inhibitors. Haemophilia. 2005;11(Suppl 1):11–7.

18. Konkle BA, Ebbesen LS, Erhardtsen E, Bianco RP, Lissitchkov T, Rusen L, et al. Randomized, prospective clinical trial of recombinant factor VIIa for secondary prophylaxis in hemophilia patients with inhibitors. J Thromb Haemost Blackwell Publishing Ltd. 2007;5:1904–13.

19. Glick HA, Doshi JA, Sonnad SS, Polsky D. Economic Evaluation in Clinical Trials. Oxford University Press; 2014.

20. Mihaylova B, Briggs A, O'Hagan A, Thompson SG. Review of statistical methods for analysing healthcare resources and costs. Health Econ. 2011;20:897–916.

21. Coughlan D, Yeh ST, Neill CO, Frick KD. Evaluating direct medical expenditures estimation methods of adults using the medical expenditure panel survey : an example focusing on head and neck cancer. Value Heal Elsevier. 2014;17:90–7.

22. Stata Statistical Software. College Station: StataCorp; 2013.

23. Blanchette VS, Key NS, Ljung LR, Manco-Johnson MJ, van den Berg HM, Srivastava A, et al. Definitions in hemophilia: communication from the SSC of the ISTH. J Thromb Haemost. 2014;12:1935–9.

24. Price VE, Hawes SA, Chan AK. A practical approach to hemophilia care in children. Paediatr Child Heal. 2007;12:381–3.

25. Donadel-Claeyssens S. European Paediatric network for Haemophilia management. Current co-ordinated activities of the PEDNET (European Paediatric network for Haemophilia management). Haemophilia. 2006;12:124–7.

26. Hanley J, McKernan A, Creagh MD, Classey S, McLaughlin P, Goddard N, et al. Guidelines for the management of acute joint bleeds and chronic synovitis in haemophilia: a United Kingdom Haemophilia Centre doctors' organisation (UKHCDO) guideline. Haemophilia. 2017;23:511–20.

8

Assessing the effects of price regulation and freedom of choice on quality: evidence from the physiotherapy market

Piia Pekola[1][*] (iD), Ismo Linnosmaa[2] and Hennamari Mikkola[1]

Abstract

In health care, many aspects of the delivery of services are subject to regulation. Often the purpose of the regulated health care system is to encourage providers to keep costs down without skimping on quality. The purpose of this paper is to analyse the effect of price regulation and free choice on quality in physiotherapy organised by the Social Insurance Institution of Finland for the disabled individuals.

We use the difference-in-differences method in our effort to isolate the effect of the regulation and for this task we have defined the regulated and non-regulated firms and their quality before and after the regulation. The variables needed in the econometric modelling were collected from several registers as well as by carrying out questionnaires on the firms.

We show that price regulation decreased quality in physiotherapy statistically significantly and the mechanism was unable to incentivise firms to invest in quality. Most likely, our results are caused by cost reduction associated with price regulation. It seems that cost reduction was carried out through quality reductions in physiotherapy instead of increasing productivity. The result is sensible because comparable quality information is not published to support patient choice in this sector.

Keywords: Competitive bidding, Financial incentives, Physiotherapy, Quality, Regulation, Service voucher

JEL codes: I11, I18, L15, L51

Background

The main purpose of the regulated health care system is to encourage providers to keep costs down without skimping on quality. Also when government agencies or insurers are purchasing health services they usually try to keep costs down without decreasing quality [1]. Yet, due to changes in the financial incentives, firms may alter their behavior regarding quality. This means that firms may have an incentive to decrease quality in order to cut the costs instead of improving productivity [2]. For previous reasons, price regulation is recommended in the literature to be linked to elements affecting competition such as free choice. In this scenario, competition will outweigh a firm's possible incentive to seek cost reductions through quality [3].

Previously mentioned plans to regulate health care prices linked with free choice have already been piloted in Finland in rehabilitation and especially in physiotherapy services organised and financed by the Social Insurance Institution (Kela). Kela has a supplemental role in the Finnish health care sector and it is a largest single organiser of rehabilitation services in Finland. Generally, Kela uses public procurement mechanisms such as competitive bidding in its effort of organising rehabilitation services. However, during the contract period 2011-2014, fixed price service vouchers were piloted in two insurance districts in physiotherapy targeted at disabled individuals. Additionally, free choice was initiated during the same period throughout the country.

Due to price regulation and free choice (henceforth also reform), the system potentially had a huge impact on the financial incentives of firms. Firms which were located in the two insurance districts where service

* Correspondence: piia.pekola@kela.fi
[1]Social Insurance Institution of Finland, PL 450, 00056 Helsinki, Finland
Full list of author information is available at the end of the article

vouchers were piloted had regulated prices. Whilst firms located in all other districts were able to define prices in their tenders during competitive bidding. Thus the reform in physiotherapy had two opposite incentives for firms: price regulation may induce firms to cut costs by decreasing quality, but free choice may lead to increased quality due to competition.

The purpose of this paper is to analyse the effects of price regulation and free choice on quality in physiotherapy organised and financed by Kela for the disabled individuals in Finland. The study is novel - it provides evidence from rehabilitation and especially physiotherapy from which there are no previous studies. Thus, we aim to broaden the literature in this respect but it is also useful for the future purposes in Finland from which there are no previous studies whatsoever in this sector. As Finland is planning to reform its health and social care sector (and especially primary health care) by introducing fixed prices and enlarging free choice to public, private and third sector providers it is useful to have knowledge from previous reforms as well.

In the previous literature, it has been shown that changes in reimbursement influence providers' incentives towards the intensity of care provided (i.e., quality of care) or patient selection [4]. Shen has analysed the effect of financial pressure on hospital quality [5]. The study demonstrated that the effect of financial pressure on quality might differ depending on the type of competition that dominates the market. Dafny on the other hand, analysed the responses of hospitals to changes in DRG (Diagnoses-related Group) pricing and found that hospitals responded to changed prices by upcoding more patients into groups in which prices had increased the most. However, the hospitals did not increase admissions differently for those diagnoses with the largest price increases and foremost, the regulator could not positively influence the quality produced by the hospitals [6].

Sood et al. analysed the change in the prospective payment system (PPS) for inpatient rehabilitation facilities (IRF) and its effect on marginal and average reimbursement. The results show that the new PPS led to a significant reduction in costs and length of stay, but had little or no impact on outcomes, e.g., mortality or the rate of return to residence in the community [7]. In a more recent study, Allen et al. analysed activity-based financing systems (Best Practice Tariffs) and found that this system incentivised hospitals to reduce unit costs and it may even facilitate patient choice and competition, but could also reduce quality if patient choice is unable to respond to quality [8]. In another study, California patient discharge data and hospital financial disclosure reports were analysed to explore the effects of competition under prospective payment on hospital costs for low and high-cost admissions within the 12 largest DRGs. With

using the DiD method, researchers were able to show that increased competition was associated with increased costs before the price regulation but the effect decreased later, especially amongst high-cost patients. Interestingly similar effects were found on high-cost patients both above and below 65 years. The findings support the idea that a fixed price scheme created an incentive to reduce expenditures on high-cost patients [3].

We are interested in the effects of price regulation and free choice on quality in physiotherapy. We use Difference-in-Differences (DiD) regression in our effort to isolate the effect of the regulation, and for this task, we have defined the regulated and non-regulated firms (666 regulated firms and 58 non-regulated firms) and their quality before and after the reform. We have also added other firm and market structure (municipality) level variables such as potential patient capacity and the amount of patients in a municipality to the analyses as control variables. We finalise our analyses with a kernel matching.

Theoretical background

Price regulation of health care providers e.g. hospitals is aimed to lower costs or at least to reduce the rate of hospital cost inflation without skimping on quality. The intuition behind prospective payment system (PPS), or any other fixed price system for that matter, is that providers will be incentivized to use less resource in treating patients and providers that have lower costs than the flat rate would benefit from the system compared to hospitals with higher costs. However, there are concerns that fixed prices such as PPS would induce hospitals to save on costs by cream skimming and/or reducing quality etc. [9]. Because of the tradeoff between intended and unintended outcomes, it is important to combine regulation and competition in health care because it has been shown that competition with non-regulated prices tends to increase costs and price regulation without competition has no financial incentive to increase quality [3].

The main purpose of the price regulation in physiotherapy in Finland was the implementation of service vouchers, which in the case of physiotherapy for disabled individuals, must not include out-of-pocket payments and were thus a fixed price system. Because also patient choice was initiated at the same time in physiotherapy, in addition to the primary function, the scheme had the capacity to support competition and increase efficiency as price regulation steers service providers to compete for patients on non-price dimensions such as quality.

When prices are regulated, prices do not have a strategic role and competition among providers is solved via quality to increase market share [10]. Prevailing theory regarding fixed prices strongly suggests that quality increases as more competitors enter the market - assuming that the regulated price is above marginal costs, that marginal costs are constant, that profit margin is positive, firms are profit maximisers and demand will be responsive to quality [11, 12].

Increased competition (with fixed prices) means that a higher density of firms are providing services in the market [13]. When the number of firms in the market increases, the demand of a firm becomes more elastic and, therefore, firms choose higher quality in order to attract more customers [14]. The magnitude of this increase in quality is defined by the quality and elasticity of the demand [15].

Despite the strong theoretical prediction with the general theory of competition and quality with fixed prices, the most recent literature shows that, e.g., a provider's altruism, increasing marginal costs and imperfect information may decrease the positive effect that competition might have on quality. In the case of altruism, firms are interested in patients' wellbeing and eventually this behavior will decrease their effort of growing profits. Brekke et al. has shown that with semi-altruistic providers there is an unambiguous relationship between increased patient choice and service quality. In this case, patient choice has two contradicting outcomes. A more quality responsive demand increases the incentives to decrease quality so that financially unprofitable patients would choose other providers. On the other hand, an altruistic provider wants to increase quality and thus patient benefit. Researchers have shown that depending on the size of the conflicting effects, competition will either decrease or increase quality [13].

The larger the profit margin, the stronger are firms' incentives to increase quality. Thus, also the increase in the regulated prices will increase the marginal net profit from higher quality. Increasing marginal costs on the other hand, diminishes firms' incentives to engage in quality competition and the reason behind increasing costs may be capacity constraints. If patient capacity is limited, firms must either abstain from quality competition (i.e., increasing volume) or invest in extra capacity which will be increasing marginal costs. Therefore, the profit margin (and thus the incentive to compete for patients) will also be greater if the level of the fixed price includes investment costs [12].

Finally, information affects patient's responsiveness towards service quality. If patients start reacting to increased quality information (i.e., quality differences) intuitively this would also affect providers' incentives towards pro-competitive direction [12]. Gravelle & Sivey (2010) have demonstrated that only if providers have similar quality and thus similar costs, increased quality information will improve quality. A similar result occurs if information is initially relatively imprecise. On the other hand, if quality differences are large between/amongst providers, cost differences also tend to be large. In this situation, with improved

information, patients are making even more accurate decisions regarding providers and with fixed prices marginal revenues are also small and thus there is no incentive to increase quality in either of the hospitals [16]. Gravelle & Masiero have studied quality incentives in a regulated market with imperfect information in their theoretical study regarding general practitioners (GPs). The study shows that for any given regulated capitation fee, quality is lower and the incentive effects on quality are smaller when there is imperfect information [17].

As can be seen from previous theoretical literature, the effect of price regulation combined with quality competition potentially leads quality in two opposite directions. Price regulation may induce firms to cut costs by reducing quality while intensified competition may incentivise firms to increase quality. As information is presumed to be imperfect in our study, the quality outcome due to reform in physiotherapy is unambiguous and by using empirical data we aim to test which effect dominates in the market.

Physiotherapy market

Public health care is universal and tax financed in Finland, but Kela has a supplementary role in the health sector as it also organises and finances health services such as rehabilitation. Kela is obliged by law to organise medical rehabilitation such as physiotherapy for disabled persons who fulfil the criteria defined in the law (Rehabilitation law 566/2005) and the institution is one of the largest organisers and financiers of rehabilitation services in Finland. In 2011, Kela had in total approximately 1,320 service providers of physiotherapy. During the same year, the annual costs of physiotherapy were approximately 50 million euros [18].

In addition to the physiotherapy services studied, there are also other ways to organise physiotherapy services in Finland. Physiotherapy may be provided as part of the public health care or by part of the occupation health care. In addition, a large part of the services are provided by private physiotherapists (firms) and patients are entitled to small subsidies from Kela. Yet, this market is not controlled by Kela and Kela is not involved in organising these services. Instead, patients using these services make the selection of providers themselves and thus the market formation is very different from the one studied. Approximately 40% of all physiotherapy firms had a contract with Kela to produce services for the disabled individuals and these services constitute about 22% of all physiotherapy provided in Finland in 2011 [19].

Kela uses public procurement mechanisms, mainly competitive bidding, when organising physiotherapy (or other rehabilitation services). Services are purchased from the private sector. In physiotherapy, during the contract period 2007-2010 all services were organised with competitive bidding, but during the contract period 2011-2014, fixed-price service vouchers were piloted in two insurance districts while 23 insurance districts continued organising competitive bidding.

A service voucher pilot, i.e. price regulation as well as the introduction of patient choice, was introduced by policy change in the procurement. Thus the fixed price system associated with patient choice was an administrative decision made by Kela. The request for registration, including information on the level of regulated prices for the pilot districts, was announced (before the pilot began) in September 2010 for the contract period 2011–2014.

Price regulation was geographically defined by Kela. The aim was to have a sufficiently competitive environment (adequate amount of supply and demand) but exclude the largest insurance districts as well as the geographically most challenging districts. During the contract period 2011–2014, a firm was able to participate in either the voucher system or in competitive bidding (depending on the insurance district they operated on) but not in both.

The chosen pilot areas had some general features: the two districts were geographically located in different parts of Finland and they could be described as medium-sized districts, which included 31 municipalities. From those 31 municipalities, Kela had service providers in 26 municipalities and there were between 1 and 22 providers in each. In 2011, the two pilot districts had 118 providers in total, which is approximately 9.5% of all firms contracted to provide services for disabled individuals. Pilot districts are presented in Fig. 1.

The procurement process is very different between competitive bidding and fixed-price service vouchers. The major difference is the pricing – the service voucher scheme had regulated prices while in competitive bidding, prices were defined by firms in their tenders. With competitive bidding, the minimum quality of the service, as well as other requirements for the service providers were defined in the request for tender. Firms set their price for a 45-min therapy session, while taking into account quality and capacity in their tenders. During the procurement process, Kela scored each firm's price and quality (education, work experience and premises, as well as its quality, the quality of the equipment and the extent to which it conformed to Kela's quality standard) in a predefined manner. After completing the procurement process, qualified firms were accepted to join a pool of firms. Patients then choose proper service providers based on their individual preferences.

With service vouchers on the other hand, separate registration processes were carried out in both of the two Kela insurance districts where fixed price service vouchers were operational. All service providers who

accepted the regulated price and who fulfilled certain predefined minimum quality criteria[1] were eligible to produce physiotherapy and these firms received written contracts with Kela for the contract period 2011-2014. A firm which declines to accept regulated prices and/or fails to meet minimum quality requirements will not be contracted with Kela and thus may not produce physiotherapy for the disabled individuals financed from NHI. The purpose of the registration process was to create a pool of eligible firms for both of the two insurance districts (or 26 municipalities). After completing registration, patients choose their service providers among eligible firms. The differences between the two different procurement mechanisms are defined in Table 1.

During the contract periods 2007–2010 and 2011–2014 medical rehabilitation was arranged by Kela if the patient fulfilled the criteria set in the rehabilitation law. A written rehabilitation plan forms the basis for medical rehabilitation services for persons with severe disabilities. The plan is drawn up with the doctor in charge of the patient's health care. Physiotherapy for disabled individuals is granted based on individual needs and requirements, the maximum being once a week for up to three years at a time.

In 2011 approximately 14,000 persons received physiotherapy services targeted at disabled individuals. In general, disabled individuals receiving physiotherapy services ranged from young children to adults up to 65 years of age. The median age of the patients was 43 years [18]. In 2011 there were approximately 1,200 (750 and 450) patients receiving these services in the two districts where fixed price service vouchers were piloted.

In physiotherapy studied, out-of-pocket payments are not required and money follows patients. Patient choice is effective throughout the country as patients may choose proper service providers from the pool of firms based on their individual preferences despite how the firms are contracted. Despite Kela covering (reasonable) travel costs to the patients, the distance to the provider is important because the service is targeted at the disabled individuals. Therefore, patients are presumed to make decisions among/between providers within their own municipalities. Based on the previously described operational environment, patients' decision-making is based on distance to the provider and quality of the service. However, Kela provides only a smidgen of information about firms to patients and information is considered imperfect in this study.

Based on recent study, over 95% of the disabled individuals (adults) receiving physiotherapy studied appreciate the right to choose a provider based on their individual preferences. Approximately 45% of the respondents pointed out that they are able choose a provider individually. Thus, despite of disabilities,

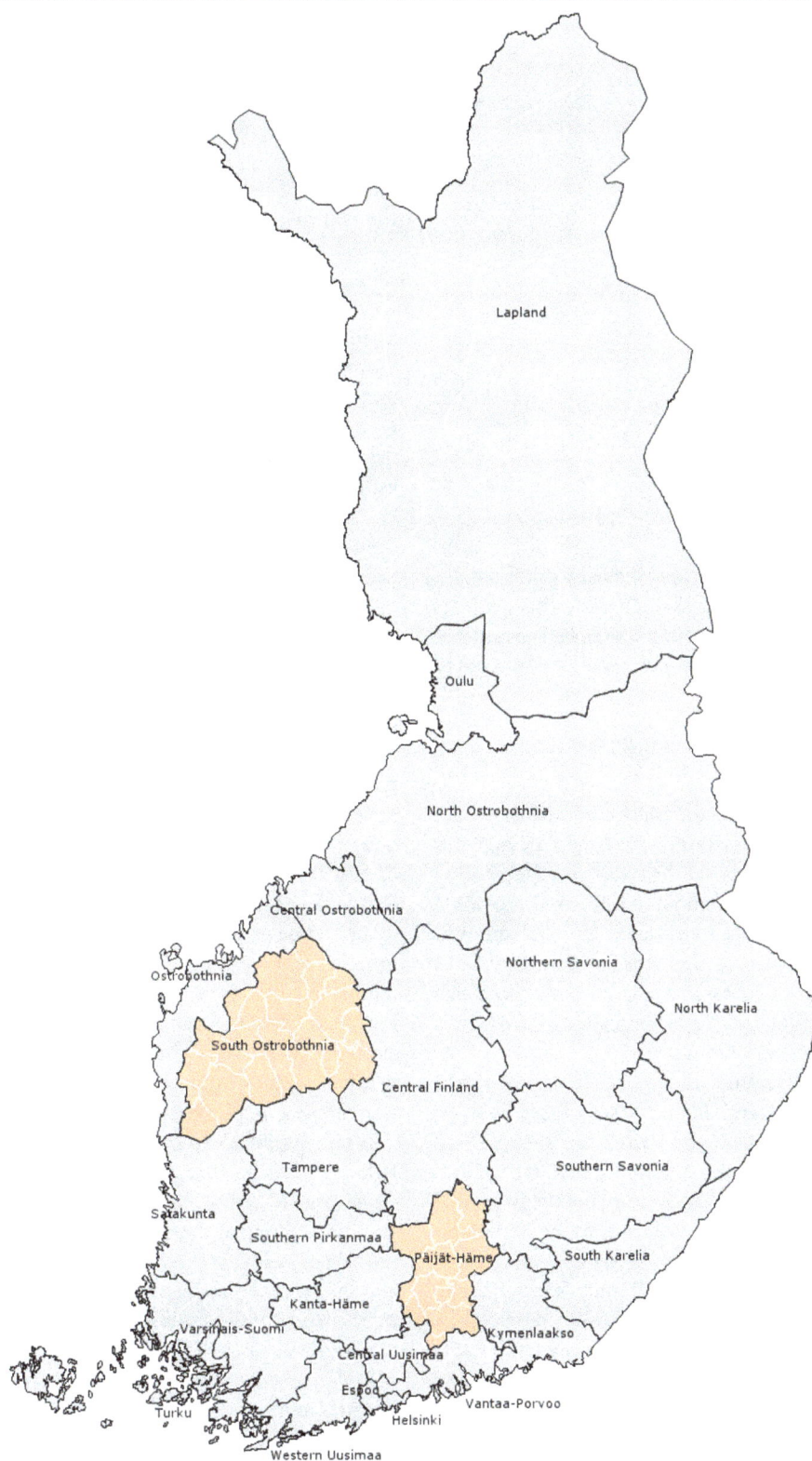

Fig. 1 Kela insurance districts in 2011. Service voucher was piloted in two districs – Päijät-Häme and South Ostrobothnia

Table 1 The differences between competitive bidding and service vouchers as procurement mechanisms

Process	Competitive bidding	Service voucher
Price	Defined by firms in their tenders	Regulated by Kela
Minimum quality and other criteria	Controlled by Kela	Controlled by Kela
Excess quality	Scored during the procurement process	Not scored or evaluated during registration
Contracting	Completed with firms based on quality-price ratio	Completed with all firms fulfilling minimum criteria
Patient choice	Patients may choose a local provider that has a contract with Kela	Patients may choose a local provider that has a contract with Kela
Out-of-pocker payments required	No	No

this patient group must be considered as any other patient or customer group in the market. In fact, this patients group could be considered as an experienced group because the therapy is very intense including weekly visits to therapists for many years [20].

Data
Sample
The variables needed in econometric modelling were collected from several registers as well as carrying out questionnaires to the firms. During the contract period of 2007 to 2010, there were about 1,460 firms providing physiotherapy for disabled individuals and the amount decreased to 1,320 firms for the contract period of 2011 to 2014. In 2011 a total of 118 firms participated Kela's service voucher pilot and approximately 1200 firms participated competitive bidding.

We used the DiD method in our effort to isolate the effect of the regulation, and, for purposes of this task, we have defined the regulated and unregulated firms and their quality before (the year 2007) and after the reform (the year 2011). We were able to gather data from 724 firms that had a contract with Kela during both periods. Our study group includes firms (n = 58) that were participating in competitive bidding in 2007 and were subject to price regulation in 2011. The control group (n = 666) includes firms that had determined their prices and quality in the tenders for both contract periods (2007-2010 and 2011-2014).

In order to control unobservable factors that could have an influence on the outcome, we have added other firm and market structure (municipality) level variables to the analyses. Our control variables are competition, potential patient capacity (describing firm size), average rental rate (a cost shifter) and the amount of disabled individuals receiving physiotherapy (a demand shifter). All of our control variables are justifiable and we face no bad control problem [21], because we are dealing with individual-level panel data and, e.g., competition (entry and exit of firms) is assessed not to be an outcome of the regulation[2]. By examining reimbursements before and after the regulation, Kela reimbursed physiotherapy (in the two pilot districts) for 112 firms in 2007 and for 105 firms in 2011. To avoid a possible bias regarding competition as a control variable, we also estimate the model without competition. In order to control possible changes in management styles etc. we also added firms types as dummy variables to the analyses[3]. For propensity score matching, we have also included the amount of population in a municipality, and firms' risk rate (1-3) describing firms' financial risk as additional controls to the estimation.

Data sources
Data regarding quality was collected after conducting questionnaires on the firms in 2013 and 2014 (fixed prices) or from Kela's procurement department (market-determined prices). However, quality was scored by using the same scaling and hence quality is comparable despite different procurement and procuring mechanisms in 2007 and 2011. During competitive bidding, Kela evaluated and scored each tender's price and quality information in a predefined manner. With service vouchers, on the other hand, only minimum quality requirements were verified by Kela, but excess quality of the service was not analysed or scored during the registration and, therefore, information on quality had to be gathered by conducting questionnaires on the firms. From a total of five questionnaires (and six reminders) that were sent to the firms in 2013 (January, February, March, April, November) – three of them were electronic and two of them were traditional post questionnaires. To gather more data, a total of 33 service providers were interviewed by phone in April 2014 [19].

Data regarding capacity and price were obtained from Kela, as was the data on the number of disabled individuals receiving physiotherapy in municipalities. The amount of population and the average level of rent in the municipalities were provided by Statistics Finland [22, 23], and information on the number of physiotherapists in the local market and firm level risk rates were obtained from Suomen Asiakastieto Oy.

Table 2 presents the average qualities and prices of regulated and unregulated firms. Table 3 provides descriptive statistics of the variables included in the estimation separately for the treatment and control groups.

I. Dependent variable
The quality scoring was based on the same scoring as was conducted during competitive bidding organised by

Table 2 Mean quality and price of the regulated and unregulated firms

Year	Quality		Price	
	Regulated	Unregulated	Regulated	Unregulated
2007	73.34 (n = 58)	68.78 (n = 666)	41.79 (n = 58)	42.68 (n = 666)
2011	70.93 (n = 58)	82.67 (n = 666)	44.81 (n = 58)	47.81 (n = 666)

Kela in 2010 for the contract period 2011-2014 for physiotherapists not providing services with service vouchers. The quality scoring of price-regulated firms was carried by the researcher between January 2014 and April 2014. This ensured that the quality analysed was the same for both regulated and non-regulated firms. Firms that did not receive a contract with Kela were excluded. Our quality measure was previously used by Pekola et al. study - it is the sum of different quality factors and it could be described as the medium/long-term quality investments of a firm rather than as the quality of care [19]. Our quality measure includes education (max 20 points), work experience (max 30 points), the premises and their quality (max 6 points), the quality of the equipment (max 6 points) and the extent to which firms complied with Kela's quality standards (max 41 points). The maximum quality score was 103 points. The qualities of the two contract periods were made comparable by multiplying the 2007 premises and their quality score points by 0.4, the equipment score by 1.2 and firms' compliance with Kela's quality standards by 1.17 because the original scoring differed between the two periods.

We argue that the quality parameters analysed in this study are valid because the scoring is uniform to all firms. Also according to the quality assurance standards by the Charted Society of Physiotherapy, quality physiotherapy includes a multitude of different quality factors [24] and Grimmer et al., for example, note that in addition to the outcome of care, the quality evaluation of physiotherapy may include different factors, such as the organisation of the service and the way in which care is provided [25].

II. Independent and control variables

We have added several firm and market structure level-independent variables into our analyses in order to control factors that could have an effect on the outcome. Our firm-level independent variables are: pre-reform quality (contract period 2007-2010), firms' potential patient capacity for disabled individuals per year, which describes firm size and risk rating (1-3) based on, e.g., each firm's financial statement. The market-level variables are: the number of competitors (firms providing physiotherapy) operating in the municipality, the average rental rate in a municipality [23], the number of disabled individuals receiving physiotherapy in a municipality, and the amount

of population in a municipality [22]. For the final model, we also added a company-type dummy variable to the model in order to control for firm level time-invariant fixed effects. Firms producing physiotherapy are divided into six different company types. Self-employed therapists are the largest group (approximately 40%). Other company types are limited partnership, partnership, limited company, foundation and association.

Methods

When analysing the effects of regulation, one approach is to compare regulated and unregulated firms or markets [26]. Stigler and Friedland's paper on regulated electricity prices is a good example of this method of analysis [27]. We used the DiD method in our effort to isolate the effect of price regulation, and for this task we have defined the regulated and non-regulated firms and their quality before and after the reform. The coefficient of interest (the interaction term) forms after the average gain over time in the control group is subtracted from the average gain over time in the treatment group. The method basically removes biases that could either be caused by permanent differences between the two groups or biases resulting from time trends unrelated to the regulation [28].

The basic model (model 1) of interest is the following

$$y_{it} = \alpha + \beta D_i + \gamma T_t + \theta D_i \times T_t + W_{it}\tau + \varepsilon_{it} \qquad (1)$$

where y is the outcome of interest e.g. quality, α is the constant term, D_i is a dummy variable identifying (firms') treatment and control groups ($D_i = 1$ study group, $D_i = 0$ control group) to be called Price regulation, T_t is the time indicator ($T_t = 0$, if t = 2007, and $T_t = 1$, if t = 2011) to be called Time, and $D_i \times T_t$ is the main interaction variable (hereafter called quality effect) of the DiD-estimation, and ε_{it} is the error term. The control variables used in the estimation were included in the vector W_{it}.

Despite DiD regression is a fairly precise mechanism for estimating the effect of a treatment or a reform with non-experimental data, there are certain well-known caveats with the DiD analyses. Parallel trend assumption is one of the most common problems with DiD estimation and, therefore; it should be tested that the two groups did not differ before the reform was implemented. Unfortunately we did not have access to additional data regarding (multiple) periods prior and post reform to have a better understanding of the parallel trend assumption in the quality of physiotherapy. However, in spite of this we use individual-level panel data, which enables us to control factors that vary across firms and factors that are unobservable. We also aim to control factors that could have an effect on quality for other reasons than price regulation and, therefore, for the model

Table 3 Descriptive statistics

Dependent variable	Variable details	Contract period 2011-2014 (post reform) Treatment group/Control group				Contract period 2007-2010 (pre reform) Treatment group/Control group			
		Mean	S.E.	Min	Max	Mean	S.E.	Min	Max
Quality	Sum of quality factors scored during competitive bidding (control group) or with regulated prices (study group) scoring conducted by the researcher based on questionnaires (max score 103 points)	70.93/82.67	12.69/12.43	47/29	99/103				
Quality	Sum of quality factors scored during competitive bidding (max score 103 points)					73.34/68.78	12.07/10.82	48.03/27.20	96.66/100.66
Independent variables									
Competition (municipality)	Total number of physiotherapists (firms) per municipality	26.12/74.70	20.38/110.81	1/0	50/403	17.35/56.91	12.16/87.02	1/0	31/318
Capacity	Firm's potential patient capacity per year	30.98/34.05	34.30/41.71	2/0	220/330	22.35/18.92	27.86/20.45	1/5	150/200
Average rental rate (municipality)	Average rental rate (€/square meter) in a municipality. Average rental rate includes all rent realized in a privately financed market, not just rents of physiotherapists (firms).	8.85/10.07	0.84/2.09	8.00/7.87	10.00/14.92	8.08/8.80	0.92/1.50	7.12/7.12	9.33/12.01
Disabled individuals (municipality)	Total number of disabled individuals in a municipality receiving physiotherapy	122.45/234.56	90.26/272.09	9.00/7.87	227/963	110.81/205.27	85.44/244.27	11/3	233/856
Population (municipality)	Total population in a municipality	46147.53/112489.20	38370.42/16446.70	3436/1503	102308/595384	44710/108784	36888.14/15683960	3564/1575	99308/568531
Risk rating	Firms are placed into different risk categories (1-3) based on their risk evaluation conducted by Suomen Asiakastieto Oy. Risk is calculated based on e.g. financial statement. Low risk =1, high risk =3	1.02/1.19	0.14/0.45	1/1	2/3	1.33/1.36	0.47/0.53	1/1	2/3

2 we have added previously mentioned pre-reform and time-varying control variables to increase the precision of our estimates.

Another robustness check is executed with a slightly different quality measure. As mentioned earlier, our original quality measure is the sum of different quality factors that were scored either during the procurement process (competitive bidding) or after firms replied to questionnaires that were sent during the research. One of the quality factors (firms' compliance with Kela's quality standards) was difficult to score outside the procurement process, because the scoring involves judgement and, therefore, for the model 4, we modified our quality variable by removing this particular quality indicator. Finally, we also added firm type dummy variables to the model in order to control for firm type time invariant factors in our analyses.

As there are previously mentioned deficits in DiD estimation and our data, in the final stage, we tested the robustness of our DiD estimates as well as the unobservable group-specific pre-regulation heterogeneity between the study group and the control group with Kernel Matching (KM) and balancing properties respectively. The basic idea with propensity score matching is to find matches for treated units from the control group [29]. Kernel matching uses all treated units and all controls in its estimation and thus this matching algorithm is used in this study because the number of treated firms is fairly small. To increase the precision of the matching we also bootstrapped standard errors. Based on Rosenbaum and Rubin, matching is a method of selecting units from the control group that are similar to units in the study group with respect to the distribution of observed covariates [30, 31]. The balancing test on the other hand, performs a balancing t-test of difference in means of the specified covariates between the control and treated groups during the pre-regulation period [32].

Results

Kela piloted regulated price service vouchers in two insurance districts during the contract period 2011-2014. Firms located in these districts had fixed prices and the prices needed to cover all costs of the service, as firms were not allowed to charge any extra fees from patients. On the other hand, patient choice was also initiated in 2011 for the same service. Free choice was granted to all patients despite the procurement mechanism.

Based on the previously described system, the service voucher reform could have induced firms to change their behaviour regarding quality. Based on theory regarding price regulation and quality competition, the effect on quality due to the reform is unambiguous. We have tested by using empirical data from physiotherapy, which theoretical prediction dominates the market.

We used DiD estimation techniques as well as Kernell matching in our effort to isolate the effect. We used firm level pre- and post-regulation data in our estimations. The data included both regulated and unregulated firms. We also used several control variables in the estimations.

Our results from the first model (Table 4) indicate that the quality of firms participating in service voucher pilots had decreased, but the study group and the control group differed from each other statistically significantly (at the 5% level) and thus the results could have been biased.

By adding control variables to the model, we aimed to control unit-specific changes between the periods and the results from model 2 (Table 5) show that the reform indeed had a negative and statistically significant effect on quality, and the use of the control variables diminished the difference between the two groups as the difference was no longer statistically significant. By removing the competition variable from the models, we aimed to remove the possibility of bad controls. However, the removal did not alter the results.

Our third model includes a modified quality measure because one aspect of the quality (firms' compliance with Kela's quality standards) was difficult to score outside of the procurement process and this difficulty could have caused problems in measuring the outcome. We continued to analyse only those firms that had a contract during both periods and results from the modified quality measure (Table 6) support our previous findings that the reform had a negative and statistically significant effect on quality. However, the effect is much more modest in this model. This could mean two things: either the difficulty of the scoring indeed overestimated the results (a negative effect) or firms decreased their quality most in this respect due to price regulation. The firms' compliance with Kela's quality standards is probably the easiest quality factor to decrease because other quality factors (such as a firm's

Table 4 Full results from DiD regression for quality (model 1)

Model	Coefficient	Standard error	P > |t|
Quality			
Time	13,8936	0,64	***
Price regulation	4,5663	1,60	**
Quality effect	−16,3050	2,27	***
Constant	68,7760	0,45	***

Significance level: 0,05% = *, 0,01% = **, =0.001 = ***

N	1448
F (3,1444)	160,00
Prob > F	0,0000
R-squared	0,2495
Adj R-squared	0,2479
Root MSE	11,71

Table 5 Full results from DiD regression for quality (model 2)

Model	Coefficient	Standard error	P > |t|
Quality			
Time	12,9472	1,11	***
Price regulation	0,3139	2,77	
Quality effect	−14,7613	3,10	***
Competition	−0,0072	0,02	*
Capacity	0,0537	0,01	***
Rent	0,4706	0,42	
Disabled individuals	0,0010	0,01	**
Quality 2007	0,7039	0,03	***
Constant	15,0494	2,91	***
Significance level: 0,05% = *, 0,01% = **, =0.001 = ***			
N	1065		
F (8,1056)	205,82		
Prob > F	0,0000		
R-squared	0,6093		
Adj R-squared	0,6063		
Root MSE	8,6152		

equipment or its premises) are likely to react more slowly to price regulation. Finally, we also added company-type dummy variables to our regression to control for firm level time-invariant factors, but the main result was not altered (Table 7).

Lastly, as a robustness check, we completed a kernel matching and, as background analysis for this, we first

Table 6 Full results from DiD regression for modified quality variable (model 3)

Model	Coefficient	Standard error	P > |t|
Quality			
Time	14,0588	0,51	***
Price regulation	−0,7175	1,43	
Quality effect	−6,7281	1,71	***
Competition	0,0029	0,01	
Capacity	−0,0030	0,01	***
Rent	0,2264	0,23	
Disabled individuals	−0,0030	0,00	
Quality 2007	0,5442	0,02	***
Constant	−8,1035	2,34	**
Significance level: 0,05% = *, 0,01% = **, =0.001 = ***			
N	1064		
F (9,1055)	243,35		
Prob > F	0,0000		
R-squared	0,6485		
Adj R-squared	0,6459		
Root MSE	6,9245		

Table 7 Full results from DiD regression with company type dummy variables

Model	Coefficient	Standard error	P > |t|
Quality			
Time	14,1022	0,51	***
Price regulation	−0,9338	1,43	
Quality effect	−6,6596	1,71	***
Competition	0,0007	0,01	
Capacity	0,0281	0,01	***
Rent	0,2706	0,23	
Disabled individuals	−0,0024	0,00	
Quality 2007	0,5524	0,02	***
Company type 1[a]	−2,6226	1,81	
Company type 2	−2,9991	1,53	
Company type 3	−2,3737	1,48	
Company type 4	−3,4304	1,87	
Company type 5	−3,7229	1,47	*
Constant	−5,7691	2,75	***
Significance level: 0,05% = *, 0,01% = **, =0.001 = ***			
[a] = foundation treated as a reference group			
N	1064		
F (13,1050)	151,39		
Prob > F	0,0000		
R-squared	0,6521		
Adj R-squared	0,6478		
Root MSE	6,9057		

estimated the probability of a firm's participation in price regulation with the probit regression. Results from the probit regression (Table 8) indicate that price-regulated firms are likely to have less competition in their area (market) but there are also more disabled residents receiving physiotherapy. The firms also have slightly higher quality before the reform, have somewhat lower financial risk and have more staff per firm (yet weakly). The results regarding, e.g., competition are sensible, as price regulation was implemented in medium-sized insurance districts.

As is suggested by previous literature [33], outcome values for quality after the reform are not included in the matching process. The balancing properties were also satisfied by using a set of baseline covariates. We were able to find 567 matches from the control group for 92 regulated firms. The description of the estimated propensity scores in regions of common support are presented in Table 9. Overlap between treatment and comparison groups is presented in Fig. 2. As can be seen, the density distribution of the propensity score is satisfying after the matching.

Table 8 Results from the probit regression

Model	Coefficient	Standard error	P > |t|
Pricereg			
Competition	−0,0348	0,0084	***
Disabled individuals	0,0060	0,0021	**
Population	0,0000	0,0000	
Risk rating	−0,3944	0,1574	*
Rent	−0,1420	0,0725	
Staff	0,0034	0,0015	*
Quality_2007	0,0124	0,0054	*
Constant	−0,5608	0,7438	

Significance level: 0,05% = *, 0,01% = **, =0.001 = ***

N	1054
LR chi2 (6)	74,01
Prob > chi2	0,0000
Pseudo R2	0,1185

Conversely, the results from the matching (Table 10) confirm our findings that the reform indeed had a negative and statistically significant effect on quality. The result of the average treatment effect of the treated is uniform (approximately −6 quality points) with the DiD analyses with control variables and a modified quality variable (Table 6). These additional identical results confirm that our results are unbiased and the negative effect on quality was caused by the service voucher reforms.

Table 9 Description of the estimated propensity score in region of common support

Model	Percentiles	Smallest
1%	0,0538	0,0529
5%	0,0586	0,0530
10%	0,0640	0,0531
25%	0,0815	0,0532
50%	0,1103	
Largest		
75%	0,1526	0,4220
90%	0,1998	0,4494
95%	0,2472	0,5516
99%	0,3824	0,9894

The region of common support is [0.0529, 0.9894]

Obs	656
Mean	0,1276
Stand. Dev.	0,0733
Variance	0,0054
Skewness	3,9020
Kurtosis	34,9751

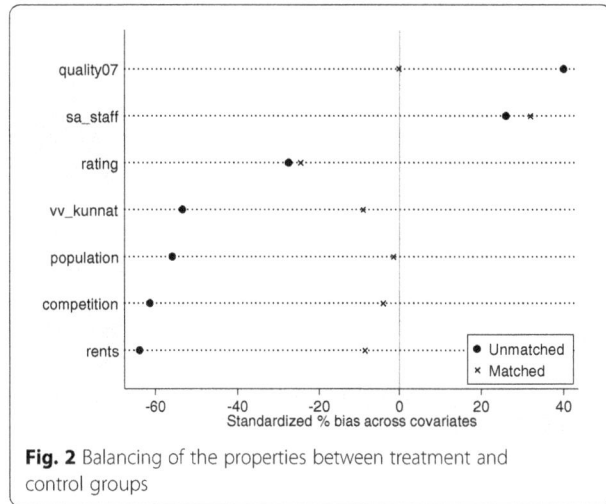

Fig. 2 Balancing of the properties between treatment and control groups

Balancing properties as well as common support of regulated and non-regulated firms are presented in Figs. 3 and 4. On a final note, it is important to mention that the balancing of the covariates describing the firms (Table 11) before the regulation is satisfactory and thus we conclude that our results are robust.

A regulatory policy that sets a price as a markup above marginal costs yields to the socially optimal price and quality if the regulator had full information about the market and its behavior [34]. If the regulated price is set under marginal costs, firms have an incentive to diminish quality. Finally, by using t-tests, we tested the differences between the average regulated prices and the prices determined by firms in the tenders before the price regulation was implemented (Table 12).

The regulated price was negligibly different statistically from the pre-regulation period prices when the earnings index was controlled. Therefore it could be stated that the quality decrease was not caused by an inappropriate level of regulated price. Most likely, our results are caused by firm's efforts to cut costs due to price regulation but it seems that this cost reduction was made by decreasing quality. We argue that competition did not incentivise firms to compete for patients on quality. It is likely that unresponsiveness of firms to quality competition is caused by imperfect information. Despite free choice having been initiated in 2011, comparable quality information is not provided for patients that would support their decision making. Therefore, the results from the empirical estimations are sensible and support theoretical findings that price regulation tends to decrease quality in health care.

Discussion

With this study, we are able to analyse price regulation combined with the free choice of patients (i.e., competition) in physiotherapy. Our findings show that quality was

Table 10 Results from the kernel matching with bootsrapped standard errors

Variable	Reps	Observed	Bias	S.E.	95% conf. Intervall	
Quality	100	−5,7311	0,049582	1,439388	−8.5872-2.8750	Normal
					−8.7314-2.3824	Percentile
					−8.7316-2.3824	Bias-corrected

decreased due to the reform. Similar reform is planned for public health care in Finland and this is the first study that uses Finnish data in analysing firms' incentives towards price regulation and free choice of patients. The aim was to test which theoretical prediction dominated in the market – price regulation and the possibility to cut costs through quality or quality competition, which by the general theory of competition with fixed prices should enhance quality unless factors such as imperfect information influence the incentives of firms.

Based on our findings, quality reduction was statistically significant in all models. All of our regression models, as well as KM, show that quality was reduced due to the service voucher reform which had fixed prices but also introduced free choice of patients. Most likely the result is caused by price regulation. Fixed prices alter the financial incentives of firms and Ellis has shown that patient selection and quality discrimination of hospitals is sometimes even boosted under competitive environment [4]. Also Meltzer et al. [3] present in their study that an increasingly competitive environment under

fixed prices has the effect of increasing quality the most for the least costly patients. Gravelle and Masiero on the other hand point out the incentive effects of providers are lower in any capitation fee when information is imperfect [17].

The more a health care provider, e.g., a hospital provides services under fixed prices, the lower the net revenue it receives. Thus, the success of the pricing must be evaluated through the interests of patients and providers [35]. Due to the imperfect information, the interest of patients is difficult to stand out despite free choice and thus the financial incentives of firms regarding price regulation is solved by reductions in quality. The result is sensible as the evaluated quality marks quality investments of firms rather that the outcome of care.

Even though our results seem solid, ideally the assessment of the regulation to the behavior and performance of firms requires a fairly lengthy time series to avoid basing conclusions on possible transitional responses [26]. Unfortunately, we did not have access to several pre- or post-treatment periods and we were unable to test, e.g., pre-treatment trends of the regulated and un-regulated groups with alternative parallel assumptions as suggested by Angrist & Pischke [21]. This is definitely a shortcoming of our study. Conversely, there are several issues that support the fact that firms were alike in both study and control groups. Firstly, all firms had to participate in competitive bidding before the implementation of the fixed-price service vouchers. Secondly, all firms had similar contracts with Kela and all firms were treating disabled individuals (criteria of the disabled were defined by Kela). Finally, all firms had to follow the minimum quality criteria defined by Kela. These issues support our understanding that the firms in both groups were similar before the reform.

Another weakness of the DiD regression lies in the unobserved temporary effect (e.g., change of study groups' behavior prior to the implementation of the price regulation) also known as Ashenfelter's dip. In our study, this means that the quality of the firms needed to decline before the price regulation, which conversely, would have overestimated the impact of price reform and biased our estimate. However, pre-regulation quality decline is not a possible option in our study because prior to the price regulation, all firms had to take part in competitive bidding and had contracts with Kela, which strongly forbids quality decline during the contract

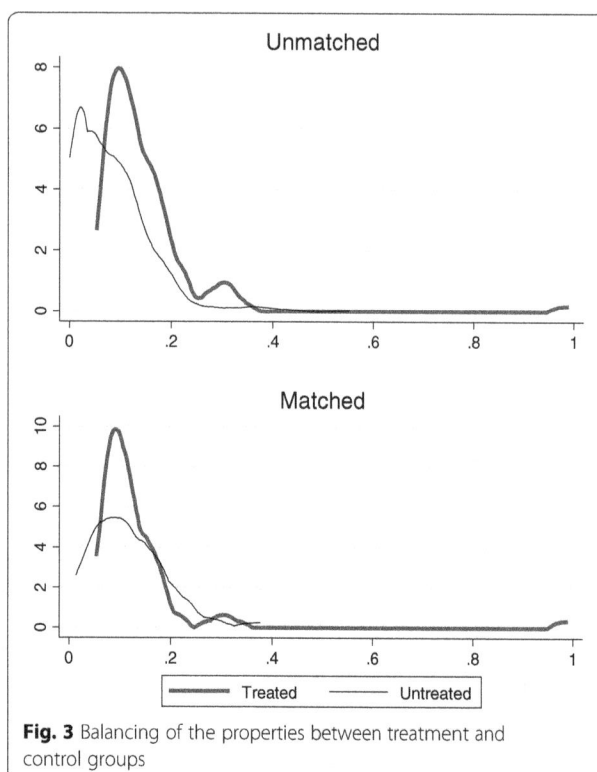

Fig. 3 Balancing of the properties between treatment and control groups

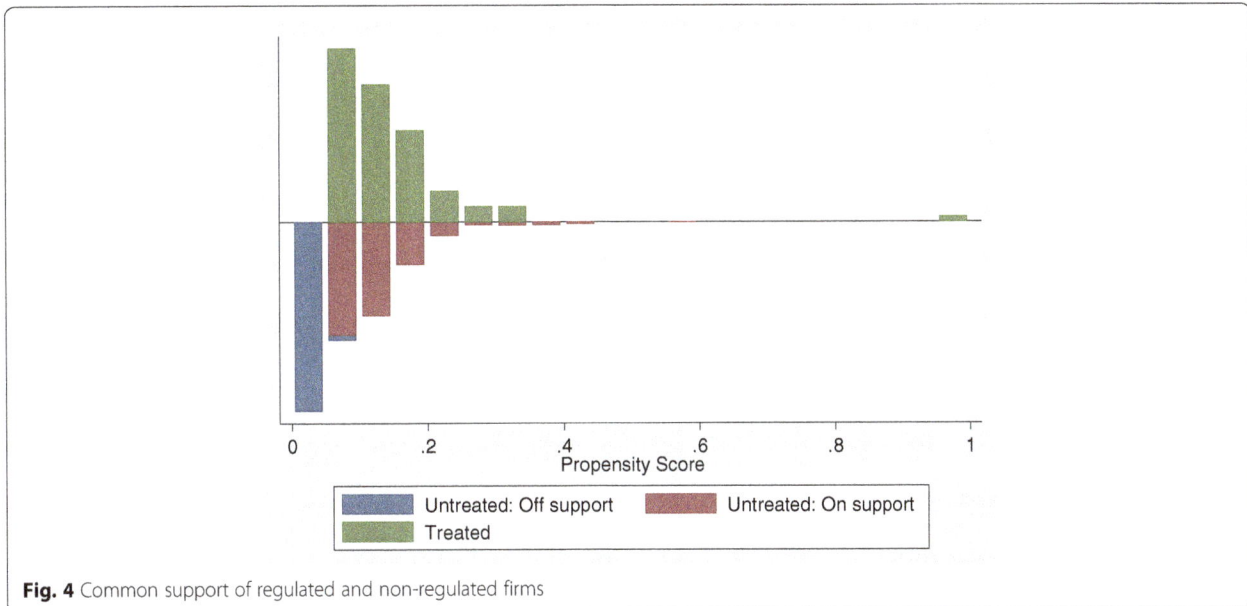

Fig. 4 Common support of regulated and non-regulated firms

period and controls it with different contractual penalty instruments. For this reason, the negative change in quality had to happen after the price regulation was implemented and was not an anticipation effect. An additionally compositional effect over time should not cause problems in this study as both regulated and unregulated firms are not going to get mixed. In our study, there is no such case in which firms with regulated insurance districts would have a chance to influence the prices or participate in competitive bidding instead and

Table 11 Results from the balancing of covariates describing the firms included in the study

| Variable | Unmatched | Mean | | | | t-test | | |
	Matched	Regulated	Non-regulated	%bias	reduct % bias	|t|	p > |t|	V (T)/V (C)
Competition	U	21,7330	65,828	−61,4		−4,74	***	0.03[a]
	M	25,3920	17,706	10,7	82,6	1,66		0,59
Disabled individuals (municipality)	U	122.4500	234.24	−53,4		−4,27	***	0.11[a]
	M	122,4500	140,16	14,5	72,9	1,39		0,62
Population	U	46148	1,10E + 05	−55,9		−4,36	***	0.05[a]
	M	46148	47888	11,1	80,2	1,6		0,70
Number of staff	U	36,7270	8,361	25,9		4,93	***	18.63[a]
	M	36,7270	4,9444	26,6	−2,4	1,09		17.12[a]
Average rental rate (municipality)	U	8,8493	10,065	−64,0		−5,39	***	0.25[a]
	M	8,8493	8,9803	15,3	76,1	1,27		0,62
Risk rating	U	1,0189	1,1913	−27,3		−2,30	*	0.55[a]
	M	1,0189	1,125	4,5	83,5	1,00		_[a]
Quality_2007	U	73,3420	68,786	40,0		4,32	***	1,23
	M	73,3420	73,36	14,2	64,6	0,72		1,45

[a] if variance ratio outside [0.69; 1.44] for U and [0.57; 1.75] for M

Results are called by using psmatch2 in Stata

	Ps R2	LR chi2	p > chi2	MeanBias	MedBias	B	R	% Var
Sample								
Unmatched	0,119	74,01	0,000	46,9	53,4	75.1[b]	0.09[b]	86
Matched	0,039	5,46	0,486	13,8	14,2	46.1[b]	0,66	29

[b] if B > 25%, R outside [0.5; 2]

Table 12 Results from t-tests regarding prices before and after the regulation

	obs	mean	se	sd	95% conf. Interval	
Pre regulation price	96	43,36	0,63	6,22	42,10	44,62
Post regulation price	118	43,89	0,34	3,70	43,21	44,57
Combined		43,65	0,34	4,99	42,98	44,32
Diff		−0,53	0,69		−1,89	0,82

t = -0.7733

degrees of freedom = 211

Ha:diff < 0	Ha:diff = 0	Ha:diff > 0
Pr (T < t) = 0.2201	Pr|T| > |t| = 0.4402	Pr (T > t) = 0.7799

therefore, before and after, comparability is not compromised.

Unfortunately due to missing data we were unable to perform proper response bias analyses on firms which participated in competitive bidding and had non-regulated prices during both periods but were not included in the study. However, firms which participated in a service voucher pilot (and had regulated prices) and were not included in the data of this study (due to missing quality data from both periods) have been previously analysed by Pekola et al. [20]. The results indicate that firms that had regulated prices but were not included in this study were smaller firms (based on potential patient capacity) and perhaps had lower than average quality.

Conclusion

Our study shows that quality was decreased due to the reform which regulated prices but also initiated free choice of patients. We aimed to analyse which of the two mechanisms dominated in the market - cost containment due to price regulation or quality competition due to free choice of patients. As all of our regression models as well as our sensitivity analyses using kernel matching present similar results, we conclude that our results are robust. However, due to the growing interest of using price regulation and competition in health care and the fact that price regulation is sometimes associated with decreased service quality it is important to discuss means aimed to target firms' unwanted behavior towards quality.

Regulators have invented different mechanisms, such as revenue-share penalties (used in different industries such as telecommunications and electric power), which are designed to eliminate this undesirable behavior, but paradoxically, they may in fact encourage firms to do just the opposite - reduce investments in quality [36]. On the other hand, even Arrow mentions in his famous 1963 paper regarding the physician market that risk and uncertainty are significant elements of health and, therefore,

information ends up having a market on its own [37]. As quality information of the service provided by the physicians is not apparent upon inspection by patients, quality deteriorates to the lowest level in the market, causing serious market failure [38].

However, by increasing information regarding the service quality of firms and initiating benchmarking has been shown to increase investments in quality [36]. We strongly believe that actions aiming to increase patients' knowledge about service providers are needed in physiotherapy. Also benchmarking could have a positive effect on quality as well. Ultimately, it is undisputed that when patient choice is more and more widely introduced, different mechanisms that enhance information must be developed in order to enhance the ability of patients to choose providers, but also to incentivise providers toward quality investments. This also presumably has an impact on the financial incentives of firms in their effort to cut costs through quality reductions when prices are fixed.

Endnotes

[1]Minimum quality criteria for firms participating in a service voucher pilot is fairly close to the minimum quality criteria for firms participating in competitive bidding. Minimum criteria linked with service voucher pilot include several issues, e.g., the firm must be entered into the prepayment register, insurance for their business (patient insurance and liability insurance) are required, their premises and equipment must be safe for disabled individuals, they must accept regulated prices and declare that they would not charge the patients any extra fees, they need to inform Kela of any changes to their business, therapists must have professional practice rights, they must have adequate first aid skills and they must be acquainted with Kela's quality standard.

[2]Due to the missing data a precise figure of firms entering and exiting the market studied may not be provided. However, based on the existing data approximately 22% of the firms exited the market after the

period 2007-2010. In contrast, approximately 16% of the firms entered the market as new providers in 2011 and the figures were similar between regulated and non-regulated areas.

[3]Approximately 48% of firms studied are self-employed, 26% are limited companies, 16% are limited partnerships and the rest (10%) are general partnerships, foundations and associations.

Abbreviations
DiD: Difference-in-Differences; DRG: Diagnosis-Related Group; GP: General Practitioner; IRF: Inpatient rehabilitation facilities; Kela: The Social Insurance Institution; KM: Kernel Matching; PPS: Prospective payment system

Acknowledgements
We would like to thank the two anonymous referees for their remarks and recommendations on how to improve the paper.

Funding
Not applicable

Authors' contributions
PP carried out the data gathering and data analyses as well as drafted the manuscript. IL substantially contributed to the data analyses, interpretation of the data, and provided comments on all drafts. HM supported the data gathering and provided comments on drafts. All authors read and approved the final manuscript. We confirm that this manuscript describes original work and has neither been published elsewhere nor is under consideration by any other journal.All authors read and approved the final manuscript.

Competing interest
We confirm that this manuscript describes original work and has neither been published elsewhere nor is under consideration by any other journal. All authors have approved the manuscript and agree with its submission to Health Economics Review. The study authors have no competing interests.

Author details
[1]Social Insurance Institution of Finland, PL 450, 00056 Helsinki, Finland.
[2]National Institute for Health and Welfare, PL 30, 00271 Helsinki, Finland.

References
1. Chalkley M, Malcomson JM. Contracting for health services with unmonitored quality*. Econ J. 1998;108:1093–110.
2. Ma Ching-to A. Health care payment systems: cost and quality incentives. J Econ Manage Strat. 1994;3(1):93–112.
3. Meltzer D, Chung J, Basu A. Does competition under medicare prospective payment selectively reduce expenditures on high-cost patients? RAND J Econ. 2002;33(3):447–68.
4. Ellis RP. Creaming, skimping and dumping: Provider competition on the intensive and extensive margins. J Health Econ. 1998;17:537–55.
5. Shen Y. The effect of financial pressure on the quality of care in hospitals. J Health Econ. 2003;22:243–69.
6. Dafny LS. How do hospitals respond to price changes? Am Econ Rev. 2005;95(5):1525–47.
7. Sood N, Buntin Beeuwkes M, Escarce JJ. Does How Much and How You Pay Matter? Evidence from the inpatient rehabilitation care prospective payment system. J Health Econ. 2008;27:1046–59.
8. Allen T, Fichera E, Sutton M. Can payers use prices to improve quality? Evidence from English hospitals. Health Econ. 2016;25:56–70.
9. Folland, S, Goodman AC, Stano M. The Economics of Health and Health Care. New Jersey: Pearson Prentice Hall; 2007.
10. Nuscheler R. Physician reimbursement, time consistency, and the quality of care. J Inst Theor Econ. 2003;159(2):302–22.
11. Gravelle H, Santos R, Siciliani L, Goudie R. Hospital Quality Competition Under Fixed Prices, CHE Research Paper 80. 2012.
12. Brekke, K. R., Gravelle, H., Siciliani, L., Straume, O. R.: Patient choice, mobility and competition among health care providers. In: Levaggi, R., Montefiori, M. (eds.) Health Care Provision and Patient Mobility – Health Integration in the European Union. Developments in health economics and public policy, Vol. 12 pp. 1-26 Springer (2014)
13. Brekke KR, Siciliani L, Straume OR. Hospital competition and quality with regulated prices. Scan J Econ. 2011;113(2):444–69.
14. Gaynor M, Town RJ: Competition in Health Care Markets, In: *Handbook of Health Economics. Volume 2.* McGuire T, Pauly M, Barros PP. (eds.) Elsevier/North-Holland; 2011;499-637.
15. Gaynor M. What do we know about competition and quality in health care markets?, Working paper 12301, National Bureau of Economic Research. 2006. http://www.nber.org/papers/w12301.
16. Gravelle H, Sivey P. Imperfect information in a quality-competitive hospital market. J Health Econ. 2010;29:524–35.
17. Gravelle G, Masiero G. Quality incentives in a regulated market with imperfect information and switching costs: Capitation in general practice. J Health Econ. 2002;19:1067–88.
18. Official Statistics of Finland. Statistical Yearbook of the Social Insurance Institution 2011, ISSN 1796-0479, Helsinki: Social Insurance Institution of Finland (referred: 19.5.2014). http://www.kela.fi/vuositilastot_kelan-kuntoutustilasto. Accessed 19 May 2014.
19. Pekola, P., Linnosmaa, I., Mikkola, H.: Competition and quality in a physiotherapy market with fixed prices. Eur. J. Health Econ., doi: 10.1007/s10198-016-0792-3 (2016)
20. Pitkänen, V & Pekola, P.: Asiakkaiden näkemykset valinnanvapaudesta. Tulokset fysioterapiaa saaville vaativan lääkinnällisen kuntoutuksen asiakkaille tehdystä kyselystä. Kela Työpapereita 95 (2016)
21. Angrist JD, Pischke J-S. Mostly Harmless Econometrics. An Empiricist's Companion: Princeton University Press; 2009.
22. Official Statistics of Finland, Population structure [e-publication], ISSN = 1797-5379, Helsinki: Statistics Finland (referred: 19.5.2014). http://www.stat.fi/til/vaerak/index.html. Accessed 19 May 2014.
23. Official Statistics of Finland, Average rents [e-publication], ISSN = 1798-100X, Helsinki: Statistics Finland (referred: 13.6.2013). http://www.tilastokeskus.fi/til/asvu/index.html. Accessed 19 May 2014.
24. Quality assurance standards for physiotherapy: service deliver, chartered society of physiotherapy (2012): 1–38. [referred 14.01.2015], http://www.csp.org.uk/publications/quality-assurance-standards. Accessed 19 May 2014.
25. Grimmer K, Beard M, Bell A, Chipchase L, Edwards E, Fulton I, Gill T. On the constructs of quality physiotherapy. Aust J Phys. 2000;46:3–7.
26. Joskow PL, Rose NL. The effects of economic regulation. In: Schmalensee R, Willig RD, editors. Handbook of Industrial Organization. 2nd ed. Amsterdam: Elsevier/North-Holland; 1989. p. 1449–506.
27. Stigler GJ, Friedland C. What can regulators regulate. The case of electricity. J Law Econ. 1962;5:1–16.
28. Imbens GW, Wooldridge JM. Recent developments in the econometrics of program evaluation. J Econ Lit. 2009;47(1):5–86.
29. Herryman M. An application of difference-in-difference and propensity score matching methods. Research paper in applied microeconometrics. The University of Sheffield. Department of Economics. 2010.

30. Rosenbaum PR, Rubin DB. The Central Role of the Propensity Score in Observational Studies for Causal Effects. Biometrika. 1983;70(1):41–55.

31. Rosenbaum PR, Rubin DB. Constructing a control group using multivariate matched sampling methods that incorporate the propensity score. Am Stat. 1985;39(1):33–8.

32. Villa JM. Simplifying the estimation of difference in differences treatment effects with Stata. In: Munich Personal RePEc Archive Paper No. 43943, vol. https://mpra.ub.uni-muenchen.de/43943/. 2012.

33. Austin PC. Balance diagnostics for comparing the distribution of baseline covariates between treatment groups in propensity-score matched samples. Stat Med. 2009;28:3083–107.

34. Baron DP. Price regulation, product quality, and asymmetric information. Am Econ Rev. 1981;71(1):212–20.

35. Ellis RP, McGuire TG. Provider behavior under prospective reimbursement. J Health Econ. 1986;5:129–51.

36. Weisman DL. Price regulation and quality. Inf Econ Policy. 2005;17:165–74.

37. Arrow KJ. Uncertainty and the welfare economics of medical care. Am Econ Rev. 1963;3(5):941–73.

38. Haas-Wilson D. Arrow and the information marker Failure in health care: The changing content and sources of health care information. J Health Polit Policy Law. 2001;26(5):1031–44.

9

Prenatal care and socioeconomic status: effect on cesarean delivery

Carine Milcent[1] and Saad Zbiri[2*]

Abstract

Cesarean deliveries are widely used in many high- and middle-income countries. This overuse both increases costs and lowers quality of care and is thus a major concern in the healthcare industry. The study first examines the impact of prenatal care utilization on cesarean delivery rates. It then determines whether socioeconomic status affects the use of prenatal care and thereby influences the cesarean delivery decision. Using exclusive French delivery data over the 2008–2014 period, with multilevel logit models, and controlling for relevant patient and hospital characteristics, we show that women who do not participate in prenatal education have an increased probability of a cesarean delivery compared to those who do. The study further indicates that attendance at prenatal education varies according to socioeconomic status. Low socioeconomic women are more likely to have cesarean deliveries and less likely to participate in prenatal education. This result emphasizes the importance of focusing on pregnancy health education, particularly for low-income women, as a potential way to limit unnecessary cesarean deliveries. Future studies would ideally investigate the effect of interventions promoting such as care participation on cesarean delivery rates.

Keywords: Cesarean delivery, Pregnancy care, Health education, Socioeconomic position

JEL classification: I12, I14, I18

Background

Health expenditures are high and continue to rise in many parts of the world, despite the financial and economic crisis that slowed the trend in some countries. This spending grew during the 2009–2016 period by 5.7% in South Korea, 2.8% in Switzerland, 2.7% in Australia, 2.1% in the United States, 1.8% in Germany and Japan, 1.1% in Canada, 0.9% in France and the United Kingdom [1]. There is therefore considerable pressure to rein in health costs. Unnecessary medical practices are usually pointed out as a cause of escalating healthcare spending [2]. Previous literature has looked into the ballooning overuse of medical services and describes it, to a large extent, as a widespread phenomenon that is difficult to address and that remains understudied [3–5]. In this research, we focus on cesareans, a mode of delivery generally considered to be overused in many industrialized countries [6, 7], and

explore the associations between cesarean delivery use, prenatal care utilization, and socioeconomic status.

Cesarean deliveries are currently one of the most common surgical procedures in the world; approximately 18 million are performed yearly worldwide, almost 6 million more than the 10–15% rate recommended by World Health Organization (WHO) [8]. Indeed, since 1985, WHO has stated that the number of cesareans should range between 10 and 15% of total deliveries, regardless of the region or the country [9]. This recommendation was reaffirmed in 2015 [10]. These presumptively unnecessary cesarean deliveries are responsible for an additional cost of more than 2 billion US dollars and for an unquantified burden on the health system through pressure on medical resources [8]. The surgical approach to delivery is associated with significantly greater economic costs than other modes of delivery. Xu et al. [11] find that estimated facility costs for low-risk childbirth are higher at hospitals with higher cesarean delivery

* Correspondence: saad.zbiri3@uvsq.fr
[2]EA 7285, Versailles Saint Quentin University, Montigny-le-Bretonneux, France
Full list of author information is available at the end of the article

rates. Similarly, Allen et al. [12] report that cesarean deliveries, especially those performed during labor, are associated with the highest hospital costs of delivery care. Moreover, when performed for first deliveries, they are associated with higher cumulative costs than other methods of delivery, regardless of the number or type of subsequent deliveries [13]. Evidence also suggests that attempted vaginal delivery (i.e., trial of labor) is a more cost-effective option for women with a previous cesarean than an elective repeat cesarean delivery, although its cost-effectiveness depends on the probability of successful vaginal delivery [14]. On the other hand, cesarean deliveries do not lead to better health outcomes for women or infants who do not require the procedure and can even cause short- and long-term adverse health effects [15–17].

The use of cesarean deliveries results from a wide array of medical and non-medical factors. Although specific medical risk factors are indications for cesarean delivery, they provide a very incomplete explanation of all cesarean deliveries [18]. Women's characteristics and preferences influence their mode of delivery [19], as do physicians' attitudes and incentives toward birth management [20, 21] and the financing and organizational structures of hospitals [22, 23].

Women's socioeconomic status is one of the individual determinants of cesarean deliveries. Many results have showed differences in the mode of delivery across socioeconomic groups, often assessed by income, occupation, or education, even after adjustment for medical risk factors. Overall, since the 2000s, analyses from developed countries have found that women of lower socioeconomic position are more likely than their better-off counterparts to have cesarean deliveries. In France, Guihard and Blondel [24] report that women with a low level of education have a higher risk of cesarean deliveries. German studies point out high rates of surgical deliveries for low-income women [25, 26]. Accordingly, Italian mothers with low education levels consistently give birth by a cesarean delivery more often than highly educated women [27]. Similarly, Lee et al. [28] describe lower cesarean delivery rates in South Korea for women with higher education or occupational levels. In a population of US Defense Department personnel, higher cesarean delivery rates were significantly associated with lower socioeconomic status [29]. From 1967 to 2004, women with the lowest level of education in Norway had the highest probability of cesarean deliveries [30]. Finally, Joseph et al. [31] find that the most affluent Canadian women are less likely to have a cesarean delivery than those in the lowest income category. The existing literature explains the high rates of cesarean deliveries for low-income patients in several ways, including by a greater preference for cesarean deliveries and a low access to obstetric care [25, 30]. However, no consensus has been reached on the underlying reasons.

Prenatal care is an important preventive healthcare service throughout pregnancy. Besides routine health evaluations, it provides education and counseling, as well as any necessary treatment [32]. WHO [33] in its *Standards for Maternal and Neonatal Care* recommends that all pregnant women have at least four antenatal assessments, starting as early as possible in the first trimester, conducted under the supervision of a skilled attendant, and spaced at regular intervals. Previous studies have examined the potential effect of organized prenatal care on perinatal health and showed it to be effective in reducing maternal mortality and serious morbidity [34]. Yan [35] reports that poor prenatal care increases the risks of many maternal complications and poor health habits during pregnancy as well as after delivery. Specifically, the increased adverse health outcomes are: insufficient gestational weight gain, prenatal smoking, premature rupture of membranes, preterm labor, no breastfeeding, postnatal underweight, and postpartum smoking. Moreover, the receipt of prenatal care is linked to different positive neonatal outcomes, in particular, reduced rates of both preterm birth and low birth weight. Blondel and Marshall [36] in France and Krueger and Scholl [37] in the United States report a higher probability of preterm deliveries among women with poor attendance at prenatal visits. Rous et al. [38] find that each additional prenatal visit is associated with higher birth weight. More broadly, Partridge et al. [39] observe that the risk of prematurity, stillbirth, and neonatal or infant death increases linearly with decreasing prenatal care utilization. Accordingly, Raatikainen et al. [40] find significantly more low-birth-weight infants and more fetal and neonatal deaths among woman with inadequate prenatal care. Finally, beyond its clear medical benefits, prenatal care may also have a psychological effect, preparing women for childbirth and motherhood [41].

While much of the research attention has focused on the relation between pregnancy care and maternal morbidity and mortality, several other health outcomes may be modified by prenatal care and require further investigation. The effect of prenatal care on method of delivery has not yet been adequately investigated. The primary objective of our study is thus to investigate the impact of routine prenatal care on cesarean delivery rates while simultaneously verifying the influence of socioeconomic conditions on these rates. A complementary objective of the analysis is to identify the socioeconomic determinants of the use of any type of prenatal care that significantly affects mode of delivery.

Our paper proceeds as follows. After this brief introduction to the conceptual framework of the study and previous literature, we describe the data used and explain our econometric strategy. We then present the descriptive analysis, provide the empirical findings, and discuss the results. Finally, we draw a general conclusion from the study.

Methods

Data

We have access to data that allow us to determine: *i)* women's use of prenatal care, *ii)* their socioeconomic position, and *iii)* many other patient and hospital characteristics. Specifically, our analysis uses unique French delivery data of all births recorded in the Yvelines administrative district for the period of 2008–2014. The dataset comes from the infant first health certificates (The *Premiers Certificats de Santé (PCS)*). Some supplementary information is secondarily extracted from an additional health certificate. This dataset contains patient demographic information; socioeconomic status of the household; detailed information about the pregnancy and delivery including prenatal care utilization, hospital stays, date and place of birth, type of delivery and procedures performed; and full information about maternal, fetal, and neonatal health. Because the certificates do not provide complete information about the hospital where the woman gave birth, we use a dataset of French annual hospital statistics (The *Statistique Annuelle des Etablissements de santé (SAE)*), a national survey conducted by the Ministry of Health and covers all French hospitals. Hence, we have information for each hospital in the Yvelines on its type, activity, organization, and medical staff configuration. Staffing is reported in terms of full-time equivalents (FTEs), except that private-practice physicians in private hospitals are reported only by number of individuals per hospital. We therefore apply a hypothetical average to take the level of work of these physicians working part-time in hospitals into account by considering that they devote 50% of their time to that practice. This method has been used by previous studies [42]. We also check that all our results are robust to the more extreme assumptions of 25% and 75%. Full tables of these results are not presented, in view of their similarity to those using the average assumption, but are available upon request.

Our analysis covers all live deliveries performed in the 11 hospitals of the Yvelines district from January 2008 to the end of December 2014. Thus, our full sample includes 102,236 observations. However, information on prenatal care use and socioeconomic status is missing for some women, thereby restricting the corresponding analyses to 68,314 and 58,324 observations, respectively. Because the two characteristics studied, prenatal care and socioeconomic status are generally highly correlated with the patient's health status, we also identify a subsample of low-risk women. To study cesarean delivery use, our low-risk subsample comprises nulliparous women aged 20–34 years, without any diagnosis or co-morbidity, giving birth at full term, during labor, without induction, to a singleton infant in cephalic presentation, and with a normal birth weight

(20,683 observations). Prenatal care participation is also studied separately in the same low-risk sample but which includes only vaginal deliveries (10,947 observations). The definition of the low-risk population is based on the medical criteria generally used [43, 44]. The quality of the data extracted is high: the medical information is completed by health professionals and data collection is regularly checked. To verify the reliability of its information, the dataset undergo a double quality control that enables the correction of false and missing data. In addition, hospital information extracted from the French annual statistics for hospitals is checked and supplemented with data from hospitals. Furthermore, the data are reported to the French data protection authority (The *Commission Nationale de l'Informatique et des Libertés (CNIL)*), de-identified, and routinely used for health statistics; accordingly, French law does not require specific written informed consent from patients. The summary statistics of the key variables of our analysis are reported in Tables 1 and 2. The mean cesarean delivery rate for the full sample is 23.9% over the study period. The French national rate was around 21% in 2010 [45].

Empirical strategy

To study the effects of both prenatal care and socioeconomic status on cesarean delivery rates, we use the following empirical specification to model the probability of cesarean delivery as:

$$P\left(Y_{ijt}\right) = f\left(P_{ijt}, S_{ijt}/X_{ijt}, V_{ijt}, e_{ijt}\right) \tag{1}$$

where i indexes individuals, j hospitals, and t years. Y is equal to one if the delivery is cesarean and zero otherwise. P denotes a vector of observable characteristics of prenatal care use with its clinical, ultrasonographic, and educational components; S is a vector of observable socioeconomic conditions: familial situation of the woman, her healthcare coverage, her educational level, her occupation and work status, and her partner's occupation and work status; X is a vector of observable epidemiologic characteristics that affect cesarean delivery use including demographics of the woman: age and parity (i.e., number of previous deliveries), and her medical risk factors: previous cesarean delivery, diabetes, hypertension, eclampsia or preeclampsia, intrauterine growth restriction, placental bleeding, other obstetric pathology (i.e., all diseases or co-morbidities not individually considered such as infection, premature rupture of membranes, obesity, or amniotic fluid abnormality), multiple delivery, term at delivery, fetal presentation, induced labor, and birth weight; V denotes a vector of observable characteristics of hospitals, including their type: ownership status, level of

Table 1 Cesarean delivery rates according to prenatal care utilization and household socioeconomic characteristics

	Full sample (N = 102,236)			Low-risk subsample (N = 20,683)		
	Deliveries, %	Cesarean rate, %	Chi-square test	Deliveries, %	Cesarean rate, %	Chi-square test
Prenatal care						
First antenatal visit	(n = 100,672)			(n = 20,357)		
First trimester	98.5	23.9	3.7	98.7	11.4	7.3[b]
Second trimester	1.2	23.0		1.0	14.7	
Third trimester	0.3	19.8		0.3	21.1	
Obstetric ultrasounds	(n = 94,686)			(n = 19,276)		
< 3	1.7	20.6	1000.0[a]	1.1	11.5	0.7
= 3	68.3	20.8		76.1	11.4	
≥ 4	30.0	30.4		22.8	11.9	
Nuchal translucency ultrasound	(n = 98,643)			(n = 19,972)		
Yes	97.1	23.9	12.5[a]	97.5	11.5	0.5
No	2.9	21.1		2.5	12.5	
Morphology ultrasound	(n = 98,334)			(n = 19,885)		
Yes	98.9	24.0	28.2[a]	99.1	11.5	0.8
No	1.1	17.0		0.9	9.3	
Early prenatal interview	(n = 88,690)			(n = 17,882)		
Yes	20.4	22.3	15.1[a]	27.9	10.6	2.6
No	79.6	23.7		72.1	11.4	
Prenatal education	(n = 82,417)			(n = 17,159)		
Yes	54.9	21.9	99.1[a]	75.8	10.9	15.6[a]
No	45.1	24.9		24.2	13.2	
Woman's socioeconomic level						
Familial situation	(n = 100,411)			(n = 20,328)		
Married or cohabiting	98.0	23.8	1.4	97.8	11.6	1.1
Single	2.0	25.0		2.2	10.0	
Healthcare coverage	(n = 100,146)			(n = 20,253)		
Insured	98.5	23.9	1.3	98.5	11.6	0.8
Uninsured	1.5	22.7		1.5	9.9	
Education	(n = 79,428)			(n = 16,080)		
Primary school	2.7	24.9	62.1[a]	1.3	16.2	45.4[a]
Some secondary school	14.0	25.2		10.4	13.0	
Completed secondary school	21.9	25.4		21.8	13.3	
College or university	61.4	22.8		66.5	9.8	
Occupation	(n = 70,201)			(n = 14,818)		
Manual worker	1.4	26.7	45.6[a]	1.1	13.8	26.7[a]
Office, sales, or service staff	55.2	24.9		57.8	12.0	
Farmer	0.3	24.4		0.3	18.2	
Crafts/trades worker or entrepreneur	2.9	25.5		2.8	11.4	
Intermediate (technical)	9.2	23.4		9.6	10.8	
Managerial or higher intellectual	31.0	22.7		28.4	9.1	
Work status	(n = 83,351)			(n = 16,838)		
Working	69.6	24.0	22.4[a]	75.8	10.9	2.2

Table 1 Cesarean delivery rates according to prenatal care utilization and household socioeconomic characteristics *(Continued)*

	Full sample (N = 102,236)			Low-risk subsample (N = 20,683)		
	Deliveries, %	Cesarean rate, %	Chi-square test	Deliveries, %	Cesarean rate, %	Chi-square test
Unemployed	6.7	25.1		7.3	10.9	
Not in labor force	23.7	22.6		16.9	11.9	
Partner's socioeconomic level						
Occupation	(n = 78,712)			(n = 15,826)		
Manual worker	9.3	24.5	19.0[a]	8.2	11.7	17.4[a]
Office, sales, or service staff	40.1	24.2		43.6	11.8	
Farmer	0.4	24.8		0.3	17.3	
Crafts/trades worker or entrepreneur	7.3	23.6		6.5	10.2	
Intermediate (technical)	6.2	23.2		6.6	8.5	
Manager or higher intellectual	36.7	22.8		34.8	10.2	
Work status	(n = 79,154)			(n = 16,148)		
Working	89.8	23.6	6.3[b]	89.8	10.9	2.2
Unemployed	4.4	24.7		4.1	12.8	
Not in labor force	5.8	24.9		6.1	10.8	

The full sample is composed of all live deliveries performed in the hospitals of the French administrative district of Yvelines in 2008–2014. The low-risk subsample only includes those deliveries of nulliparous women aged 20–34 years, without any diagnosis or co-morbidity, giving birth at full term, during labor, without induction, to a singleton infant in cephalic presentation, and with a normal birth weight
[a] = 1% significance level, [b] = 5%

equipment assessed based on the level of neonatal care, and teaching status, their organization: day of delivery, obstetrician availability, and size expressed as annual volume of deliveries, and their staff: FTEs midwives, obstetricians, and anesthetists per occupied bed; and e is the error term.

To explore whether the effect (if any) of participation in prenatal care on mode of delivery varies by socioeconomic status, we specify the following model of prenatal care utilization:

$$P\left(P_{ijt}\right) = f\left(S_{ijt}/X_{ijt}, e_{ijt}\right) \qquad (2)$$

where i indexes individuals, j hospitals, and t years. P is a dummy for prenatal care; X is a set of individual epidemiologic factors that may impact prenatal care use including demographics of the woman: age and parity, and her medical characteristics: previous cesarean delivery, diabetes, hypertension, eclampsia or preeclampsia, intrauterine growth restriction, placental bleeding, other obstetric pathology, multiple delivery, term at delivery, fetal presentation, onset of labor, mode of delivery, and birth weight; S is the set of socioeconomic conditions of the woman and her partner: familial situation, healthcare coverage, educational level, occupation, and work status; and e is the error term.

All models are estimated by multilevel logistic regressions and include heteroscedasticity-robust standard errors that account for within-hospital dependencies across observations. Because our panel consists of women giving

birth in different years and different hospitals, we include year of delivery and hospital fixed effects in each model, to capture the heterogeneity in time and among hospitals. Moreover, we also use hospital random effects for model 1, to consider invariant hospital characteristic variables while we assume that the hospital characteristics not explicitly taken into account in the model are not correlated with any explanatory variables.

Results and discussion
Descriptive statistics
Table 1 reports the distribution of cesarean deliveries according to prenatal care utilization characteristics. French prenatal care includes at least 7 prenatal visits, which begin during the first trimester. Hence, a woman who has her first prenatal care visit in the second or third trimester starts clinical care late and thus has less prenatal care. Three ultrasounds are recommended: the first trimester ultrasound estimates nuchal translucency thickness to assess the probability of chromosomal abnormalities, while the second or third trimester scan screens for morphologic malformations and anomalies. Prenatal educational services include a prenatal interview offered during the first trimester and prenatal education sessions that usually take place during the third trimester. Cesarean delivery rates do not differ significantly according to the trimester of the first prenatal visit. Among women who have more than the 3 recommended ultrasounds during their pregnancy, 30.4% have cesarean deliveries, significantly higher than the rate around 21% for

Table 2 Prenatal education attendance rates according to household socioeconomic characteristics

	Full sample (N = 82,417)			Low-risk subsample (N = 10,947)		
	Deliveries, %	Attendance rate, %	Chi-square test	Deliveries, %	Attendance rate, %	Chi-square test
Woman's socioeconomic level						
Familial situation	(n = 81,062)			(n = 10,769)		
Married or cohabiting	97.9	55.2	188.4[a]	97.7	75.5	58.9[a]
Single	2.1	38.4		2.3	54.2	
Healthcare coverage	(n = 80,889)			(n = 10,724)		
Insured	98.5	55.1	35.0[a]	98.4	75.3	8.2[a]
Uninsured	1.5	46.6		1.6	65.9	
Education	(n = 65,006)			(n = 8673)		
Primary school	2.7	21.9	4200.0[a]	1.4	38.8	602.3[a]
Some secondary school	13.8	32.7		10.4	51.9	
Completed secondary school	21.7	45.0		21.1	64.3	
College or university	61.8	63.3		67.1	82.2	
Occupation	(n = 57,115)			(n = 7906)		
Manual worker	1.3	35.4	1100.0[a]	1.0	60.8	217.6[a]
Office, sales, or service staff	54.7	53.3		58.5	73.7	
Farmer	0.3	40.9		0.2	62.5	
Craft/trades worker or entrepreneur	3.0	56.2		2.7	76.1	
Intermediate (technical)	8.9	59.4		9.2	81.6	
Managerial or higher intellectual	31.8	67.1		28.4	88.5	
Work status	(n = 67,502)			(n = 8977)		
Working	69.8	60.8	3500.0[a]	75.7	80.7	533.5[a]
Unemployed	6.6	47.4		7.5	62.0	
Not in labor force	23.6	34.0		16.8	53.9	
Partner's socioeconomic level						
Occupation	(n = 63,959)			(n = 8454)		
Manual worker	9.1	35.6	2000.0[a]	8.3	57.0	363.7[a]
Office, sales, or service staff	39.7	50.0		44.2	71.1	
Farmer	0.4	43.3		0.3	70.8	
Craft/trades worker or entrepreneur	7.3	51.5		6.5	74.6	
Intermediate (technical)	5.9	58.5		6.7	81.1	
Managerial or higher intellectual	37.6	64.4		34.0	86.3	
Work status	(n = 64,121)			(n = 8606)		
Working	89.9	56.3	688.3[a]	89.9	77.5	149.5[a]
Unemployed	4.3	37.5		3.9	57.9	
Not in labor force	5.8	40.5		6.2	59.2	

The full sample is composed of all live deliveries performed in the hospitals of the French administrative district of Yvelines in 2008–2014. The low-risk subsample only includes those deliveries of nulliparous women aged 20–34 years, without any diagnosis or co-morbidity, giving birth at full term, by vaginal delivery, without induction, to a singleton infant in cephalic presentation, and with a normal birth weight

[a] = 1% significance level

women who undergo 3 or fewer ultrasounds. Women with no nuchal translucency scan or no morphologic ultrasound have significantly lower cesarean delivery rates, respectively 21.1% and 17%. Women who do not attend an early prenatal interview have a cesarean delivery rate of 23.7%, significantly higher than the 22.3% rate for women who do. Similarly, the cesarean delivery rate for women not attending prenatal education is significantly higher: 24.9% versus 21.9% for those who did. In the subsample of low-risk women, the only difference according to prenatal care use that remains significant in the cesarean delivery rates for this subsample is that based on participation in prenatal education.

Table 1 also shows the variations in the cesarean delivery rates as a function of the socioeconomic characteristics of the women and their partners. Available socioeconomic data apply the official socioeconomic classification of the French national institute of statistics and economic studies (Institut National de la Statistique et des Etudes Economiques (INSEE)) and thus identify the socioeconomic level of each household accurately. The cesarean delivery rates do not differ significantly by family situation or healthcare coverage. However, women with lower educational levels have significantly higher rates of cesarean deliveries: 24.9% for those who only completed primary school, 25.2% for those who did some secondary school, and 25.4% for those who did complete secondary school (i.e., women having reached the final year of secondary school, whether or not they obtained the baccalaureate degree), while the most highly educated women (i.e., post-secondary education) have a cesarean delivery rate of only 22.8%. Similarly, this rate is significantly higher among women working jobs requiring lower skills: 26.7% for manual workers and 24.9% for office, sales, or service staff; compared with higher skills: 23.4% for intermediate (i.e., technical and associate professional) occupations, and 22.7% for managers and higher intellectual workers. The cesarean delivery rate is 25.1% for unemployed women but 24% for working patients. The number of cesarean deliveries also differs according to the partner's socioeconomic level. Cesarean delivery rates are significantly higher for women whose partners are not working: 24.9% for women with partners that are not in the labor force (i.e., students, apprentices, homemakers, retirees, those on parental leave, and others neither working nor looking for work), and 24.7% when partners are unemployed, whereas 23.6% when partners are working; or have low-skilled jobs: more than 24% when partners have low-skilled jobs, while around 23% when partners have a high-skilled occupation. Moreover, the preliminary statistics for the low-risk subsample are similar, which means epidemiologic factors alone do not explain the socioeconomic factors affecting cesarean delivery use.

As shown above, the only cesarean rates that differ significantly in both the full and low-risk subsamples are those related to participation in prenatal education (Table 1). Moreover, nearly half the women in our entire population do not participate in this care (Table 1). We present these participation rates according to socioeconomic characteristics in Table 2. Single women have a significantly lower participation rate: 38.4% compared

with 55.2%. Similarly, uninsured patients participate significantly less often, at rates of 46.6% versus 55.1%, as do women with lower versus higher educational levels. Prenatal education participation rates are 21.9% for women with a primary school education, 32.7% for those with some secondary education, 45% for those who did complete secondary school, and 63.3% for those with some post-secondary education. Similarly, low-skilled women participate at significantly lower rates: 35.4% for manual workers, 40.9% for farmers, and 53.3% for office, sales, or service staff, but 67.1% for women in managerial and higher intellectual/professional occupations. Women out of (versus in) the labor market have significantly lower rates of prenatal education participation: 34% for women not in the labor force, 47.4% for those unemployed, while 60.8% for working women. Results are similar for partners: participation is significantly lower when the partner is not working nor has a low-skilled job. Specifically, the prenatal education participation rate is 35.6% when partners are manual workers, 43.3% when farmers, and 50% when office, sales, or service staff, but 64.4% when they have managerial and higher intellectual occupations; 37.5% and 40.5% when partners are unemployed and out of the labor force, respectively, while 56.3% when they work. The same disparities in prenatal education participation according to socioeconomic variables appear in the low-risk subsample.

Regression results

We present, first, the effects of regular prenatal care on the cesarean delivery rate. Controlling for epidemiologic and hospital characteristics in columns 1 and 2 of Table 3, we find that prenatal care utilization affects the probability of cesarean deliveries. The period of the first prenatal clinical visit does not affect this probability. Ultrasound care does, however: women undergoing more than 3 ultrasounds have a 31% higher probability of cesarean deliveries. The nuchal translucency ultrasound does not appear to affect cesarean delivery rates. However, women who do not have the morphologic ultrasound have a cesarean delivery probability 25% lower than those who do. Interestingly, women who do not participate in prenatal education are 33% more likely to have cesarean deliveries, although attendance at the early prenatal interview has no clear effect on this probability. When we use the subsample with available socioeconomic variables, which enables us to take these characteristics into account, the results are the same, in both hospital fixed and random effects specifications (columns 5 and 6 of Table 3).

Table 3 Effects of prenatal care and socioeconomic status on cesarean delivery use, logit model 1 (odds ratios)

	Full sample						Low-risk subsample			
	(1)	(2)	(3)	(4)	(5)	(6)	(7)	(8)	(9)	(10)
Prenatal care										
First prenatal visit										
Second trimester	1.10 (0.129)	1.09 (0.129)			1.06 (0.174)	1.05 (0.169)	1.75[c] (0.509)	1.67[c] (0.464)	1.40 (0.573)	1.34 (0.524)
Third trimester	1.06 (0.252)	1.05 (0.249)			0.46 (0.259)	0.46 (0.258)	1.92 (1.379)	1.93 (1.386)	2.24 (1.528)	2.27 (1.543)
Obstetric ultrasounds										
< 3	1.02 (0.062)	1.02 (0.061)			1.05 (0.190)	1.05 (0.190)	1.04 (0.329)	1.06 (0.337)	0.87 (0.326)	0.88 (0.334)
≥ 4	1.31[a] (0.057)	1.31[a] (0.058)			1.32[a] (0.090)	1.32[a] (0.091)	1.12 (0.113)	1.11 (0.110)	1.10 (0.121)	1.09 (0.118)
No nuchal translucency ultrasound	0.98 (0.076)	0.99 (0.074)			0.96 (0.130)	0.97 (0.129)	0.95 (0.293)	1.00 (0.289)	1.01 (0.355)	1.06 (0.345)
No morphology ultrasound	0.75[b] (0.108)	0.75[b] (0.108)			0.69[a] (0.076)	0.69[a] (0.076)	0.82 (0.221)	0.78 (0.205)	0.71 (0.235)	0.67 (0.218)
No early prenatal interview	1.06[b] (0.049)	1.06 (0.049)			1.05 (0.048)	1.05 (0.047)	1.00 (0.079)	1.01 (0.077)	0.97 (0.093)	0.98 (0.092)
No prenatal education	1.33[a] (0.022)	1.33[a] (0.022)			1.39[a] (0.038)	1.39[a] (0.038)	1.25[a] (0.068)	1.26[a] (0.062)	1.22[b] (0.098)	1.22[a] (0.092)
Woman's socioeconomic level										
Single			0.77[a] (0.071)	0.77[a] (0.072)	0.72[c] (0.129)	0.72[c] (0.131)	0.44[a] (0.113)	0.44[a] (0.115)	0.48[a] (0.119)	0.48[a] (0.122)
Uninsured			1.06 (0.078)	1.06 (0.078)	1.10 (0.094)	1.10 (0.094)	0.91 (0.306)	0.92 (0.311)	0.67 (0.247)	0.68 (0.251)
Education										
Primary school			1.23[c] (0.140)	1.22[c] (0.141)	1.19 (0.172)	1.19 (0.173)	1.45 (0.578)	1.45 (0.582)	1.47 (0.603)	1.46 (0.595)
Some secondary school			1.33[a] (0.059)	1.33[a] (0.059)	1.29[a] (0.083)	1.29[a] (0.084)	1.34[b] (0.161)	1.35[b] (0.164)	1.32[b] (0.151)	1.34[b] (0.155)
Completed secondary school			1.29[a] (0.039)	1.29[a] (0.039)	1.24[a] (0.035)	1.24[a] (0.034)	1.27[a] (0.081)	1.28[a] (0.084)	1.29[a] (0.082)	1.30[a] (0.085)
Occupation										
Manual worker			1.26[a] (0.097)	1.26[a] (0.097)	1.33[a] (0.131)	1.33[a] (0.131)	1.55 (0.492)	1.55 (0.495)	1.47 (0.553)	1.50 (0.570)
Office, sales, or service staff			1.13[a] (0.042)	1.13[a] (0.042)	1.12[a] (0.041)	1.12[a] (0.041)	1.14[c] (0.080)	1.14[c] (0.081)	1.12[c] (0.072)	1.12[c] (0.071)
Farmer			1.24 (0.455)	1.25 (0.457)	1.03 (0.426)	1.04 (0.431)	1.29 (0.877)	1.32 (0.892)	1.80 (1.186)	1.82 (1.194)
Craft/trades worker or entrepreneur			1.10 (0.080)	1.10 (0.080)	1.14[c] (0.090)	1.14[c] (0.090)	1.16 (0.281)	1.15 (0.275)	1.18 (0.354)	1.17 (0.347)
Intermediate (technical)			1.13[a] (0.052)	1.13[a] (0.052)	1.13[c] (0.075)	1.13[c] (0.074)	1.19[a] (0.058)	1.20[a] (0.064)	1.25[a] (0.078)	1.26[a] (0.085)
Work status										
Unemployed			1.14[b] (0.066)	1.14[b] (0.066)	1.14[c] (0.080)	1.14[c] (0.080)	0.81 (0.111)	0.81 (0.114)	0.74[b] (0.099)	0.74[b] (0.101)
Not in labor force			0.94 (0.041)	0.94 (0.041)	0.91 (0.058)	0.91 (0.058)	1.01 (0.111)	1.01 (0.108)	1.01 (0.113)	1.01 (0.116)

Table 3 Effects of prenatal care and socioeconomic status on cesarean delivery use, logit model 1 (odds ratios) *(Continued)*

	Full sample						Low-risk subsample			
	(1)	(2)	(3)	(4)	(5)	(6)	(7)	(8)	(9)	(10)
Partner's socioeconomic level										
Occupation										
Manual worker			1.15[a]	1.15[a]	1.08	1.08				
			(0.057)	(0.057)	(0.067)	(0.067)				
Office, sales, or service staff			1.13[a]	1.13[a]	1.11[a]	1.11[a]				
			(0.033)	(0.033)	(0.043)	(0.043)				
Farmer			1.06	1.06	1.05	1.05				
			(0.218)	(0.217)	(0.273)	(0.271)				
Craft/trades worker or entrepreneur			1.10	1.10	1.06	1.06				
			(0.075)	(0.074)	(0.087)	(0.086)				
Intermediate (technical)			1.07	1.07	1.09	1.09				
			(0.054)	(0.055)	(0.095)	(0.096)				
Work status										
Unemployed			1.01	1.01	1.11	1.11				
			(0.080)	(0.080)	(0.114)	(0.115)				
Not in labor force			1.17[a]	1.17[a]	1.12[b]	1.12[b]				
			(0.050)	(0.050)	(0.064)	(0.064)				
Epidemiologic controls	Yes	Yes	Yes	Yes	Yes	Yes	No	No	No	No
Hospital controls	Yes	Yes	Yes	Yes	Yes	Yes	Yes	Yes	Yes	Yes
Year fixed effects	Yes	Yes	Yes	Yes	Yes	Yes	Yes	Yes	Yes	Yes
Hospital effects	Fixed	Random	Fixed	Random	Fixed	Random	Fixed	Random	Fixed	Random
Residence fixed effects	No	No	No	No	No	No	No	No	Yes	Yes
N (observations)	68,314	68,314	58,324	58,324	41,141	41,141	9507	9507	8020	8020

Columns 1–6 use the full sample of women while columns 7–10 use the subsample of low-risk women (nulliparous, aged 20–34 years, without any diagnosis or co-morbidity, giving birth at full term, during labor, without induction, to a singleton infant in cephalic presentation, and with a normal birth weight). Epidemiologic control variables include woman's demographics (age and parity) and medical risk factors (previous cesarean, diabetes, hypertension, eclampsia or preeclampsia, fetal growth restriction, placental bleeding, other obstetric pathology, plurality, term at delivery, fetal presentation, induced labor, and birth weight). Hospital control variables include hospital type (ownership status, equipment level, and teaching status), organization (day of delivery, obstetrician availability, and size), and staff (midwives, obstetricians, and anesthetists in FTEs per bed). Hospital invariant control variables (ownership status, equipment level, and teaching status) are only included in regressions with hospital random effects. Robust standard errors in parentheses
[a] = 1% significance level, [b] = 5%, [c] = 10%

Table 3 also shows in columns 3 and 4 the effects of the socioeconomic status of each partner on the use of cesarean deliveries while controlling for epidemiologic and hospital characteristics. Familial situation has a significant effect: single women are 23% more likely to have a cesarean delivery compared to those who do not. Insurance coverage, however, does not affect this probability. More interestingly, compared with the most highly educated women, patients with primary, some secondary, or completed secondary education are respectively 22–23%, 33% and 29% more likely to have a cesarean delivery. Similarly, women working at low-skilled jobs have a higher probability of cesarean deliveries: compared with the most highly qualified women, this probability is 26% higher for manual workers, and 13% higher for office, sales, or service staff as well as for workers with intermediate occupations. Moreover, unemployed women have a probability of a cesarean delivery 14% higher than that of working women. Likewise, the partner's socioeconomic level affects the

woman's probability of a cesarean delivery, which is 15% higher for women whose partners are manual workers, and 13% higher when they are service workers. This probability is 17% higher when the partner is not in the labor force, versus is working. Adjustment for hospitals' fixed or random effects does not change these results, which are similar even in the subsample with available prenatal care variables (columns 5 and 6 of Table 3). According to our study, low socioeconomic status significantly and substantially increases the probability of cesarean deliveries. Our results are therefore consistent with the previous literature from high-income countries, as detailed above in the Introduction.

Table 6 in Appendix presents the effects of the epidemiologic and hospital control variables on cesarean delivery use. Many epidemiologic control risk factors are significantly associated with a higher probability of cesarean deliveries: age, nulliparity, previous cesarean, diabetes, hypertension, eclampsia or preeclampsia, fetal growth restriction, placental bleeding, other obstetric pathology, preterm and post-term delivery, abnormal presentation, induced labor, low and high birth weight; as are some hospital control characteristics: private ownership status, high equipment level, working-day delivery, low hospital size, and low FTE obstetricians per bed. As expected, the effects of these variables are similar to those found in previous studies.

Our results clearly demonstrate that, all else being equal, both prenatal care and socioeconomic position influence the cesarean decision. Because the data have been anonymized, women are not identifiable within the study period. We cannot thus use the fixed effects for women that would allow us to control for the unobservable heterogeneity between them, which may correlate with cesarean delivery use and either prenatal care utilization or socioeconomic status. However, we do control for many observed characteristics of women and their partners. Furthermore, we also performed several additional sensitivity analyses to consider potential relevant confounding factors. First, one natural and straightforward explanation of our results might be the epidemiologic factors: the low-income women and those with high utilization rates of ultrasound care or low rates of prenatal educational care may also be the at-risk population. For example, women with various epidemiologic risk factors require more obstetric ultrasounds than traditionally recommended. Furthermore, the low-income population is also the population most at risk in terms of co-morbidity and diagnosis. As a robustness check, we examine the low-risk subsample to further control for medical severity (see details on the low-risk subsample for cesarean delivery use above in the Methods). These results are presented in columns 7 and 8 of Table 3. In this subsample with fewer observations, we include woman's socioeconomic characteristics only, to avoid the consequences of the very likely collinearity between the socioeconomic variables of the woman and her partner on the efficiency of the estimates. When we focus on low-risk women, the effects of the obstetric ultrasound care are no longer significant, but the effects of prenatal education remain significantly associated with a higher probability of a cesarean delivery for nonparticipants. In addition, the woman's socioeconomic position has the same effects on the cesarean delivery probability in this subsample as in the overall population: the lower the socioeconomic indicator, the higher the cesarean delivery rate. Using the partner's socioeconomic variables produces similar findings (Table 7 in Appendix).

Woman's preferences are another important factor to consider: those who choose to undergo substantial ultrasonographic examinations as well as those who prefer not to attend prenatal education may also prefer a cesarean delivery. To control for the woman's preference, we can use unplanned deliveries, assuming that if the woman has a preference for a cesarean delivery, the obstetrician would plan this. The data available here do not provide any information about women's preferences. This assumption can be debated, but appears reasonable to us. The existing literature reports that women's preferences affect the rates of elective cesarean deliveries [19, 46–48]. Reasons identified as influencing a woman's decision to request an elective cesarean delivery include cultural factors, fear of pain during labor and delivery, previous experience, and interactions with health care professionals [47]. The woman's choice can be a primary indication for planned elective cesarean deliveries, but is not an indication for those that are not planned [48].

Unplanned deliveries also include only deliveries for which the patient did not know her mode of delivery in advance. Because most women still perceive prenatal education simply as preparation for vaginal delivery, women with a planned cesarean delivery may choose not to attend. Focusing on unplanned deliveries may thus control for these two factors. Columns 7 and 8 of Table 3 report the effects of prenatal care utilization on cesarean delivery use in the low-risk subsample that includes only unplanned deliveries. Even when the mode of delivery is not planned, prenatal education is still a highly significant variable. Therefore, neither women's preference nor their advance knowledge of their mode of delivery explains the effects of prenatal education on cesarean deliveries.

Furthermore, income level is a factor that explains woman's access to prenatal care [25, 49], and women with low socioeconomic positions may face constraints in their access to health care that may explain their high use of cesarean deliveries. Since no healthcare access variable is available in our data, we use the woman's town of residence, available for some observations. We do not include town of residence fixed effects in the first regressions because this variable is not available for all observations. Columns 9 and 10 of Table 3 show the effects of socioeconomic status on the probability of a cesarean delivery for low-risk women, with dummy variables included for town of residence. Cesarean delivery is still most prevalent for women with low, compared with high, socioeconomic status. We therefore cannot interpret lack of access to obstetric care as the explanation for the effects of socioeconomic status on cesarean delivery use. Moreover, including fixed effects for town of residence also allows us to control for area-based socioeconomic differences. Individual and area-based socioeconomic conditions are different aspects of socioeconomic position, and both dimensions may affect the probability of a cesarean delivery [50]. Indeed, individual socioeconomic characteristics may capture some effects of area-based socioeconomic conditions, as women with low socioeconomic positions mostly live in less affluent areas. When we include dummy variables for the woman's town of residence, the effects of socioeconomic status on the probability of cesarean deliveries persist. Individual socioeconomic status is thus an independent socioeconomic factor affecting cesarean delivery rates. The results are again the same even when we use the partner's socioeconomic characteristics (Table 7 in Appendix).

Because prenatal education participation significantly affects cesarean deliveries, we sought to assess in column 1 of Table 4 whether or not socioeconomic conditions affect its utilization during pregnancy, while taking epidemiologic characteristics into account. Familial situation and healthcare coverage do not significantly affect the probability of this participation, but educational level does. Specifically, compared to the women with the most education, the probability of attendance at prenatal education for those with primary schooling only, some secondary school, and who completed secondary school is respectively 47%, 42%, and 27% lower. Likewise, the women with the fewest skills are least likely to participate in prenatal education. Compared with the managers (i.e., the most highly skilled women), women who are crafts/trades workers or entrepreneurs are 13% less likely to participate, and those working as office, sales, or service staff 11% less likely. Further, compared with working women, those who are not in the labor force as well as unemployed ones are respectively 29% and 14% less likely to participate. The same is true for women whose partners have low-skilled jobs or do not work: the probability of participation is 26% lower when the partner is a manual worker or a farmer, and 15% lower if he is an office, sales, or service worker, as well as 26% lower if unemployed, and 22% lower if he is not in the labor force.

Table 8 in Appendix presents the effects of the epidemiologic control variables on prenatal education participation. Several epidemiologic control factors are significantly associated with a lower probability of prenatal education attendance: younger and older age, multiparity, diabetes, fetal growth restriction, other obstetric pathology, preterm delivery, non-spontaneous onset of labor, cesarean delivery, and low birth weight.

Again, to better control for differences in epidemiologic characteristics that may explain these findings, we perform the same estimates in the low-risk subsample (see details on the low-risk subsample for prenatal care participation above in the Methods). The results are presented in column 2 of Table 4. When we focus on low-risk patients, women in low socioeconomic positions remain less likely to participate in prenatal education.

Moreover, we also include the woman's town of residence as a fixed effect in column 3 of Table 4, which made it possible to take geographic differences across women into account, including those related to health care access and to area-based socioeconomic status. Indeed, individual socioeconomic variables can capture disparities in healthcare access as well as the variables based on area-based socioeconomic conditions. Our finding show that, regardless of differences in prenatal care access and area-based socioeconomic situation, women with low, compared with high, socioeconomic status are less likely to use prenatal education. Results using partner's socioeconomic variables are very similar (Table 9 in Appendix).

Because our results show that socioeconomic status significantly affects prenatal education participation (Table 4), we went on to examine the effects of interaction terms for both of these variables on cesarean delivery use. We thus study whether or not the effects of prenatal education vary by socioeconomic status, which we are unable to study from the results of Table 3. For each occupation, we seek to compare the impact of socioeconomic status on those with and without prenatal education. Therefore, we add dummy variables for prenatal education crossed with the dummy variables for the woman's occupation, as well as dummy variables for no prenatal education crossed with the dummy variables for the woman's occupation. This exclude from the regression the global effects of prenatal education and of occupation type; when we consider all types of occupation and the constant, however, it introduce a strict collinearity problem. We therefore include a constraint in the model: the sum of all the crossed occupation and prenatal education variables equals 0. The results are presented as odds ratios. Table 10 in Appendix provides the results as coefficients. This model also enables us to answer the question: Do the effects of prenatal education vary for different occupation types? We do so by comparing the coefficient values between different occupation types crossed with prenatal education. Table 5 reports the results for model 1 with the variables described here. In low and intermediate occupational category (manual workers, office, sales, or service staff, and intermediate (technical) occupations), the women who do not participate in prenatal education are more likely to have cesarean deliveries than those who do participate. Moreover, in response to the question of whether the effects of prenatal education vary for different occupation types, we see that for managerial or higher intellectual occupations as well as intermediate (technical) occupations, prenatal education has a negative cumulative effect with socioeconomic status on the probability of cesarean deliveries (compared to the average effect of the sample). Interaction terms for prenatal education and other available socioeconomic variables

Table 4 Effects of socioeconomic status on prenatal education utilization, logit model 2 (odds ratios)

	Full sample	Low-risk subsample	
	(1)	(2)	(3)
Woman's socioeconomic level			
Single	1.07	0.52[a]	0.50[a]
	(0.134)	(0.087)	(0.088)
Uninsured	1.06	1.37	1.34
	(0.111)	(0.475)	(0.578)
Education			
Primary school	0.53[a]	0.61	0.72
	(0.106)	(0.189)	(0.221)
Some secondary school	0.58[a]	0.43[a]	0.45[a]
	(0.054)	(0.088)	(0.117)
Completed secondary school	0.73[a]	0.62[a]	0.60[a]
	(0.038)	(0.086)	(0.098)
Occupation			
Manual worker	0.90	0.63	0.45
	(0.128)	(0.279)	(0.231)
Office, sales, or service staff	0.89[a]	0.65[a]	0.63[a]
	(0.023)	(0.041)	(0.049)
Farmer	0.75	0.49	0.51
	(0.170)	(0.358)	(0.382)
Craft/trades worker or entrepreneur	0.87[a]	0.58[a]	0.60[a]
	(0.046)	(0.062)	(0.081)
Intermediate (technical)	0.94	0.84	0.77[c]
	(0.061)	(0.152)	(0.118)
Work status			
Unemployed	0.86[a]	0.77[c]	0.80[c]
	(0.032)	(0.107)	(0.095)
Not in labor force	0.71[a]	0.57[a]	0.62[a]
	(0.034)	(0.043)	(0.080)
Partner's socioeconomic level			
Occupation			
Manual worker	0.74[a]		
	(0.050)		
Office, sales, or service staff	0.85[a]		
	(0.027)		
Farmer	0.74[b]		
	(0.109)		
Craft/trades worker or entrepreneur	0.91[c]		
	(0.045)		
Intermediate (technical)	0.92[b]		
	(0.039)		
Work status			
Unemployed	0.74[a]		
	(0.051)		
Not in labor force	0.78[a]		
	(0.052)		
Epidemiologic controls	Yes	No	No
Year fixed effects	Yes	Yes	Yes

Table 4 Effects of socioeconomic status on prenatal education utilization, logit model 2 (odds ratios) *(Continued)*

	Full sample	Low-risk subsample	
	(1)	(2)	(3)
Hospital effects	Fixed	Fixed	Fixed
Residence fixed effects	No	No	Yes
N (observations)	48,042	7064	6033

Column 1 uses the full sample of women while columns 2 and 3 use the subsample of low-risk women (nulliparous, aged 20–34 years, without any diagnosis or co-morbidity, giving birth at full term, by vaginal delivery, without induction, to a singleton infant in cephalic presentation, and with a normal birth weight). Epidemiologic control variables include woman's demographics (age and parity) and medical factors (previous cesarean, diabetes, hypertension, eclampsia or preeclampsia, fetal growth restriction, placental bleeding, other obstetric pathology, plurality, term at delivery, fetal presentation, onset of labor, mode of delivery, and birth weight). Robust standard errors in parentheses
[a] = 1% significance level, [b] = 5%, [c] = 10%

yield the same results (Table 11 in the Appendix presents the results as odds ratios. However, the results as coefficients are available upon request).

Discussion

We investigate a rarely studied question in this paper: how patient care throughout pregnancy affects mode of delivery. We use a rich and large database of delivery information for the years 2008–2014, which allows us to take many patient- and hospital-level characteristics that may affect obstetric practices into account. We estimate multilevel logit models, first to study the effects of prenatal care on cesarean delivery and then to assess whether socioeconomic status influences prenatal care and specifically participation in prenatal education, which appears to affect mode of delivery significantly.

Our primary results show that prenatal education affects cesarean delivery rates. The probability of a cesarean delivery increases by 20 to 40% for women who do not participate in prenatal education. Two mechanisms may explain this finding. On the one hand, prenatal education may improve women's knowledge about mode of delivery. Several studies report that women are not aware of the risks and benefits of birth procedures, and that this lack of knowledge results in some of them choosing cesarean rather than vaginal delivery [51, 52]. Indeed, a substantial proportion of women continue to consider the cesarean as the safest method of delivery, especially for the child, even though epidemiologic studies demonstrate conclusively that cesarean, compared to vaginal, deliveries increase maternal morbidity in this and future pregnancies and do not improve infant health. On the other hand, prenatal education may have positive psychological effects on pregnant women, who are often anxious about giving birth. Indeed, fear of childbirth is strongly associated with performance of cesarean deliveries [53].

Table 5 Effects of prenatal care and socioeconomic status on cesarean delivery use, interaction terms for prenatal care and socioeconomic status, logit model 1 (odds ratios)

	(1)	(2)
Crossed dummy variables for woman's occupation and prenatal education participation		
Manual worker × No prenatal education	1.28[b] (0.131)	1.28[b] (0.130)
Manual worker × Prenatal education	1.16 (0.196)	1.16 (0.198)
Office, sales, or service staff × No prenatal education	1.16[c] (0.097)	1.16[c] (0.097)
Office, sales, or service staff × Prenatal education	0.86[c] (0.069)	0.85[c] (0.069)
Farmer × No prenatal education	1.10 (0.621)	1.11 (0.629)
Farmer × Prenatal education	0.76 (0.227)	0.76 (0.228)
Craft/trades worker or entrepreneur × No prenatal education	1.11 (0.187)	1.11 (0.187)
Craft/trades worker or entrepreneur × Prenatal education	0.91 (0.131)	0.90 (0.131)
Intermediate (technical) occupation × No prenatal education	1.20[b] (0.102)	1.20[b] (0.101)
Intermediate (technical) occupation × Prenatal education	0.84[a] (0.050)	0.84[a] (0.050)
Managerial or higher intellectual occupation × No prenatal education	1.10 (0.067)	1.10 (0.066)
Managerial or higher intellectual occupation × Prenatal education	0.74[a] (0.060)	0.74[a] (0.059)
Epidemiologic and hospital controls	Yes	Yes
Other prenatal care and socioeconomic variables	Yes	Yes
Year fixed effects	Yes	Yes
Hospital effects	Fixed	Random
N (observations)	41,141	41,141

All regressions use the full sample of women and include a constraint: the sum of all the crossed variables equals 0. Epidemiologic control variables include woman's demographics (age and parity) and medical risk factors (previous cesarean, diabetes, hypertension, eclampsia or preeclampsia, fetal growth restriction, placental bleeding, other obstetric pathology, plurality, term at delivery, fetal presentation, induced labor, and birth weight). Hospital control variables include hospital type (ownership status, equipment level, and teaching status), organization (day of delivery, obstetrician availability, and size), and staff (midwives, obstetricians, and anesthetists in FTEs per bed). Hospital invariant control variables (ownership status, equipment level, and teaching status) are only included in the regression with hospital random effects. Other prenatal care variables are trimester of the first antenatal visit, number of obstetric ultrasounds, nuchal translucency ultrasound, morphology ultrasound, and early prenatal interview. Other socioeconomic variables include woman's familial situation, healthcare coverage, education and work status, and her partner's occupation and work status. Robust standard errors in parentheses
[a] = 1% significance level, [b] = 5%, [c] = 10%

Since a significant proportion of obstetricians are willing to proceed with a cesarean delivery if requested [54, 55], the woman's choice is an important determinant of cesarean deliveries to consider: the number of patient-request cesarean deliveries is currently estimated at 4–18% of the total [56]. Women attending prenatal education may be more aware of the risks of cesarean deliveries and less affected by fear of giving birth, and may therefore ask less often for a cesarean delivery. Moreover, a well-informed patient is likely to be better able to respond to the information she receives from the obstetrician and to participate in the decision process about method of delivery than someone less informed. This may affect physician and hospital incentives to perform more cesarean deliveries.

Moreover, we find that socioeconomic status influences uptake of prenatal education. Using several individual socioeconomic indicators, our results confirm that low socioeconomic women are more likely to have cesarean deliveries and further show that women in this subgroup have a lower probability of participating in prenatal education. For example, compared to the women with the most education, women who have no postsecondary schooling have at least a 20% lower probability of attendance at prenatal education. The problem of socioeconomic disparities in method of delivery is the focus of much attention, especially in view of the difficulty in modifying socioeconomic differences by public policy interventions. Since utilization of prenatal education may be a factor substantially more susceptible to change, our finding is of interest.

In order to address the possible individual level self-selection into prenatal education participation, our empirical model includes a large set of available covariates. We also perform several robustness analyses that allow many potential confounding factors to be taken into account. However, we cannot fully control for all differences between women who choose to attend prenatal education and women who do not, including in their risk for cesarean delivery. Hence, our results do not allow any causal inferences. Future research exploring the effect of implementation or promotion of such care programs on mode of delivery is thus highly recommended. If our observed associations are confirmed to be causal, a straightforward implication would be that public policies promoting participation rates for prenatal education and targeting this promotion primarily at low-income women could lead to real reductions in cesarean delivery rates.

Conclusion

Overall, our analysis reinforces recent economic studies reporting that support of patient decision-making may impact the use of medical services substantially. Previous efforts to limit inappropriate medical care has mainly targeted providers, for instance, by reducing benefits or restricting eligibility, but has encountered serious political difficulties. Patient education may have an important impact on limiting medical overuse.

Appendix

Table 6 Effects of epidemiologic and hospital factors on cesarean delivery use, logit model 1 (odds ratios)

	(1)	(2)	(3)	(4)	(5)	(6)
Patient demographics						
Age (years)	1.05[a] (0.002)	1.05[a] (0.002)	1.06[a] (0.003)	1.06[a] (0.003)	1.06[a] (0.002)	1.06[a] (0.002)
Nulliparous	3.57[a] (0.283)	3.57[a] (0.283)	3.34[a] (0.250)	3.33[a] (0.250)	3.82[a] (0.277)	3.81[a] (0.277)
Medical risk factors						
Previous cesarean	20.60[a] (1.934)	20.59[a] (1.928)	21.75[a] (2.560)	21.73[a] (2.548)	22.06[a] (2.448)	22.03[a] (2.436)
Diabetes	1.37[a] (0.080)	1.37[a] (0.081)	1.26[b] (0.130)	1.26[b] (0.130)	1.26[a] (0.107)	1.26[a] (0.107)
Hypertension	1.91[a] (0.116)	1.91[a] (0.115)	1.67[a] (0.151)	1.67[a] (0.151)	1.75[a] (0.176)	1.75[a] (0.175)
Eclampsia or preeclampsia	3.59[a] (0.279)	3.59[a] (0.280)	3.63[a] (0.631)	3.63[a] (0.631)	4.22[a] (0.568)	4.23[a] (0.570)
Fetal growth restriction	1.80[a] (0.254)	1.80[a] (0.254)	2.18[a] (0.529)	2.18[a] (0.529)	2.10[a] (0.483)	2.11[a] (0.484)
Placental bleeding	10.49[a] (3.541)	10.52[a] (3.545)	11.67[a] (3.684)	11.73[a] (3.682)	13.42[a] (4.661)	13.46[a] (4.657)
Other obstetric pathology	0.98 (0.028)	0.98 (0.028)	1.08[a] (0.030)	1.08[a] (0.029)	1.03 (0.035)	1.03 (0.035)
Multiple delivery	1.11 (0.187)	1.11 (0.187)	1.31 (0.242)	1.30 (0.242)	1.24 (0.230)	1.24 (0.230)
Term at delivery						
Preterm (< 37 weeks of gestation)	1.39[a] (0.143)	1.39[a] (0.143)	1.37[a] (0.129)	1.38[a] (0.129)	1.27[b] (0.155)	1.27[b] (0.154)
Post-term (> 41 weeks of gestation)	2.38[a] (0.547)	2.40[a] (0.549)	3.18[a] (0.629)	3.19[a] (0.625)	2.89[a] (0.681)	2.90[a] (0.679)
Abnormal presentation (Breech or transverse)	33.19[a] (4.784)	33.17[a] (4.777)	33.99[a] (4.554)	33.97[a] (4.546)	36.40[a] (6.517)	36.37[a] (6.498)
Induced labor	1.16[b] (0.088)	1.16[b] (0.088)	1.15[c] (0.093)	1.15[c] (0.093)	1.14[c] (0.090)	1.14[c] (0.090)
Birth weight						
Low birth weight (< 2500 g)	1.69[a] (0.095)	1.69[a] (0.095)	1.65[a] (0.094)	1.65[a] (0.094)	1.49[a] (0.115)	1.49[a] (0.114)
High birth weight (> 4000 g)	1.95[a] (0.147)	1.95[a] (0.147)	2.08[a] (0.190)	2.08[a] (0.190)	2.07[a] (0.168)	2.07[a] (0.169)
Hospital type						
Private		1.79[b] (0.419)		1.79[a] (0.326)		2.21[a] (0.402)
Level of equipment						
Neonatology unit		1.26[b] (0.137)		1.22[b] (0.110)		1.31[a] (0.124)
Neonatal intensive care unit		1.52[b] (0.318)		1.46[b] (0.246)		1.65[a] (0.245)
Teaching		1.04 (0.162)		1.14 (0.140)		1.17 (0.121)
Hospital organization						
Non-working day delivery (weekend or holiday)	0.61[a] (0.029)	0.61[a] (0.029)	0.59[a] (0.029)	0.59[a] (0.029)	0.60[a] (0.032)	0.60[a] (0.032)
On-call obstetrician outside the unit	1.13 (0.105)	0.95 (0.099)	1.26[b] (0.126)	1.04 (0.106)	1.17 (0.123)	0.88 (0.095)
Size						
< 1000 deliveries per year	0.99 (0.043)	1.04 (0.050)	0.83[a] (0.033)	1.02 (0.117)	1.17[a] (0.044)	1.25[c] (0.145)
≥ 2000 deliveries per year	0.93[c] (0.038)	0.92[b] (0.035)	0.94 (0.045)	0.93[c] (0.039)	0.91[b] (0.040)	0.90[a] (0.034)
Hospital staff						
Midwives (FTEs per bed)	0.87 (0.104)	0.87 (0.097)	0.89 (0.132)	0.90 (0.126)	0.88 (0.124)	0.91 (0.112)
Obstetricians (FTEs per bed)	0.70 (0.185)	0.68[c] (0.144)	0.57[c] (0.183)	0.57[b] (0.154)	0.69 (0.229)	0.70 (0.172)
Anesthetists (FTEs per bed)	1.25 (0.480)	1.21 (0.386)	1.06 (0.354)	1.06 (0.257)	1.10 (0.450)	1.05 (0.296)
Prenatal care variables	Yes	Yes	No	No	Yes	Yes
Socioeconomic variables	No	No	Yes	Yes	Yes	Yes
Year fixed effects	Yes	Yes	Yes	Yes	Yes	Yes
Hospital effects	Fixed	Random	Fixed	Random	Fixed	Random
N (observations)	68,314	68,314	58,324	58,324	41,141	41,141

All regressions use the full sample of women. Prenatal care variables are trimester of the first antenatal visit, number of obstetric ultrasounds, nuchal translucency ultrasound, morphology ultrasound, early prenatal interview, and prenatal education. Socioeconomic variables include woman's socioeconomic level (familial situation, healthcare coverage, education, occupation, and work status), and her partner's one (occupation and work status). Robust standard errors in parentheses
[a] = 1% significance level, [b] = 5%, [c] = 10%

Table 7 Effects of prenatal care and socioeconomic status on cesarean delivery use, low-risk subsample with partner's socioeconomic variables included, logit model 1 (odds ratios)

	(1)	(2)	(3)	(4)
Prenatal care				
First prenatal visit				
Second trimester	1.09 (0.299)	1.03 (0.271)	0.69 (0.356)	0.67 (0.284)
Third trimester	3.69[b] (1.907)	3.79[a] (1.921)	3.46[b] (1.716)	3.58[a] (1.704)
Obstetric ultrasounds				
< 3	0.83 (0.301)	0.84 (0.307)	0.71 (0.310)	0.72 (0.245)
≥ 4	1.14[c] (0.088)	1.12 (0.087)	1.12 (0.090)	1.10 (0.087)
No nuchal translucency ultrasound	0.89 (0.210)	0.93 (0.202)	0.97 (0.281)	1.01 (0.232)
No morphology ultrasound	0.84 (0.314)	0.80 (0.295)	0.79 (0.327)	0.75 (0.218)
No early prenatal interview	1.01 (0.083)	1.02 (0.079)	0.99 (0.080)	1.01 (0.090)
No prenatal education	1.35[a] (0.082)	1.37[a] (0.084)	1.33[a] (0.112)	1.33[a] (0.088)
Partner's socioeconomic level				
Occupation				
Manual worker	0.99 (0.182)	1.00 (0.187)	0.88 (0.127)	0.89 (0.195)
Office, sales, or service staff	1.09 (0.089)	1.10 (0.090)	1.08 (0.088)	1.08 (0.077)
Farmer	2.14[b] (0.798)	2.14[b] (0.794)	2.57[b] (1.179)	2.56[b] (1.005)
Craft/trades worker or entrepreneur	1.05 (0.121)	1.05 (0.121)	1.01 (0.152)	1.02 (0.142)
Intermediate (technical)	0.78 (0.143)	0.79 (0.142)	0.84 (0.132)	0.85 (0.162)
Work status				
Unemployed	1.44[a] (0.118)	1.43[a] (0.115)	1.60[b] (0.293)	1.60[a] (0.169)
Not in labor force	0.90 (0.081)	0.89 (0.082)	0.88 (0.153)	0.86 (0.096)
Hospital controls	Yes	Yes	Yes	Yes
Year fixed effects	Yes	Yes	Yes	Yes
Hospital effects	Fixed	Random	Fixed	Random
Residence fixed effects	No	No	Yes	Yes
N (observations)	10,732	10,732	9197	9197

All regressions use the subsample of low-risk women (nulliparous, aged 20–34 years, without any diagnosis or co-morbidity, giving birth at full term, during labor, without induction, to a singleton infant in cephalic presentation, and with a normal birth weight). Hospital control variables include hospital type (ownership status, equipment level, and teaching status), organization (day of delivery, obstetrician availability, and size), and staff (midwives, obstetricians, and anesthetists in FTEs per bed). Hospital invariant control variables (ownership status, equipment level, and teaching status) are only included in regressions with hospital random effects. Robust standard errors in parentheses
[a] = 1% significance level, [b] = 5%, [c] = 10%

Table 8 Effects of epidemiologic characteristics on prenatal care utilization, logit model 2 (odds ratios)

	(1)
Patient demographics	
Age	
< 20 years	0.33[a] (0.041)
≥ 35 years	0.94[a] (0.021)
Parity	
= 1	0.26[a] (0.035)
≥ 2	0.14[a] (0.024)
Medical factors	
Previous cesarean	0.96 (0.047)
Diabetes	0.81[a] (0.046)
Hypertension	1.05 (0.126)
Eclampsia or preeclampsia	0.92 (0.114)
Fetal growth restriction	0.83[c] (0.092)
Placental bleeding	1.05 (0.154)
Other obstetric pathology	0.76[a] (0.035)
Multiple delivery	0.97 (0.119)
Term at delivery	
Preterm (< 37 weeks of gestation)	0.64[a] (0.030)
Post-term (> 41 weeks of gestation)	1.08 (0.337)
Abnormal presentation (Breech or transverse)	0.99 (0.128)
Onset of labor	
Induced	0.91[b] (0.036)
Cesarean before labor	0.63[a] (0.016)
Mode of delivery	
Cesarean	0.87[a] (0.030)
Birth weight	
Low birth weight (< 2500 g)	0.80[a] (0.064)
High birth weight (> 4000 g)	1.01 (0.042)
Socioeconomic variables	Yes
Year fixed effects	Yes
Hospital effects	Fixed
N (observations)	48,042

The regression uses the full sample of women. Socioeconomic variables include woman's socioeconomic level (familial situation, healthcare coverage, education, occupation, and work status), and her partner's one (occupation and work status). Robust standard errors in parentheses
[a] = 1% significance level, [b] = 5%, [c] = 10%

Table 9 Effects of socioeconomic status on prenatal education utilization, low-risk subsample with partner's socioeconomic variables included, logit model 2 (odds ratios)

	(1)	(2)
Partner's socioeconomic level		
Occupation		
Manual worker	0.37[a] (0.086)	0.36[a] (0.076)
Office, sales, or service staff	0.53[a] (0.062)	0.53[a] (0.060)
Farmer	0.46[b] (0.156)	0.62 (0.193)
Craft/trades worker or entrepreneur	0.61[b] (0.124)	0.62[b] (0.118)
Intermediate (technical)	0.90 (0.147)	0.90 (0.178)
Work status		
Unemployed	0.61[a] (0.084)	0.63[a] (0.080)
Not in labor force	0.57[a] (0.055)	0.60[a] (0.081)
Year fixed effects	Yes	Yes
Hospital effects	Fixed	Fixed
Residence fixed effects	No	Yes
N (observations)	8083	6977

All regressions use the subsample of low-risk women (nulliparous, aged 20–34 years, without any diagnosis or co-morbidity, giving birth at full term, by vaginal delivery, without induction, to a singleton infant in cephalic presentation, and with a normal birth weight). Robust standard errors in parentheses
[a] = 1% significance level, [b] = 5%

Table 10 Effects of prenatal care and socioeconomic status on cesarean delivery use, interaction terms for prenatal care and socioeconomic status, logit model 1 (coefficients)

	(1)	(2)
Crossed dummy variables for woman's occupation and prenatal education participation		
Manual worker × No prenatal education	0.25^b (0.102)	0.24^b (0.102)
Manual worker × Prenatal education	0.14 (0.170)	0.15 (0.171)
Office, sales, or service staff × No prenatal education	0.15^c (0.084)	0.15^c (0.083)
Office, sales, or service staff × Prenatal education	-0.16^c (0.081)	-0.16^c (0.081)
Farmer × No prenatal education	0.10 (0.565)	0.11 (0.566)
Farmer × Prenatal education	−0.28 (0.301)	− 0.28 (0.300)
Craft/trades worker or entrepreneur × No prenatal education	0.10 (0.169)	0.10 (0.169)
Craft/trades worker or entrepreneur × Prenatal education	−0.10 (0.144)	−0.10 (0.145)
Intermediate (technical) occupation × No prenatal education	0.18^b (0.085)	0.18^b (0.084)
Intermediate (technical) occupation × Prenatal education	-0.17^a (0.060)	-0.18^a (0.060)
Managerial or higher intellectual occupation × No prenatal education	0.09 (0.061)	0.09 (0.060)
Managerial or higher intellectual occupation × Prenatal education	-0.30^a (0.081)	-0.31^a (0.081)
Epidemiologic and hospital controls	Yes	Yes
Other prenatal care and socioeconomic variables	Yes	Yes
Year fixed effects	Yes	Yes
Hospital effects	Fixed	Random
N (observations)	41,141	41,141

All regressions use the full sample of women and include a constraint: the sum of all the crossed variables equals 0. Epidemiologic control variables include woman's demographics (age and parity) and medical risk factors (previous cesarean, diabetes, hypertension, eclampsia or preeclampsia, fetal growth restriction, placental bleeding, other obstetric pathology, plurality, term at delivery, fetal presentation, induced labor, and birth weight). Hospital control variables include hospital type (ownership status, equipment level, and teaching status), organization (day of delivery, obstetrician availability, and size), and staff (midwives, obstetricians, and anesthetists in FTEs per bed). Hospital invariant control variables (ownership status, equipment level, and teaching status) are only included in the regression with hospital random effects. Other prenatal care variables are trimester of the first antenatal visit, number of obstetric ultrasounds, nuchal translucency ultrasound, morphology ultrasound, and early prenatal interview. Other socioeconomic variables include woman's familial situation, healthcare coverage, education and work status, and her partner's occupation and work status. Robust standard errors in parentheses
^{a} = 1% significance level, ^{b} = 5%, ^{c} = 10%

Table 11 Effects of prenatal care and socioeconomic status on cesarean delivery use, further interaction terms for prenatal care and socioeconomic status, logit model 1 (odds ratios)

	(1)	(2)	(3)	(4)	(5)	(6)	(7)	(8)
Crossed dummy variables for woman's education and prenatal education participation								
Primary school × No prenatal education	1.01 (0.137)	1.01 (0.137)						
Primary school × Prenatal education	1.12 (0.278)	1.12 (0.281)						
Some secondary school × No prenatal education	1.16[b] (0.071)	1.16[b] (0.071)						
Some secondary school × Prenatal education	1.03 (0.047)	1.03 (0.047)						
Completed secondary school × No prenatal education	1.14[b] (0.067)	1.14[b] (0.067)						
Completed secondary school × Prenatal education	0.92 (0.051)	0.92 (0.053)						
College or university × No prenatal education	1.03 (0.053)	1.03 (0.052)						
College or university × Prenatal education	0.68[a] (0.023)	0.68[a] (0.023)						
Crossed dummy variables for woman's work status and prenatal education participation								
Unemployed × No prenatal education			1.28[a] (0.083)	1.28[a] (0.084)				
Unemployed × Prenatal education			0.98 (0.079)	0.98 (0.078)				
Not in labor force × No prenatal education			0.95 (0.057)	0.95 (0.056)				
Not in labor force × Prenatal education			0.86 (0.094)	0.87 (0.094)				
Working × No prenatal education			1.19[a] (0.036)	1.19[a] (0.035)				
Working × Prenatal education			0.82[a] (0.019)	0.82[a] (0.019)				
Crossed dummy variables for partner's occupation and prenatal education participation								
Manual worker × No prenatal education					1.11 (0.073)	1.11[c] (0.072)		
Manual worker × Prenatal education					0.94 (0.062)	0.94 (0.063)		
Office, sales, or service staff × No prenatal education					1.22[a] (0.092)	1.22[a] (0.091)		
Office, sales, or service staff × Prenatal education					0.88[a] (0.039)	0.88[a] (0.039)		
Farmer × No prenatal education					1.07 (0.185)	1.06 (0.186)		
Farmer × Prenatal education					0.91 (0.365)	0.90 (0.362)		

Table 11 Effects of prenatal care and socioeconomic status on cesarean delivery use, further interaction terms for prenatal care and socioeconomic status, logit model 1 (odds ratios) *(Continued)*

	(1)	(2)	(3)	(4)	(5)	(6)	(7)	(8)
Craft/trades worker or entrepreneur × No prenatal education					1.09 (0.098)	1.10 (0.098)		
Craft/trades worker or entrepreneur × Prenatal education					0.89 (0.068)	0.88 (0.068)		
Intermediate (technical) occupation × No prenatal education					1.33[b] (0.171)	1.33[b] (0.170)		
Intermediate (technical) occupation × Prenatal education					0.82[c] (0.089)	0.82[c] (0.090)		
Managerial or higher intellectual occupation × No prenatal education					1.13[a] (0.052)	1.13[a] (0.051)		
Managerial or higher intellectual occupation × Prenatal education					0.78[a] (0.045)	0.78[a] (0.045)		
Crossed dummy variables for partner's work status and prenatal education participation								
Unemployed × No prenatal education							1.20 (0.238)	1.20 (0.239)
Unemployed × Prenatal education							0.88 (0.079)	0.88 (0.079)
Not in labor force × No prenatal education							1.13 (0.099)	1.13 (0.100)
Not in labor force × Prenatal education							0.96 (0.117)	0.96 (0.118)
Working × No prenatal education							1.10[b] (0.047)	1.10[b] (0.048)
Working × Prenatal education							0.78[a] (0.028)	0.78[a] (0.028)
Epidemiologic and hospital controls	Yes	Yes	Yes	Yes	Yes	Yes	Yes	Yes
Other prenatal care and socioeconomic variables	Yes	Yes	Yes	Yes	Yes	Yes	Yes	Yes
Year fixed effects	Yes	Yes	Yes	Yes	Yes	Yes	Yes	Yes
Hospital effects	Fixed	Random	Fixed	Random	Fixed	Random	Fixed	Random
N (observations)	41,141	41,141	41,141	41,141	41,141	41,141	41,141	41,141

All regressions use the full sample of women and include a constraint: the sum of all the crossed variables equals 0. Epidemiologic control variables include woman's demographics (age and parity) and medical risk factors (previous cesarean, diabetes, hypertension, eclampsia or preeclampsia, fetal growth restriction, placental bleeding, other obstetric pathology, plurality, term at delivery, fetal presentation, induced labor, and birth weight). Hospital control variables include hospital type (ownership status, equipment level, and teaching status), organization (day of delivery, obstetrician availability, and size), and staff (midwives, obstetricians, and anesthetists in FTEs per bed). Hospital invariant control variables (ownership status, equipment level, and teaching status) are only included in regressions with hospital random effects. Other prenatal care variables are trimester of the first antenatal visit, number of obstetric ultrasounds, nuchal translucency ultrasound, morphology ultrasound, and early prenatal interview. Other socioeconomic variables include woman's familial situation, healthcare coverage, occupation, education except for columns 1–2 and work status except for columns 3–4, and her partner's occupation except for columns 5–6 and work status except for columns 7–8. Robust standard errors in parentheses
[a] = 1% significance level, [b] = 5%, [c] = 10%

Abbreviations

CNIL: Commission Nationale de l'Informatique et des Libertés, French data protection commission authority; FTE: Full-time equivalent; *INSEE: Institut National de la Statistique et des Etudes Economiques*, French national institute of statistics and economic studies; *PCS: Premiers Certificats de Santé*, infant first health certificates; *SAE: Statistique Annuelle des Etablissements de santé*, French annual hospital statistics; US: United States; WHO: World Health Organization

Acknowledgements

We would like to thank Patrick Rozenberg for access to data, and for his helpful support and comments. Thanks also to the seminar participants at the 2016 London International Health Conference and the 2016 Barcelona EuHEA Conference for their constructive comments.

Funding

Not applicable.

Authors' contributions

CM was responsible for the study design. SZ participated in the study design, analyzed the data, interpreted the results, and wrote the first draft of the manuscript. CM supervised the analysis and interpretation of data, and reviewed the manuscript. Both authors approved the final manuscript.

Competing interests

The authors declare that they have no competing interests.

Author details

[1]Paris-Jourdan Sciences Economiques, French National Center for Scientific Research, Paris, France. [2]EA 7285, Versailles Saint Quentin University, Montigny-le-Bretonneux, France.

References

1. Organization for Economic Cooperation and Development. Health at a Glance: OECD Indicators. http://www.oecd-ilibrary.org/social-issues-migration-health/health-at-a-glance_19991312. Accessed on 12 Jan 2018.
2. Emanuel EJ, Fuchs VR. The perfect storm of overutilization. JAMA. 2008; 299(23):2789–91.
3. Keyhani S, Siu AL. The underuse of overuse research. Health Serv Res. 2008; 43(6):1923–30.
4. Korenstein D, Falk R, Howell EA, Bishop T, Keyhani S. Overuse of health care services in the United States: an understudied problem. Arch Intern Med. 2012;172(2):171–8.
5. Nassery N, Segal JB, Chang E, Bridges JF. Systematic overuse of healthcare services: a conceptual model. Appl Health Econ Health Policy. 2015;13(1):1–6.
6. Betrán AP, Merialdi M, Lauer JA, Bing-Shun W, Thomas J, Van Look P, Wagner M. Rates of caesarean section: analysis of global, regional and national estimates. Paediatr Perinat Epidemiol. 2007;21(2):98–113.
7. Villar J, Valladares E, Wojdyla D, Zavaleta N, Carroli G, Velazco A, Shah A, Campodónico L, Bataglia V, Faundes A, Langer A, Narváez A, Donner A, Romero M, Reynoso S, de Pádua KS, Giordano D, Kublickas M, Acosta A. WHO 2005 global survey on maternal and perinatal health research group. Caesarean delivery rates and pregnancy outcomes: the 2005 WHO global survey on maternal and perinatal health in Latin America. Lancet. 2006; 367(9525):1819–29.
8. Gibbons L, Belizan JM, Lauer JA, Betran AP, Merialdi M, Althabe F. Inequities in the use of cesarean section deliveries in the world. Am J Obstet Gynecol. 2012;206(4):331–e1.
9. World Health Organization. Appropriate technology for birth. Lancet. 1985; 2(8452):436–7.
10. World Health Organization. WHO Statement on Caesarean Section Rates. 2015. http://apps.who.int/iris/bitstream/10665/161442/1/WHO_RHR_15.02_eng.pdf?ua=1. Accessed on 5 Aug 2017.
11. Xu X, Gariepy A, Lundsberg LS, Sheth SS, Pettker CM, Krumholz HM, Illuzzi JL. Wide variation found in hospital facility costs for maternity stays involving low-risk childbirth. Health Aff. 2015;34(7):1212–9.
12. Allen VM, O'Connell CM, Farrell SA, Baskett TF. Economic implications of method of delivery. Am J Obstet Gynecol. 2005;193(1):192–7.
13. Allen VM, O'Connell CM, Baskett TF. Cumulative economic implications of initial method of delivery. Obstet Gynecol. 2006;108(3, Part 1):549–55.
14. Gilbert SA, Grobman WA, Landon MB, Varner MW, Wapner RJ, Sorokin Y, Sibai BM, Thorp JM, Ramin SM, Mercer BM, Eunice Kennedy Shriver National Institute of Child Health and Human Development Maternal-Fetal Medicine Units Network. Lifetime cost-effectiveness of trial of labor after cesarean in the United States. Value Health. 2013;16(6):953–64.
15. Belizán JM, Althabe F, Cafferata ML. Health consequences of the increasing caesarean section rates. Epidemiology. 2007;18(4):485–6.
16. Hyde MJ, Mostyn A, Modi N, Kemp PR. The health implications of birth by caesarean section. Biol Rev. 2012;87(1):229–43.
17. Villar J, Carroli G, Zavaleta N, Donner A, Wojdyla D, Faundes A, Velazco A, Bataglia V, Langer A, Narváez A, Valladares E, Shah A, Campodónico L, Romero M, Reynoso S, de Pádua KS, Giordano D, Kublickas M, Maternal AA. Neonatal individual risks and benefits associated with caesarean delivery: multicentre prospective study. BMJ. 2007;335(7628):1025.
18. O'Leary CM, De Klerk N, Keogh J, Pennell C, De Groot J, York L, Mulroy S, Stanley FJ. Trends in mode of delivery during 1984-2003: can they be explained by pregnancy and delivery complications? BJOG. 2007;114(7):855–64.
19. Mazzoni A, Althabe F, Liu NH, Bonotti AM, Gibbons L, Sánchez AJ, Belizán JM. Women's preference for caesarean section: a systematic review and meta-analysis of observational studies. BJOG. 2011;118(4):391–9.
20. Grant D. Physician financial incentives and cesarean delivery: new conclusions from the healthcare cost and utilization project. J Health Econ. 2009;28(1):244–50.
21. Epstein AJ, Nicholson S. The formation and evolution of physician treatment styles: an application to cesarean sections. J Health Econ. 2009;28(6):1126–40.
22. Lin HC, Xirasagar S. Institutional factors in cesarean delivery rates: policy and research implications. Obstet Gynecol. 2004;103(1):128–36.
23. Milcent C, Rochut J. Hospital payment system and medical practice: the cesarean section in France. Rev Economique. 2009;60(2):489–506.
24. Guihard P, Blondel B. Trends in risk factors for caesarean sections in France between 1981 and 1995: lessons for reducing the rates in the future. BJOG. 2001;108(1):48–55.
25. Kottwitz A. Mode of birth and social inequalities in health: the effect of maternal education and access to hospital care on cesarean delivery. Health Place. 2014;27:9–21.
26. Simoes E, Kunz S, Bosing-Schwenkglenks M, Schmahl FW. Occupation and risk of cesarean section: study based on the perinatal survey of Baden-Württemberg, Germany. Arch Gynecol Obstet. 2005;271(4):338–42.
27. Cesaroni G, Forastiere F, Perucci CA. Are cesarean deliveries more likely for poorly educated parents? A brief report from Italy. Birth. 2008;35(3):241–4.
28. Lee SI, Khang YH, Yun S, Jo MW. Rising rates, changing relationships: caesarean section and its correlates in South Korea, 1988–2000. BJOG. 2005;112(6):810–9.
29. Linton A, Peterson MR, Williams TV. Effects of maternal characteristics on cesarean delivery rates among US Department of defense healthcare beneficiaries, 1996-2002. Birth. 2004;31(1):3–11.
30. Tollånes MC, Thompson JM, Daltveit AK, Irgens LM. Cesarean section and maternal education; secular trends in Norway, 1967–2004. Acta Obstet Gynecol Scand. 2007;86(7):840–8.
31. Joseph KS, Dodds L, Allen AC, Jones DV, Monterrosa L, Robinson H, Liston RM, Young DC. Socioeconomic status and receipt of obstetric services in Canada. Obstet Gynecol. 2006;107(3):641–50.

32. Alexander GR, Kotelchuck M. Assessing the role and effectiveness of prenatal care: history, challenges, and directions for future research. Public Health Rep. 2001;116(4):306.

33. World Health Organization. Provision of effective antenatal care. 2006. http://www.who.int/reproductivehealth/publications/maternal_perinatal_health/effective_antenatal_care.pdf. Accessed 10 Aug 2017.

34. Carroli G, Rooney C, Villar J. How effective is antenatal care in preventing maternal mortality and serious morbidity? An overview of the evidence. Paediatr Perinat Epidemiol. 2001;15(s1):1–42.

35. Yan J. The effects of prenatal care utilization on maternal health and health behaviors. Health Econ. 2017;26(8):1001–18.

36. Blondel B, Marshall B. Poor antenatal care in 20 French districts: risk factors and pregnancy outcome. J Epidemiol Community Health. 1998;52(8):501–6.

37. Krueger PM, Scholl TO. Adequacy of prenatal care and pregnancy outcome. J Am Osteopath Assoc. 2000;100(8):485–92.

38. Rous JJ, Jewell RT, Brown RW. The effect of prenatal care on birthweight: a full-information maximum likelihood approach. Health Econ. 2004;13(3):251–64.

39. Partridge S, Balayla J, Holcroft CA, Abenhaim HA. Inadequate prenatal care utilization and risks of infant mortality and poor birth outcome: a retrospective analysis of 28,729,765 US deliveries over 8 years. Am J Perinatol. 2012;29(10):787.

40. Raatikainen K, Heiskanen N, Heinonen S. Under-attending free antenatal care is associated with adverse pregnancy outcomes. BMC Public Health. 2007;7(1):1.

41. Sieber S, Germann N, Barbir A, Ehlert U. Emotional well-being and predictors of birth-anxiety, self-efficacy, and psychosocial adaptation in healthy pregnant women. Acta Obstet Gynecol Scand. 2006;85(10):1200–7.

42. Clark AE, Milcent C. Public employment and political pressure: the case of French hospitals. J Health Econ. 2011;30(5):1103–12.

43. Robson MS. Classification of caesarean sections. Fetal Mater Med Rev. 2001; 12(01):23–39.

44. Coulm B, Ray C, Lelong N, Drewniak N, Zeitlin J, Blondel B. Obstetric interventions for low-risk pregnant women in France: do maternity unit characteristics make a difference? Birth. 2012;39(3):183–91.

45. Blondel B, Lelong N, Kermarrec M, Goffinet F, National Coordination Group of the National Perinatal Surveys. Trends in perinatal health in France from 1995 to 2010. Results from the French National Perinatal Surveys. J Gynécol Obstét Biol Reprod. 2012;41(4):e1–e15.

46. Hildingsson I. How much influence do women in Sweden have on caesarean section? A follow-up study of women's preferences in early pregnancy. Midwifery. 2008;24(1):46–54.

47. O'Donovan C, O'Donovan J. Why do women request an elective cesarean delivery for non-medical reasons? A systematic review of the qualitative literature. Birth. 2017; https://doi.org/10.1111/birt.12319.

48. Quinlivan JA, Petersen RW, Nichols CN. Patient preference the leading indication for elective caesarean section in public patients–results of a 2-year prospective audit in a teaching hospital. Aust N Z J Obstet Gynaecol. 1999;39(2):207–14.

49. Beeckman K, Louckx F, Putman K. Determinants of the number of antenatal visits in a metropolitan region. BMC Public Health. 2010;10(1):1.

50. Fairley L, Dundas R, Leyland AH. The influence of both individual and area based socioeconomic status on temporal trends in caesarean sections in Scotland 1980-2000. BMC Public Health. 2011;11(1):1.

51. Chen MM, Hancock H. Women's knowledge of options for birth after caesarean section. Women Birth. 2012;25(3):e19–26.

52. Loke AY, Davies L, Li SF. Factors influencing the decision that women make on their mode of delivery: the health belief model. BMC Health Serv Res. 2015;15(1):1.

53. Räisänen S, Lehto SM, Nielsen HS, Gissler M, Kramer MR, Heinonen S. Fear of childbirth in nulliparous and multiparous women: a population-based analysis of all singleton births in Finland in 1997-2010. BJOG. 2014;121(8): 965–70.

54. Cotzias CS, Paterson-Brown S, Fisk NM. Obstetricians say yes to maternal request for elective caesarean section: a survey of current opinion. Eur J Obstet Gynecol Reprod Biol. 2001;97(1):15–6.

55. Wax JR, Cartin A, Pinette MG, Blackstone J. Patient choice cesarean-the Maine experience. Birth. 2005;32(3):203–6.

56. Wax JR, Cartin A, Pinette MG, Blackstone J. Patient choice cesarean: an evidence-based review. Obstet Gynecol Surv. 2004;59(8):601–16.

10

Does birth under-registration reduce childhood immunization? Evidence from the Dominican Republic

Steve Brito[1], Ana Corbacho[1] and Rene Osorio[2*]

Abstract

The consequences of lacking birth certificates remain largely unexplored in the economic literature. We intend to fill this knowledge gap studying the effect of lacking birth certificates on immunization of children in the Dominican Republic. This is an interesting country because a significant number of children of Haitian descent face the consequences of lacking proper documentation. We use the distance to the civil registry office and the mother's document of identification as instrumental variables of the child's birth certificate. After controlling for distance to immunization services and other determinants, this paper finds that children between 0 and 59 months of age that do not have birth certificates are behind by nearly one vaccine (out of a total of nine) compared to those that have birth certificates.

Keywords: Immunization, Under-registration, Health access

Background

Birth registration, which provides legal proof of a child's existence and nationality, is considered a fundamental human right according to the Convention on the Rights of the Child (1989). In many countries, identity documents are required to access benefits such as school diplomas, health care services, conditional cash transfers, pensions, banking services, civil rights, adoption, divorce, marriage and inheritance.

This paper to sheds light on the effect of birth under-registration on health access. Childhood immunizations, a key component of health care services, are intended to be administered to all children on a standardized schedule. The paper focuses on the effect of under-registration of births on childhood immunization in the Dominican Republic, the country with the second highest percentage (22%) of children under the age of 5 without birth certificates in Latin American and Caribbean (LAC) countries (UNICEF [39]) (Fig. 1).

Studying the factors that affect immunization in the region is important because proper vaccination can reduce infant morbidity (Aaby et al.[1]; Bishar et al. [10]; Breiman et al. [16]). Vaccination is also crucial in reducing infant mortality under 5, according to the fourth Millennium Development Goal (MDG4). Furthermore, vaccinating communities reduces the risk of disease outbreaks and their spread to neighboring communities. Many studies have shown that vaccination at the appropriate age has positive effects on cognitive development, educational achievement, and productivity in developing countries (Bloom et al. [12]; Canning et al. [17]).

Another reason to study immunization determinants is that increasing vaccination coverage is cost-effective. According to the World Health Organization (WHO), polio eradication saved governments US$1.5 billion per year in treatment and rehabilitation costs (Bloom et al. [11]). The Institute of Medicine reports that for every dollar spent on the MMR vaccine, US$21 is saved (Bloom et al.[11]). Extensive literature on the economics of immunization finds good reasons for vaccination due to its cost-benefit and/or cost-effectiveness (WHO [40]).

After controlling for well-established socioeconomic determinants of immunization and endogeneity, this

* Correspondence: reneosorio77@gmail.com
[2]Inter-American Development Bank, 1300 New York Avenue NW, Washington, DC 20577, USA
Full list of author information is available at the end of the article

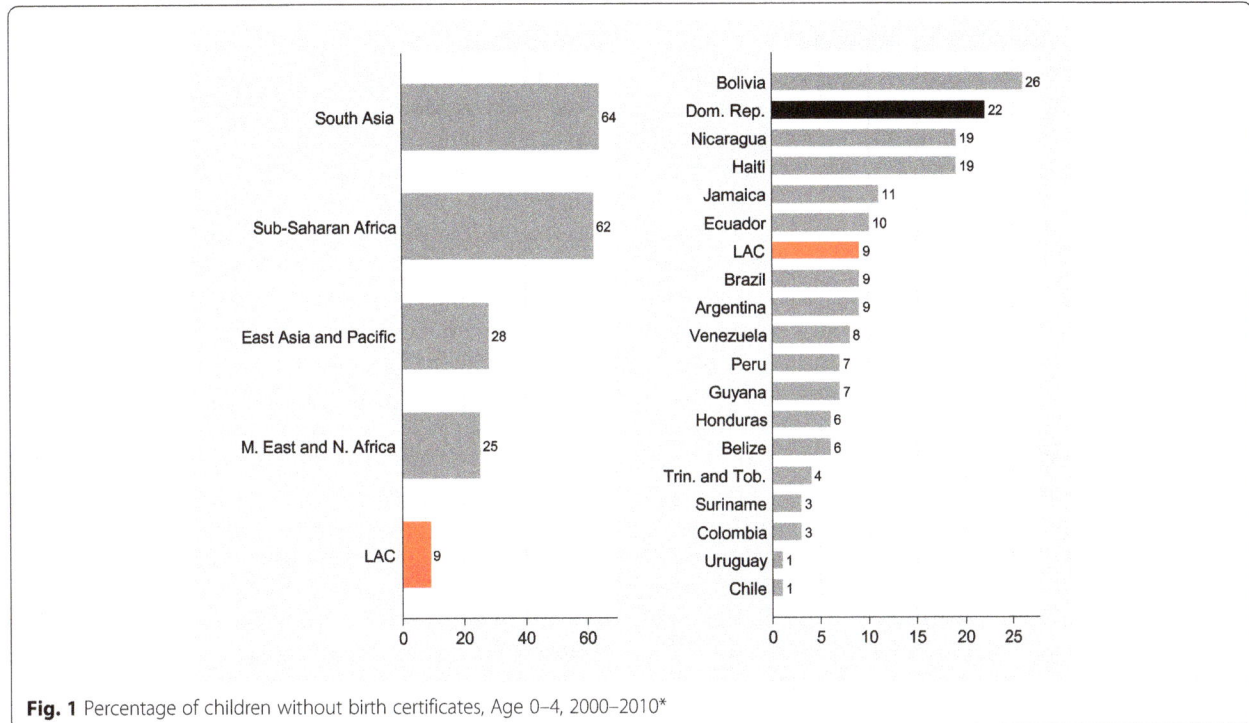

Fig. 1 Percentage of children without birth certificates, Age 0–4, 2000–2010*

study found that those children without birth certificates have 0.7 vaccines fewer than children with birth certificates. As variables were included that might be correlated to the instruments, the results were found to be robust to threats to the exclusion restriction of the instrumental variables such as location of immunization centers and mobile immunization campaigns.

The reason that undocumented children receive fewer vaccinations is because they cannot be registered in the Dominican social security system, which guarantees access to public vaccination facilities or reimburses costs incurred in private health facilities. Moreover, the lack of a birth certificate makes it difficult to prove age, and most countries, including the Dominican Republic, follow WHO's immunization schedule, which is based on the age of the child. The two vaccines that have lower probability of being delivered are the first doses of polio (OPV1), and pertussis, tetanus, and diphtheria (DTP1). The result is reduced immunization rates and/or delays in vaccine administration.

The rest of the paper is organized as follows. Section 2 reviews the related literature and examines factors associated with the registration of children's births and immunization. Section 3 presents the data used and the methodology and potential econometric difficulties, and Section 4 analyzes the results and provides conclusions.

Literature review

Qualitative studies in the LAC region have shown that children without identity documents have more difficulty accessing public services, including health services.

Bracamonte and Ordonez [15] cover the effects of the lack of a birth certificate in Chile, Colombia, Honduras, Ecuador, Nicaragua, and Peru on access to education, health services, and conditional cash transfers. Harbitz and Tamargo [32] explore the factors that contribute to under-registration of births and lack of legal identity. Harbitz and Boekle-Giuffrida [31] document the diverse challenges faced by those lacking legal identity documents. Cody [21] finds that birth registration is a prerequisite for accessing health services in many developing regions.

But the consequences of the lack of birth certificates are only beginning to be studied. In this regard, Castro and Rud [18] find a correlation between education and identity documents in children and adults. Brito et al. [23] study the effects of the lack of birth certificates on educational attainment and conclude that birth under-registration reduces educational attainment. Gine and Yang [29] link the development of fingerprinting in Malawi, a very accurate technology of personal identification, with improvements in borrowers' creditworthiness, repayment rates, and expansion of the credit received. Fagernas [27] finds increased enforcement of child labor laws and educational attainment in the early 20th century in the United States, after birth registration laws were approved.

This paper examines the consequences of the lack of birth certificates on immunization. Immunization is studied rather than other health care services due to the availability of data, but other health-related programs, such as maternal care, may also be affected by the lack of a legal identity. Immunization programs have been more successful in reaching segments of the most disadvantaged populations in developing countries. In fact, according to WHO, by 2010, LAC countries had achieved coverage above 90% of measles vaccines (MCV) and the three recommended doses of DTP among children aged 12-23 months. Worldwide, coverage rates are typically above 75%, even in the least developed regions.

Notwithstanding these high coverage rates, they are not complete. The lack of services due to system failures, poor public awareness, and misconceptions even in well-developed countries are among the reasons behind incomplete immunization schedules (Schmitt [37]; Discover Magazine [24]). Other factors associated with under-immunization are race, ethnicity, birth order, marital status of the respondent, number of children in the household, access to public or private health insurance, decentralization of public services, and conditional cash transfers, among others (Adler et al. [3]; Feilden and Nielsen [28]; Barker et al. [8]; Khalegian [34]; Bardenheier et al. [6]; Chaui et al. [19]; Berman et al. [9]; Bakirci and Torun [5]; Acemoglu et al. [2]; Barham and Maluccio [7]).

Vaccine coverage is the most frequently used indicator of immunization among children between 12 and 23 months of age, but delays in delivery are overlooked (Chu et al. [20]; Faustini et al. [30]; Hull et al. [33]; Akmatov et al. [4]). Vaccines have the highest effectiveness during the recommended age range, and yet show lower compliance than uptake rates. Therefore, timely vaccination rather than coverage may be more important when the timing of delivery is crucial (Bolton et al. [14]). Factors affecting delay are similar to those affecting uptake. Single parenting, parental education, large family size, insurance coverage, and birth order have been documented as affecting delays in vaccination (Bobo et al. [13]; Essex et al. [26]; Dombkowski et al. [25]). This analysis encompasses both immunization coverage and timely vaccination.

Data

The data come from the 2007 Demographic and Health Survey (DHS) of the Dominican Republic. The DHS includes extensive information on health and education outcomes, as well as household socioeconomic characteristics. It is among the few surveys with information on identity documents.[1] The DHS of the Dominican Republic contains data on geographic location of clusters of households. The data collection was done in the year 2007 between March and August using face to face interviews completed in 97% of the houses selected of a total of 33,437. The questionnaire used during the interview was answered by mostly females (aged 15-19) although efforts were made to interview males (aged 15-59). This DHS survey was collected while the people were present in their homes. Hence, data from hospitals, health centers or immunization records did not form part of the survey

to avoid problems with self-selection issues. The two other sources of data are global positioning system (GPS) data on civil registry offices and on immunization centers.

The main variables of interest are immunization outcomes. All children with complete or incomplete vaccinations and those who had never been vaccinated were included in the econometric analysis. Only those children who died before the data was collected are not part our sample. Of the 5,157 children in our sample 4% reported that a child had died, however we do not have information on the immunization records or birth registration of the deceased children. The survey does not contain information about the cause of death which might include unvaccinated children dying from diseases that vaccination might have prevented. For this reason, it is difficult to say anything about the type of bias or censoring this might introduce to our analysis. More problematic could be inaccurate recall of the immunization records of the children without immunization cards. For these children, their parents might have stated incorrectly the number of doses received of a given vaccine included, causing inconsistent estimations in our econometric analysis. Fortunately, the survey recorded information from immunization cards, which were available in 71% of the children in our sample. We used information from vaccination cards for a robustness check in Table 8.

The focus is on the nine vaccines recommended by the WHO in its extended program of immunization (EPI) worldwide. Hence, the vaccines analyzed in this paper are the following:

- one dose of Bacillus Calmette-Guerin (BCG) and one of hepatitis b (HEPB)
- three doses of Diphtheria Tetanus Pertussis (DTP) or three doses of pentavalent which includes five vaccines in one shot against diphtheria, tetanus, pertussis, hepatitis B and haemophilus influezae b
- three doses of Polio (OPV)
- one dose of measles (MCV) or one dose of triple viral containing vaccines against measles, mumps and rubella (MMR) in one shot

Figure 2 shows the number of vaccines as well as the age range recommended to receive them.

During the survey, mothers were asked to show the vaccination card (70% compliance) to verify whether or not the children had been vaccinated. The cards also contained the day, month, and year of vaccination. Those mothers who reported not having their children's vaccination card responded from memory but did not provide the date of vaccination. Some literature has found that data using parental recall slightly underreports immunization rates (see Simpson et al. [38]; Langsten and Hill [35]). To check the robustness of the results to this potential measurement

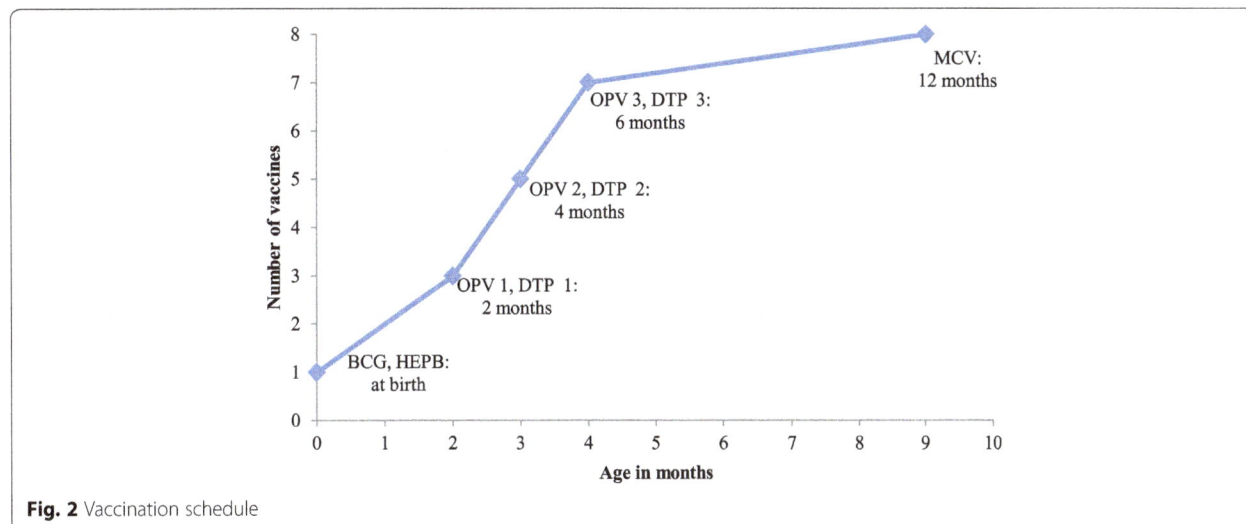

Fig. 2 Vaccination schedule

error, we repeated the analysis described below with the subsample of children with vaccination cards and obtained similar results. Comparisons with the study's main results are reported in the Appendix.

The DHS 2007 contains information on the current age in months of the children at the moment of the interview. We used this information to construct Fig. 3. This figure shows the age distribution for administration of the BCG, DTP1, DTP3 and MCV vaccines. We excluded from the figure the age distribution corresponding to the HEPB and the OPV vaccines because the former is superimposed with the distribution of the BCG and the latter with those of the DTPs. All data in Fig. 3 are from the subsample with vaccination cards the delay in age-appropriate vaccination for those without cards cannot be calculated.

All distributions peak around the recommended age, indicating that most children receive their vaccines when they are due, but they also have long right-sided tails, indicating delays. On the other hand, shorter left tails suggest that premature delivery is less frequent. The distribution of the BCG that is administered after birth shows the least prominent tail, perhaps because it is delivered at birth. The distributions for those vaccines administered after birth show more significant delays.

Table 1 contains the summary statistics. The BCG, delivered usually at birth, shows the highest percentage of compliance (98%). This is consistent with the fact that 98% of the children are born in hospitals, health centers, or with medical attention. The data show that the administration of vaccines diminishes monotonically after

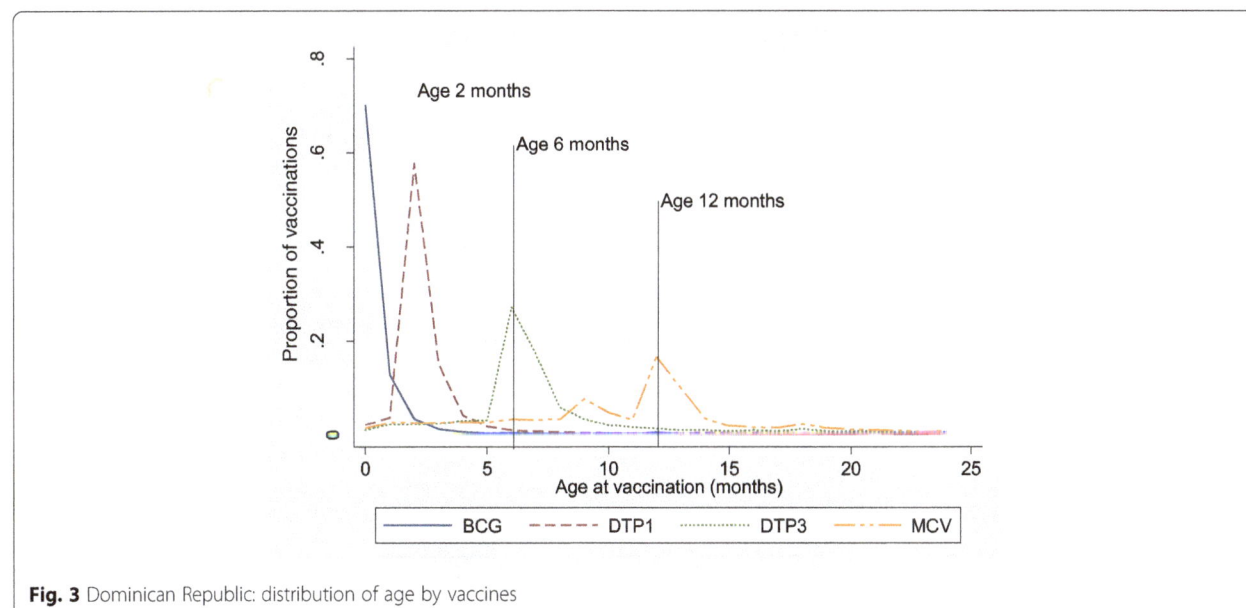

Fig. 3 Dominican Republic: distribution of age by vaccines

birth, so the first vaccines have higher uptake rates, while the MCV, given at 9–12 months, has the lowest.

Our outcome variables capture both total uptake and timely vaccination. Total uptake is simply the total number of vaccines received by a child 0–59 months old. We also looked at uptake on individual vaccines. Several other dependent variables that seek to measure delays in vaccination were also constructed. The first variable on timely vaccination is the proportion of age-due vaccines actually delivered. This variable seeks to control not only for the number of vaccines received but also for those vaccines which are due in relation to the age of the child. This variable, in contrast with the total number of vaccines, does not take into account the vaccines outside the recommended age range but only those that had to be delivered within a certain time frame. The second variable is a dummy that measures complete vaccination at 7 months; another variable measures complete vaccination at 13 months. These ages were chosen because at 6 months a child ought to have received eight vaccines, and at 12 months ought to have received the full set of nine vaccines.

Table 1 also reports that around 30% of the households in the sample responded that the nearest health center is too far away. However, self-reported distances are prone to measurement error. Data were therefore collected on the exact location of immunization centers in the country and the distance from the cluster of households was calculated. The linear distance between health immunization centers and the cluster of households is only 2.4 kilometers on average, with a maximum of 18 kilometers. The Appendix: Figures 5 and 6) contains information on the location of each immunization center in the Dominican Republic in various provinces distinguished in colors and symbols and the frequency distribution of this linear GPS-measured distance. The different symbols and colors in the map of Figure A1 illustrate the location of immunization centers. We calculate the minimum distance to the nearest immunization center regardless of the location of the latter, as the parents are not bound or legally constrained to vaccinate their children in their home province. Very few households are located more than 10 kilometers from the nearest immunization center, and the immunization centers cover the entire national territory reasonably well. Moreover, around 70% of them offer services all day rather than only half a day.

(a) The dominican health system

The Dominican health system has both public and private sector components. In the public sector, immunization is provided free of charge to all, regardless of possession of identity documents. However, access to the private health care system and reimbursement by the state social security system requires proof of identity.

Otherwise, Dominicans must pay out of pocket for private health services, including vaccines and shots.

Thus, the lack of documents may affect those children who are uninsured in remote areas where the state has little presence and who cannot afford the fees charged by private health care providers, reducing their access to immunization services. This hypothesis is tested by exploiting data on access to immunization centers, using self-reported perception of distance to health centers in the DHS[2] and the GPS-measured linear distance to the nearest immunization center.

With regard to the legal framework, the two laws that define the structure of the health system in the Dominican Republican are the General Law on Health (*Ley 42-01*) and the Law on the Dominican Social Security System (*Ley 87-01*), both passed in 2001. They divide the health system into public and private providers. Figure 4 illustrates the provision of health care services in the Dominican Republic.

Article 3 of Law 42-01 grants Dominican citizens and foreign legal residents the right to health care. Law 87-01 also states that the Social Security System must serve all Dominicans and legal residents in the country without discrimination. In theory, these laws do not exclude undocumented people from public access to health care. In practice, the fact that 98% of women give birth in a health center or a hospital seems to corroborate what the laws state.

Methods

This paper answers several questions. Does lacking a birth certificate reduce the number of vaccines delivered? Which vaccines are primarily affected? What are the potential mechanisms? Does birth under-registration reduce timely vaccination?

To address these questions, we ran several econometric models using the dependent variables described above on uptake and timely vaccination. The empirical strategy uses different limited dependent-variable models that relate vaccine outcomes to birth registration, children's characteristics, mother's characteristics, and other controls frequently used in the immunization literature.

Our empirical strategy takes into account potential endogeneity of our variable of interest, lack of a birth certificate. Vaccination may increase the incentive to register a child's birth, generating reverse causation. In this case, the association between immunization and birth certificates would increase if vaccination increased the number of children with birth certificates. In such cases, children vaccinated will be more likely to have birth certificates. Nonetheless, the direction of the bias is jointly determined by the other factor that causes endogeneity. The association of omitted factors with vaccination and their correlation with birth registration

Table 1 Summary Statistics for the Dominican Republic 2007 for Children aged 0–59 Months

	(1.1)	(1.2)	(1.3)	(1.4)	(1.5)
Variables	N	mean	sd	min	max
Dependent variables:					
Number of vaccines	5,157	7.630	1.990	0	9
BCG uptake	5,157	0.984	0.127	0	1
HEPB uptake	5,157	0.943	0.232	0	1
DTP1 uptake	5,157	0.925	0.264	0	1
DTP2 uptake	5,157	0.843	0.364	0	1
DTP3 uptake	5,157	0.730	0.444	0	1
OPV1 uptake	5,157	0.948	0.222	0	1
OPV2 uptake	5,157	0.859	0.348	0	1
OPV3 uptake	5,157	0.699	0.459	0	1
MCV uptake	5,157	0.699	0.459	0	1
Proportion of age-due vaccines (age > 12 months)	3,478	0.589	0.291	0	1
Complete vaccination at 7 months of age	4,314	0.235	0.424	0	1
Complete vaccination at 13 months of age	4,315	0.231	0.422	0	1
Endogenous variable:					
Child without birth certificate	5,157	0.188	0.390	0	1
Instrumental variables:					
Distance to nearest registry in km	5,157	4.849	4.147	0.036	28.6
Mother without document of identification	5,157	0.107	0.309	0	1
Rest of controls:					
Child is a girl	5,157	0.474	0.499	0	1
Card (seen)	5,157	0.709	0.454	0	1
Current age of the child (months)	5,157	30.03	17.54	0	59
Aged 0-2 months	5,157	0.02	0.141	0	1
Aged 3-6 months	5,157	0.09	0.291	0	1
Aged 7-12 months	5,157	0.100	0.301	0	1
Birth order	5,157	2.519	1.313	1	5
Born in hospital/health center	5,157	0.982	0.134	0	1
Mother's schooling in years	5,157	8.344	4.391	0	19
Mother works	5,157	0.291	0.454	0	1
One parent born abroad	5,157	0.042	0.201	0	1
Wealth index	5,157	2.333	1.302	1	5
Rural área	5,157	0.440	0.496	0	1
No water/electricity	5,157	0.033	0.179	0	1
Vaccinated in a campaign	5,157	0.354	0.478	0	1
Health center far away	5,157	0.296	0.456	0	1
Distance to nearest immunization center in km	5,157	2.360	2.375	0.008	18.4
Immunization center attends morning and afternoon	5,157	0.705	0.456	0	1

Source: Dominican Republic DHS (2007)

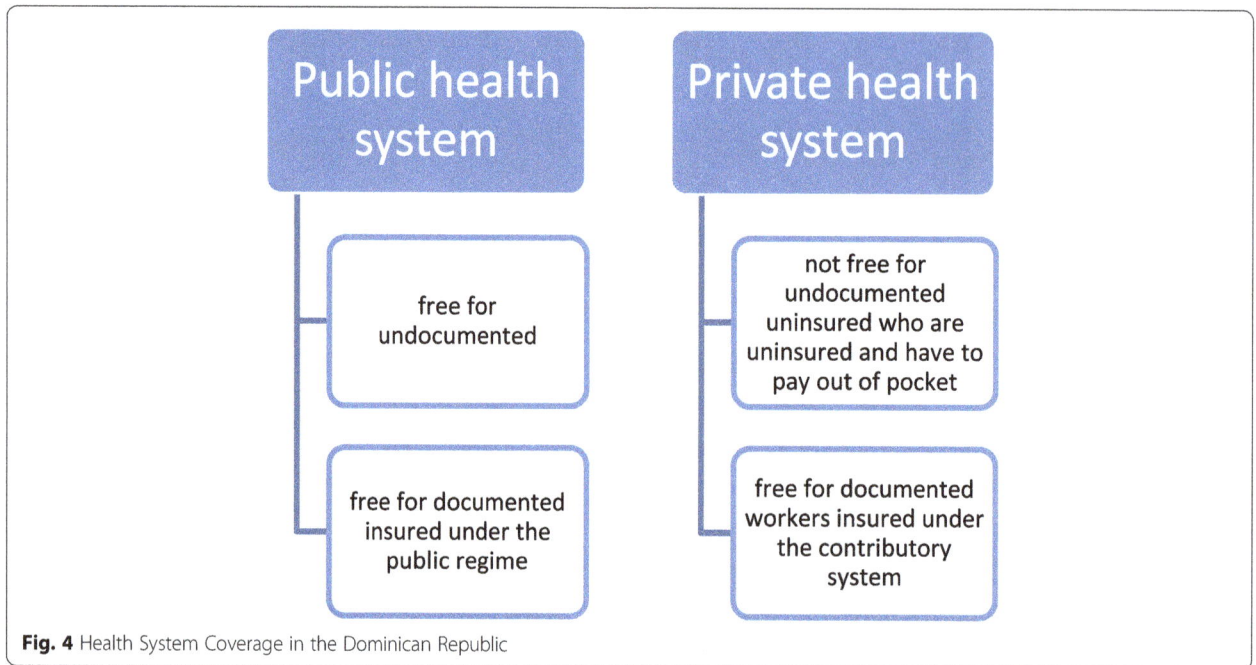

Fig. 4 Health System Coverage in the Dominican Republic

is unknown. These omitted factors could include preference for health care services, in particular attitudes on vaccination, and birth registration. Thus, the bias of the coefficient is a priori unknown.

To address this potential endogeneity, we used two instrumental variables: (i) distance from the household cluster to the civil registry office, and (ii) whether or not the mother has an identity document *(cédula de identidad)*. Following Corbacho and Osorio [22] and Brito et al. [23], we use GPS-measured distance from the cluster of households to the civil registry office as an instrumental variable of whether or not a child has a birth certificate.[3] There are several mechanisms through which distance to the registry office may decrease chances of a parent registering the child's birth. An obvious one is transportation costs. Another may be lower access to information about the necessary steps and requirements to obtain a birth certificate. Corbacho and Osorio [22] also find that lack of legal identity of the mother explains the lack of birth certificates for her children, since it is one of the prerequisites to register a child's birth. However, it is important to clarify that all children born on Dominican soil have the right to be Dominicans and receive identity documents regardless of their parents' origin (the principle of jus solis), but in practice the requirement to present the parents' documents of identification conflicts with this principle.

We explore the validity of these instrumental variables using a battery of econometric tests and by adding controls that might be correlated with the instrumental variables. For example, the distance to civil registry offices and the mother not having an identity document could be negatively correlated with the existence of health care

services such as immunization centers. Thus, to our basic specification, we add as a control the distance to immunization centers to check for the stability of the coefficients in the presence of controls likely correlated with our instruments. After controlling for other determinants of vaccination, our two instrumental variables should not be expected to have an independent effect on vaccines, while being good predictors of birth registration. We also checked in Appendix: Table 8 if the instrumental variables were correlated with the outcomes of interest.

Results

(i) First stage: correlation of birth certificates with distance and mother's ID

In the first stage, we explored the relationship between birth certificates, distance to civil registries, and mother's identity document after controlling for other socioeconomic characteristics. Table 2 reports the marginal results for children aged 0-59 months of the regression:

$$NoBirthCert_i^* = \beta_1 + mindist_i\beta_2 + MotherID_i\beta_3 + X_i\beta_4 + \gamma_j + \varepsilon_i \quad (1)$$

We used as the dependent variable whether or not the child had a birth certificate and, as predictors, the distance from each cluster of household where child i lives to the nearest civil registry office, a dummy variable indicating whether or not his/her mother lacked an identity document, controls X_i, and household dummies in some cases and province or municipality dummies in others. The

Dominican Republic is divided into provinces, including the national district where the capital city is located. The next political subdivision is municipalities. We denote these political subdivisions as γ_i in our regressions.

Columns 1 through 4 show a strong and significant effect of both intended instrumental variables on the probability of not possessing a birth certificate. The marginal effects show that every kilometer is associated with an increase in the probability of a child not having a birth certificate of 0.01 percentage points. The mother possessing an identity document increases the probability of registering a child's birth by at least 0.35 percentage points.

(ii) Second stage: impact of birth registration on immunization

The second stage of our analysis looked at the question: *What is the impact of birth registration on immunization?* The basic empirical specification is:

$$Vacc_i = \beta_0 + NoBirthCert_i\beta_1 + X_i\beta_2 + \gamma_j + \varepsilon_i \qquad (2)$$

where $Vacc_i$ is any of the immunization variables listed in the summary statistics above for child i; $NoBirthCert_i$ is a binary variable that indicates if child i does not have a birth certificate; X_i is a list of controls; γ_j are household dummies in some regressions and province or municipality dummies in others; and ε_i is the error of the equation. We used a combination of linear and non-linear models such as OLS, 2SLS and MLE[4] models to account for endogeneity of birth certificates and for the fact that $Vacc_i$ is a discrete variable.

The results of the regressions are reported in Table 3. There $Vacc_i$ is the number of vaccines for children aged 0-59 months. MLE is a maximum likelihood estimator that derives a two-step estimator. In the first stage of the MLE, regression (1) is estimated, with $NoBirthCert_i^*$ being an unobserved probability. The only thing observed is when the child has a birth certificate, in which case the variable used in the first and second stage $NoBirthCert_i$ is equal to 1 and is 0 otherwise. Marginal coefficients are reported as they are easier to interpret in the case of non-linear models.

The first OLS estimate in Table 3, with household dummies, shows that not having a birth certificate has no statistically significant effect on the number of vaccines. However, when we specified the age of the child in linear form, we obtained a significant estimate even with household dummies. Since having or not having a birth certificate is likely to be a household characteristic, we dropped household dummies to avoid problems with multicollinearity. As a result, the OLS regressions without household dummies in Table 3 then show coefficients around 0.5. These estimates suggest that the variation in the number of vaccines is associated with the lack of a birth certificate even after accounting for those unobservable factors

correlated with not possessing a birth certificate. The instrumental variables are used in columns 3 and 4. The 2SLS specification in column 3 shows an effect of 0.57 fewer vaccines, but the MLE in column 4 shows a larger effect of nearly 0.65. The difference may be explained by the econometric specification because 2SLS treats the endogenous variable as linear, whereas the MLE treats it as binary.

With respect to other determinants, we find that children with their vaccination cards receive around 0.2 more vaccines than others. Those born in hospitals and health centers receive more vaccines than those born elsewhere, although the significance is not robust across the econometric specifications. This could be associated with the fact that it may be affecting only the BCG and HEPB vaccines, both given during the first two months of life, usually after birth. This is also consistent with the fact that these first vaccines have the highest uptake rates, as explored in further detail below.

One of the most robust findings in the literature on vaccines is that birth order affects the immunization of children in the same households. Older children receive more vaccines than their younger siblings, even after accounting for the difference attributable to their age. In fact, these results are statistically significant across most econometric specifications, except in the case when household dummies are introduced in column 1.

Mothers' education increases vaccination, but the effect is small compared to other determinants. Children born of parents born abroad (the majority of whom are Haitian) receive at least 0.3 fewer vaccines than children whose parents are Dominicans. This could be due to myriad factors, such as language barrier, discrimination, or lack of awareness of the importance of vaccination. With regard to household characteristics, only two are significant: (i) lack of water or electricity; and (ii) wealth, but this characteristic is not robust across specifications, therefore we omitted it. It is also surprising that rural areas do not have lower immunization records than urban areas.

The next step was to add more controls in order to check the robustness of the results. The most immediate threat to the exclusion restriction is that parents who live far from health facilities may also live farther from civil registry offices and lack identity documents. If this threat to the exclusion restriction is real and the variables that capture access to immunization centers are unobserved, the coefficients in columns 3 and 4 would be biased despite using instrumental variables. Fortunately, we found information on access to health centers, mobile immunization campaigns, and location of permanent immunization centers.

The variables added were: i) *vaccinated in a campaign,* which measures if the child was vaccinated in any mobile vaccination campaign; ii) *health center far away,* which captures self-reported perception of distance to the health center; iii) *distance to nearest immunization center in km,*

Table 2 First Stage –Correlation of birth registration with instrumental variables

Dependent variable:	(2.1)	(2.2)	(2.3)	(2.4)
1 if child does not have birth certificate, 0 otherwise	OLS	PROBIT	OLS	PROBIT
Distance to nearest registry in km	0.010***	0.009***	0.011***	0.010***
	(0.002)	(0.002)	(0.002)	(0.002)
Mother without document of identification	0.376***	0.348***	0.376***	0.377***
	(0.017)	(0.026)	(0.018)	(0.028)
Aged 0-2 months	0.266***	0.327***	0.247***	0.314***
	(0.035)	(0.055)	(0.035)	(0.058)
Aged 3-6 months	0.084***	0.098***	0.068***	0.086***
	(0.017)	(0.022)	(0.017)	(0.023)
Aged 7-12 months	0.074***	0.086***	0.072***	0.088***
	(0.016)	(0.021)	(0.016)	(0.022)
Child is a girl	-0.018*	-0.017*	-0.015	-0.017
	(0.010)	(0.010)	(0.010)	(0.011)
Birth order	0.013***	0.012***	0.011***	0.011**
	(0.004)	(0.004)	(0.004)	(0.004)
Born in hospital/health center	-0.089**	-0.067	-0.060	-0.038
	(0.037)	(0.045)	(0.037)	(0.043)
Mother's schooling in years	-0.013***	-0.015***	-0.013***	-0.015***
	(0.001)	(0.001)	(0.001)	(0.002)
Mother works	-0.013	-0.024**	-0.017	-0.030**
	(0.011)	(0.012)	(0.011)	(0.012)
One parent born abroad	0.102***	0.075**	0.118***	0.102***
	(0.026)	(0.030)	(0.026)	(0.035)
Rural area	0.014	0.022	-0.001	0.014
	(0.013)	(0.014)	(0.015)	(0.017)
No water/electricity	0.018	-0.004	0.063**	0.027
	(0.029)	(0.027)	(0.031)	(0.034)
Health center far away	0.013	0.013	0.011	0.012
	(0.011)	(0.012)	(0.011)	(0.013)
Vaccinated in a campaign	-0.003	-0.005	-0.013	-0.014
	(0.011)	(0.012)	(0.011)	(0.012)
Dist to immun center in km	-0.004	-0.005	-0.003	-0.004
	(0.003)	(0.003)	(0.003)	(0.004)
Immun cent attends morning/ afternoon	0.003	0.005	-0.000	-0.003
	(0.011)	(0.011)	(0.012)	(0.013)
Constant	0.177***		0.182***	
	(0.034)		(0.034)	
Household dummies	No	No	No	No
Province dummies	Yes	Yes	No	No
Municipality dummies	No	No	Yes	Yes
Observations	5157	5157	5157	5157
R^2	0.232		0.282	
Pseudo R^2		0.219		0.258

Notes: Marginal effects. Robust standard errors in parentheses. * $p < 0.1$, ** $p < 0.05$, *** $p < 0.01$

Table 3 Effect of lack of birth certificate on number of vaccines (Age 0-59 months)

Dependent variable	(3.1)	(3.2)	(3.3)	(3.4)	(3.5)	(3.6)	(3.7)
Number of vaccines received by the child	OLS	OLS	2SLS	MLE	OLS	2SLS	MLE
Child without birth certificate	-0.276	-0.303***	-0.572***	-0.649***	-0.544**	-0.299***	-0.755***
	(0.214)	(0.059)	(0.204)	(0.152)	(0.224)	(0.060)	(0.156)
Card (seen)	0.016	0.217***	0.207***	0.214***	0.191***	0.237***	0.233***
	(0.291)	(0.047)	(0.047)	(0.043)	(0.050)	(0.047)	(0.042)
Aged 0-2 months	-4.950***	-6.040***	-5.956***	-5.935***	-5.855***	-5.992***	-5.852***
	(0.780)	(0.098)	(0.113)	(0.141)	(0.116)	(0.103)	(0.141)
Aged 3-6 months	-3.800***	-3.915***	-3.886***	-3.879***	-3.836***	-3.923***	-3.875***
	(0.282)	(0.076)	(0.078)	(0.068)	(0.083)	(0.077)	(0.067)
Aged 7-12 months	-1.304***	-1.269***	-1.244***	-1.237***	-1.194***	-1.278***	-1.235***
	(0.220)	(0.071)	(0.074)	(0.064)	(0.078)	(0.072)	(0.064)
Child is a girl	-0.085	0.026	0.022	0.020	-0.055	0.011	0.002
	(0.110)	(0.037)	(0.037)	(0.037)	(0.049)	(0.037)	(0.036)
Birth order	-0.016	-0.055***	-0.055***	-0.055***	-0.044***	-0.051***	-0.050***
	(0.087)	(0.017)	(0.017)	(0.015)	(0.017)	(0.017)	(0.015)
Born in hospital/health center	0.613	0.455**	0.427**	0.417***	0.495**	0.540***	0.494***
	(0.706)	(0.199)	(0.199)	(0.141)	(0.198)	(0.203)	(0.142)
Mother's schooling in years		0.026***	0.021***	0.019***	0.020***	0.027***	0.017***
		(0.005)	(0.006)	(0.006)	(0.006)	(0.005)	(0.006)
Mother Works		-0.006	-0.011	-0.011	-0.097	0.012	0.006
		(0.042)	(0.041)	(0.042)	(0.070)	(0.042)	(0.042)
One parent born abroad	0.119	-0.502***	-0.430***	-0.414***	-0.366***	-0.450***	-0.336***
	(0.180)	(0.134)	(0.141)	(0.102)	(0.141)	(0.133)	(0.103)
Rural area		0.025	0.039	0.042	-0.147	0.053	0.077
		(0.042)	(0.044)	(0.043)	(0.134)	(0.047)	(0.047)
No water/electricity		-0.696***	-0.679***	-0.676***	-0.693***	-0.787***	-0.768***
		(0.150)	(0.151)	(0.108)	(0.164)	(0.165)	(0.115)
Health center far away		-0.120***	-0.117***	-0.115***	-0.076	-0.124***	-0.118***
		(0.043)	(0.043)	(0.042)	(0.051)	(0.045)	(0.043)
Vaccinated in a campaign	0.221	0.059	0.056	0.057	0.117**	0.074*	0.072*
	(0.222)	(0.042)	(0.042)	(0.042)	(0.052)	(0.043)	(0.042)
Dist to immun center in km		-0.006	-0.005	-0.005	-0.018	-0.020	-0.019
		(0.010)	(0.010)	(0.010)	(0.012)	(0.012)	(0.012)
Immun cent attends morning/afternoon		0.050	0.051	0.051	-0.006	0.032	0.034
		(0.041)	(0.041)	(0.041)	(0.052)	(0.045)	(0.043)
Constant	7.307***	7.012***	7.098***	7.117***	6.288***	6.981***	7.118***
	(0.277)	(0.136)	(0.149)	(0.136)	(0.485)	(0.138)	(0.135)
Household dummies	Yes	No	No	No	No	No	No
Province dummies	No	Yes	Yes	Yes	No	No	No
Municipality dummies	No	No	No	No	Yes	Yes	Yes
Observations	5157	5157	5157	5157	5157	5157	5157
R^2	0.948	0.556	0.553		0.653	0.581	

Table 3 Effect of lack of birth certificate on number of vaccines (Age 0-59 months) *(Continued)*

Under-identification test:		
Kleibergen-Paap rk LM stat	220.9	220.4
Weak identification tests:		
Cragg-Donald Wald F stat	255.4	244.3
Kleibergen-Paap rk Wald F	154.5	147.5
Over identification test:		
Hansen P-value	0.788	

Notes: Marginal effects. Robust standard errors in parentheses. * $p < 0.1$, ** $p < 0.05$, *** $p < 0.01$

which involved collecting data on the location of more than 800 permanent immunization centers in the Dominican Republic; and iv) *immunization center open morning/afternoon.* To obtain data related to variables iii and iv, the address, hours of operation, and latitude and longitude of the immunization centers were collected. The results appear in columns 2 through 7 in Table 3. They still show the lack of a birth certificate has a negative and significant effect on vaccinations. Hence, the instrumental variables were robust to the addition of these crucial controls.

We used the standard battery of econometric tests performed to assess the validity of instruments. The tests at the bottom of Table 3 generally indicate that there are no reasons to cast doubt on the validity of the instrumental variables. This is so because they are sufficiently correlated with the endogenous variable and they are not correlated with the error term of regression (2). Column 7 is likely the most robust specification, with instrumental variables and dummies at the municipal level. This estimate suggests that lacking a birth certificate is associated with a reduction of 0.7 vaccines. Thus, not having this document seems to be an impediment to have complete vaccine coverage.

With regard to the new controls added to check for robustness of the basic specifications, we find that vaccination campaigns are strongly associated with immunization. Specifically, a child vaccinated in a mobile vaccination campaign receives 0.07 more vaccines than children vaccinated only at permanent immunization centers. The fact that the mother considers the health center far away is associated with a reduction in the number of vaccines by 0.12. Finally, the actual linear distance to the immunization center was not significant.

(iii) Effect on individual vaccines

The results so far established that lacking a birth certificate reduces the number of vaccines in children under 59 months of age. But, what can be said about the effect on each individual vaccine? We explore this in Table 4, which shows regressions for the BCG, HEPB, DTP1, DTP2, DTP3, OPV1, OPV2, OPV3 and MCV vaccines. The results presented come from IV-PROBIT specifications following the procedure described in Rivers and

Vuong [36] to correct for endogeneity in a PROBIT model where the endogenous variable is also binary.

Three vaccines seem to be affected by the lack of a birth certificate: the DTP1, OPV1 and MCV. The coefficients were statistically significant also when we included dummy variables at the household level in OLS regressions (except for the MCV). Children without birth certificates have 13, 11, and 30 percentage points less likelihood of being vaccinated with DTP1, OPV1, and MCV, respectively. These results should be of great concern to national authorities and civil society because polio destroys motor neurons and causes muscle weakness, resulting in permanent physical damage. Diphtheria, tetanus, and pertussis are highly contagious and develop into epidemics quickly in large, populated areas. According to the WHO, measles is a leading cause of vaccine-preventable child mortality.

We also repeated the analysis using the sample of children with vaccination cards. The results are contained in the Appendix: Table 7. The results change but only slightly. For example, the impact of not having birth certificate on the number of vaccines changes from -0.76 to -0.69 and remains statistically significant. As for DTP1, OPV1 and MCV the effects are similar with the exception of the one for OPV1 which becomes not significant. The difference between these results and the ones obtained with the whole sample could be attributed to unobservable attributes that are correlated with the possession of a vaccination card, and to the reduction of degrees of freedom because only 70% of the children have these cards.

Discussion

(a) Why does the lack of a birth certificate affect vaccination?

One mechanism of transmission could be related to the need to prove a child's age in order to receive a specific vaccine. Given that in the Dominican Republic there is a schedule of vaccinations that recommends that vaccines be given at a particular age, not having proof of age-appropriateness could be one channel of transmission. The vaccination schedule is based on the fact that the immune system's response is optimal at the recommended age. Undocumented immigrants are also afraid to enter public services facilities,

Table 4 Effect of Lack of Birth Certificate on Individual Vaccines

Dependent variable:	(4.1)	(4.2)	(4.3)	(4.4)	(4.5)	(4.6)	(4.7)	(4.8)	(4.9)
1 if child took vaccine, 0 otherwise	BCG	HEPB	DTP1	DTP2	DTP3	OPV1	OPV2	OPV3	MCV
Child without birth certificate	-0.031	-0.037	-0.131**	-0.117*	-0.088	-0.107**	-0.007	-0.135*	-0.299***
	(0.032)	(0.038)	(0.053)	(0.060)	(0.072)	(0.049)	(0.045)	(0.076)	(0.083)
Card (seen)	0.029***	-0.029***	0.027***	0.089***	0.175***	0.005	0.172***	0.426***	-0.143***
	(0.007)	(0.006)	(0.008)	(0.014)	(0.018)	(0.005)	(0.014)	(0.017)	(0.017)
Aged 0-2 months	0.010	0.026	-0.926***	-0.875***	-0.742***	-0.944***	-0.897***		-0.719***
	(0.012)	(0.017)	(0.023)	(0.009)	(0.008)	(0.024)	(0.007)		(0.013)
Aged 3-6 months	0.000	0.013	-0.268***	-0.646***	-0.772***	-0.166***	-0.634***	-0.793***	-0.776***
	(0.008)	(0.011)	(0.027)	(0.024)	(0.010)	(0.023)	(0.026)	(0.008)	(0.009)
Aged 7-12 months	0.013**	0.018*	-0.018	-0.103***	-0.268***	-0.007	-0.075***	-0.276***	-0.705***
	(0.005)	(0.010)	(0.013)	(0.023)	(0.027)	(0.009)	(0.022)	(0.028)	(0.014)
Child is a girl	-0.000	-0.004	0.005	0.006	0.004	-0.006	-0.003	-0.006	0.004
	(0.004)	(0.007)	(0.006)	(0.010)	(0.014)	(0.004)	(0.010)	(0.015)	(0.016)
Birth order	-0.002	0.001	-0.006***	-0.009**	-0.012**	-0.003	-0.008**	-0.009	-0.015**
	(0.002)	(0.003)	(0.002)	(0.004)	(0.006)	(0.002)	(0.004)	(0.006)	(0.006)
Born in hospital/health center	0.059**	0.096**	0.054*	0.075	0.130**	-0.003	-0.015	-0.011	0.168***
	(0.028)	(0.038)	(0.031)	(0.046)	(0.056)	(0.014)	(0.031)	(0.057)	(0.064)
Mother's schooling in years	0.001*	0.002*	0.001	0.004**	0.008***	-0.001	0.005***	0.008***	0.005**
	(0.001)	(0.001)	(0.001)	(0.002)	(0.002)	(0.001)	(0.002)	(0.002)	(0.003)
Mother works	-0.001	0.007	-0.000	-0.005	0.003	0.002	-0.002	0.016	-0.000
	(0.005)	(0.007)	(0.007)	(0.012)	(0.016)	(0.005)	(0.011)	(0.017)	(0.018)
One parent born abroad	-0.004	-0.050**	-0.010	-0.079**	-0.058	-0.001	-0.082**	-0.055	-0.041
	(0.012)	(0.023)	(0.017)	(0.036)	(0.042)	(0.011)	(0.035)	(0.043)	(0.048)
Rural area	0.013**	0.024**	0.014*	0.026*	0.018	0.006	0.022	0.015	0.035
	(0.006)	(0.010)	(0.009)	(0.015)	(0.021)	(0.006)	(0.014)	(0.022)	(0.023)
No water/electricity	-0.065**	-0.100***	-0.037	-0.112***	-0.248***	-0.001	-0.064*	-0.130**	-0.116**
	(0.028)	(0.035)	(0.024)	(0.043)	(0.049)	(0.012)	(0.036)	(0.054)	(0.057)
Health center far away	0.007	-0.004	-0.024***	-0.023*	-0.050***	-0.008	-0.004	-0.023	-0.028
	(0.004)	(0.008)	(0.008)	(0.012)	(0.017)	(0.005)	(0.011)	(0.017)	(0.019)
Vaccinated in a campaign	-0.011**	-0.014*	0.003	0.020*	0.018	-0.003	0.020*	0.026	0.027
	(0.005)	(0.008)	(0.007)	(0.012)	(0.016)	(0.005)	(0.011)	(0.016)	(0.018)
Dist to immun center in km	-0.002	-0.006***	0.003	-0.003	-0.006	0.000	-0.005*	-0.008*	-0.003
	(0.001)	(0.002)	(0.002)	(0.003)	(0.005)	(0.001)	(0.003)	(0.005)	(0.005)
Immun cent attends morning/ afternoon	-0.006	0.009	0.006	0.017	-0.004	-0.000	-0.003	-0.031*	-0.008
	(0.005)	(0.008)	(0.007)	(0.013)	(0.017)	(0.005)	(0.012)	(0.018)	(0.018)
Observations	5157	5157	5157	5157	5157	5157	5157	5157	5157

Notes: All coefficients are marginal effects from regressions IV-PROBIT. Robust standard errors in parentheses. * $p < 0.1$, ** $p < 0.05$, *** $p < 0.01$. All regressions also include controls for municipality dummies

where proof of documentation is needed, in order to avoid problems with their immigration status. Therefore, it is highly likely that mothers whose children lack identity documents avoid visiting immunization centers.

(b) Does the lack of a birth certificate produce delays in vaccination?

We also examined the effect of lack of birth certificates on delays in immunization delivery. The results are reported in Table 5. The sample is composed of children with vaccination cards because these cards are the source of information about the vaccination date. The regressions control for all of the determinants that appear in the tables above.

Table 5 Effect of Lack of Birth Certificate on Timely Vaccination

	(5.1) Proportion of age-due vaccines (children aged 0-59 months)	(5.2) Up to date vaccinations at 7 months (children aged >7 months)	(5.3) Up to date vaccinations at 12 months (children aged > 12 months)
Child without birth certificate	-0.108**	-0.020	-0.265***
	(0.054)	(0.093)	(0.080)
Card (seen)	2.181***		
	(0.088)		
Aged 0-2 months	0.121***		
	(0.046)		
Aged 3-6 months	-0.164***		
	(0.015)		
Aged 7-12 months	-0.033*	-0.040	
	(0.019)	(0.027)	
Child is a girl	0.023**	0.032*	0.016
	(0.012)	(0.018)	(0.021)
Birth order	-0.021***	-0.023***	-0.018**
	(0.005)	(0.008)	(0.009)
Born in hospital/health center	0.031	-0.037	-0.041
	(0.051)	(0.090)	(0.099)
Mother's schooling in years	0.002	0.001	-0.004
	(0.002)	(0.003)	(0.004)
Mother works	0.002	0.015	0.020
	(0.014)	(0.021)	(0.024)
One parent born abroad	-0.078**	-0.123***	-0.121*
	(0.035)	(0.047)	(0.064)
Rural area	-0.009	-0.018	-0.003
	(0.015)	(0.027)	(0.031)
No water/electricity	-0.087***	-0.132**	-0.151**
	(0.033)	(0.058)	(0.070)
Health center far away	-0.002	-0.021	0.016
	(0.013)	(0.022)	(0.025)
Vaccinated in a campaign	-0.050***	-0.051**	-0.052**
	(0.014)	(0.020)	(0.022)
Dist to immun center in km	-0.000	-0.002	-0.007
	(0.003)	(0.006)	(0.007)
Immun cent attends morning/afternoon	0.033**	0.051**	0.022
	(0.013)	(0.021)	(0.024)
Constant	-1.551***		
	(0.087)		
Observations	3478	3066	2594

Notes: Coefficients are marginal effects from regressions IV-TOBIT for column (5.1) and from regressions IV-PROBIT for columns (5.2) and (5.3). Robust standard errors in parentheses. All regressions include municipality dummies
* $p < 0.1$, ** $p < 0.05$, *** $p < 0.01$

Among children without birth certificates, the proportion of age-due vaccines decreases by about 10% according to the estimate in column 1. Up to date vaccinations at 7 months is not affected by the lack of a birth certificate. However, the probability of having complete, up-to-date vaccinations at 12 months is reduced by 27 percentage points if the child lacks a birth certificate, as suggested by the IVPROBIT regression in column 3.

Conclusions

Healthy children do better in school, and as adults they are more productive at work. Health care at an early age, including immunization, is thus a crucial component of long-term economic prosperity. However, while much research on the socioeconomic characteristics of infant vaccination has been conducted, nothing has been said about the effect of the lack of legal identity on access to health services. This is the first study that aims to quantify a causal impact of the lack of a birth certificate on infant vaccination. The Dominican Republic is a highly relevant case because it is one of the few countries in Latin America and the Caribbean where under-registration birth is considerable.

We found that children without birth certificates are behind by 0.7 vaccines compared to those with birth certificates. In addition, the probability of vaccination with DTP1, OPV1, and MCV is reduced by 8, 7, and 19 percentage points respectively. Moreover, timely vaccination is less likely to occur when a child lacks a birth certificate. The proportion of age-due vaccines for children of a given age is reduced by 10 percent, and the probability of vaccination in due time at 12 months of age is reduced by 23 percentage points.

These findings have important policy implications. Around 98% children are born in hospitals and health centers and more than 90% receive at least the first two vaccines, BCG and HEPB. Given that health services have better coverage and far more outreach activities than civil registries, there is an opportunity to integrate their work in order to reduce the percentage of children without birth certificates and increase immunization rates.

Endnotes

[1] The DHS was not designed to study legal identity issues. Fortunately for the Dominican Republic, the 2006 ENHOGAR household survey asked about birth certificates. This provided a secondary and independent source of data to cross-check the accuracy of birth registration rates in the DHS. We were able to confirm that birth registration rates in both datasets coincide, being 22 percent for children under the age of 5.

[2] Health centers may not coincide with immunization centers, but they may serve as a proxy for the actual location of immunization centers, as they generally include a unit devoted to immunizations.

[3] The DHS contains a random error in the position of the cluster of households. This is done to protect the confidentiality of the household members. See http://dhsprogram.com/faq.cfm for more details.

[4] We used the treatreg command in STATA.

Appendix

Table 6 Permanent Immunization Centers

Province	Open Morning	Open Morning/ Afternoon	Number
Azua	11	26	37
Bahoruco	3	9	12
Barahona	8	17	25
Dajabon	5	14	19
Distrito Nacional	26	70	96
Duarte	7	17	24
El Seybo	3	9	12
Elias Pina	5	14	19
Espalliat	9	20	29
Hato Mayor	6	12	18
Hermanas Mirabal	6	18	24
Independencia	2	7	9
La Altagracia	2	7	9
La Romana	3	5	8
La Vega	12	32	44
Maria Trinidad Sanchez	4	10	14
Monseñor Noel	7	17	24
Monte Christi	5	15	20
Monte Plata	2	5	7
Pedernales	2	3	5
Peravia	6	18	24
Puerto Plata	9	22	31
Samana	5	12	17
San Cristobal	10	25	35
San Jose Ocoa	4	11	15
San Juan de la Maguan	13	37	50
San Pedro de Macoris	8	22	30
Sanchez Ramirez	8	22	30
Santiago	21	52	73
Santiago Rodriguez	5	12	17
Santo Domingo	23	57	80
Valverde	5	15	20
Total	245	632	877

Source: Health Ministry of the Dominican Republic

Table 7 Effect of Lack of Birth Certificate on Vaccination using Data from Vaccination Cards

Dependent variable	(A2.1) MLE2 number of vaccines	(A2.2) IVPROBIT DTP1	(A2.3) IVPROBIT OPV1	(A2.4) IVPROBIT MCV
Child without birth certificate	-0.694***	-0.292***	-0.077	-0.278**
	(0.180)	(0.107)	(0.054)	(0.114)
Aged 0-2 months	-6.155***		-0.986***	-0.600***
	(0.147)		(0.004)	(0.017)
Aged 3-6 months	-4.111***	-0.283***	-0.175***	-0.744***
	(0.069)	(0.031)	(0.028)	(0.010)
Aged 7-12 months	-1.370***	-0.021	-0.010	-0.694***
	(0.066)	(0.014)	(0.010)	(0.015)
Child is a girl	0.023	0.001	-0.009**	0.018
	(0.041)	(0.007)	(0.005)	(0.024)
Birth order	-0.070***	-0.009***	-0.003	-0.038***
	(0.018)	(0.003)	(0.002)	(0.010)
Born in hospital/health center	0.303	0.048	-0.008	0.135
	(0.194)	(0.044)	(0.012)	(0.102)
Mother's schooling in years	0.003	-0.003**	-0.001	-0.001
	(0.007)	(0.001)	(0.001)	(0.004)
Mother works	-0.010	0.010	0.000	-0.001
	(0.048)	(0.007)	(0.005)	(0.027)
One parent born abroad	-0.566***	-0.009	-0.013	-0.057
	(0.125)	(0.019)	(0.014)	(0.074)
Rural area	0.047	0.007	-0.007	0.009
	(0.060)	(0.010)	(0.007)	(0.033)
No water/electricity	-0.576***	0.006	0.006	-0.060
	(0.146)	(0.019)	(0.009)	(0.088)
Health center far away	-0.047	-0.002	-0.000	-0.031
	(0.049)	(0.008)	(0.005)	(0.028)
Vaccinated in a campaign	-0.059	-0.008	-0.007	-0.024
	(0.049)	(0.009)	(0.006)	(0.026)
Dist to immun center in km	-0.001	0.004*	0.002	0.001
	(0.013)	(0.002)	(0.001)	(0.008)
Immun cent attends morning/afternoon	0.027	0.003	-0.005	-0.006
	(0.049)	(0.008)	(0.005)	(0.028)
Household dummies	No	No	No	No
Province dummies	No	No	No	No
Municipality dummies	Yes	Yes	Yes	Yes
Observations	3654	3654	3654	3654

Notes: Marginal effects; Standard errors in parentheses. * $p < 0.1$, ** $p < 0.05$, *** $p < 0.01$

Table 8 Effect of Instrumental Variables on Vaccinations

	(A3.1)	(A3.2)	(A3.3)	(A3.4)
Dependent variable:	Number of vaccines	DTP1	DTP3	MCV
Child without birth certificate	-0.263***	-0.028***	-0.039**	-0.042***
	(0.062)	(0.011)	(0.016)	(0.014)
Distance to nearest registry in km	-0.017	-0.001	-0.002	-0.003
	(0.010)	(0.002)	(0.002)	(0.002)
Mother without birth certificate	-0.115	-0.024	-0.011	-0.030
	(0.085)	(0.020)	(0.022)	(0.020)
Card (seen)	0.233***	-0.002	0.062***	-0.121***
	(0.047)	(0.007)	(0.013)	(0.012)
Aged 0-2 months	-5.984***	-0.912***	-0.816***	-0.780***
	(0.104)	(0.023)	(0.019)	(0.022)
Aged 3-6 months	-3.918***	-0.240***	-0.790***	-0.784***
	(0.077)	(0.021)	(0.014)	(0.013)
Aged 7-12 months	-1.275***	-0.023**	-0.212***	-0.703***
	(0.072)	(0.011)	(0.022)	(0.017)
Child is a girl	0.012	0.003	0.008	0.008
	(0.037)	(0.006)	(0.010)	(0.009)
Birth order	-0.054***	-0.008***	-0.010**	-0.011***
	(0.017)	(0.003)	(0.005)	(0.004)
Born in hospital/health center	0.524***	0.075**	0.123**	0.092**
	(0.202)	(0.037)	(0.048)	(0.044)
Mother's schooling in years	0.024***	0.001	0.005***	0.003**
	(0.005)	(0.001)	(0.001)	(0.001)
Mother works	0.012	0.001	0.006	0.001
	(0.042)	(0.007)	(0.012)	(0.010)
One parent born abroad	-0.408***	-0.038*	-0.052*	-0.043
	(0.137)	(0.023)	(0.031)	(0.031)
Rural area	0.135**	0.014	0.017	0.015
	(0.059)	(0.010)	(0.016)	(0.014)
No water/electricity	-0.746***	-0.048*	-0.216***	-0.068*
	(0.165)	(0.028)	(0.039)	(0.037)
Health center far away	-0.118***	-0.023***	-0.035***	-0.016
	(0.045)	(0.008)	(0.012)	(0.011)
Vaccinated in a campaign	0.075*	0.005	0.012	0.014
	(0.043)	(0.006)	(0.012)	(0.011)
Dist to immun center in km	-0.009	0.002	-0.005	0.002
	(0.013)	(0.002)	(0.004)	(0.003)
Immun cent attends morning/afternoon	0.033	0.011	0.010	-0.003
	(0.045)	(0.008)	(0.012)	(0.011)
Household dummies	No	No	No	No

Table 8 Effect of Instrumental Variables on Vaccinations *(Continued)*

Province dummies	No	No	No	No
Municipality dummies	Yes	Yes	Yes	Yes
Observations	5157	5157	5157	5157
R^2	0.582	0.343	0.393	0.539

Notes: Coefficients from OLS regressions. Robust standard errors in parentheses. * $p < 0.1$, ** $p < 0.05$, *** $p < 0.01$

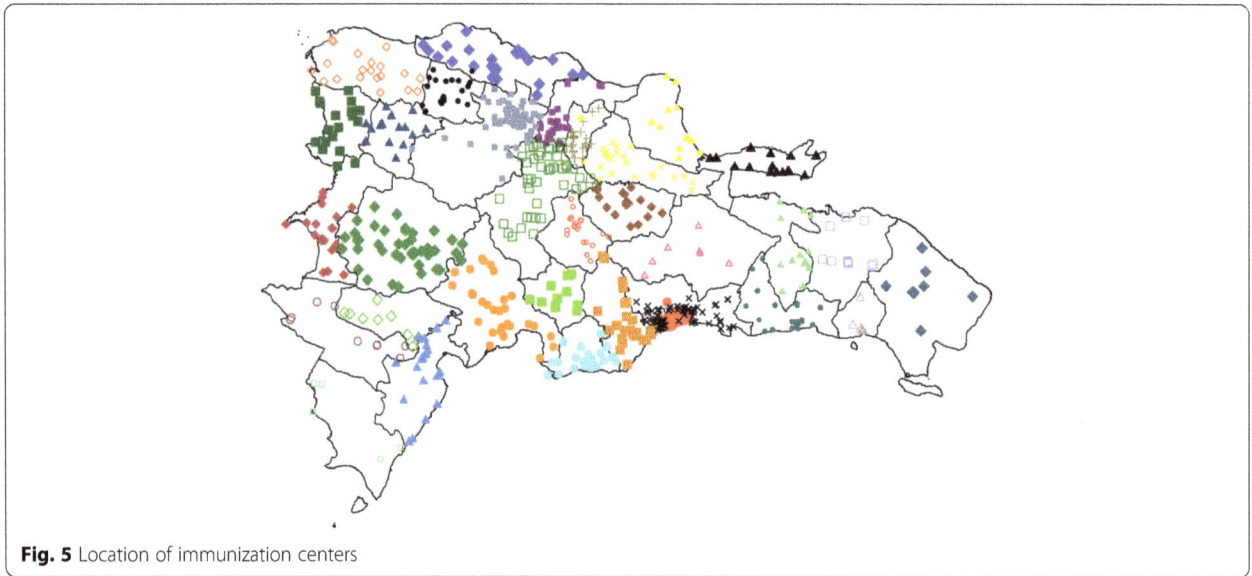

Fig. 5 Location of immunization centers

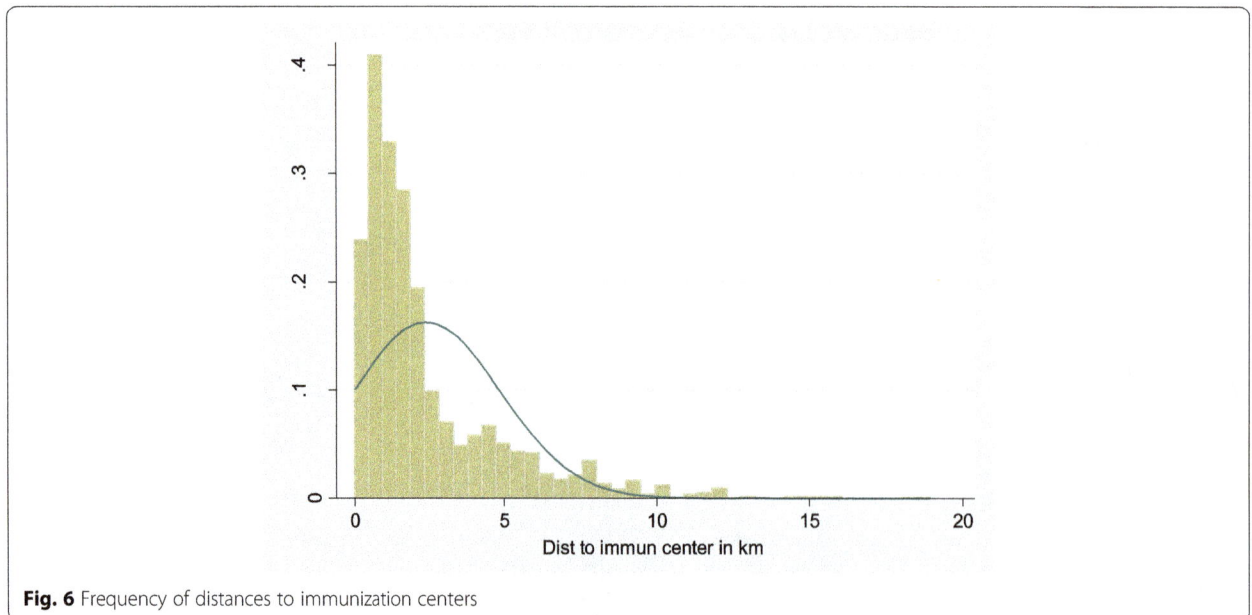

Fig. 6 Frequency of distances to immunization centers

Acknowledgements

The authors thank Nils Handler for valuable research assistance and the Junta Central Electoral of the Dominican Republic for data on the location of civil registries. Mia Harbitz, Senior Specialist at the IDB, United Nations Development Programme, United Nations Children's Fund, Pan American Health Organization, Organization of American States, participants of the Fifth Bolivian Conference on Development Economics 2013 and the Latin American Economic Association Conference 2013 for useful comments.

Disclaimer

This article was prepared when Ana Corbacho was Sector Economic Advisor and Steve Brito was research fellow at the Inter-American Development Bank. The views expressed in this paper are those of the author(s) and do not necessarily represent the views of the IMF, its Executive Board, or IMF management. The views expressed in this paper are those of the author(s) and do not necessarily represent the views of the IDB, its Executive Board, or management.

Authors' contributions

All authors contributed equally. All authors read and approved the final manuscript.

Competing interests

The authors declare that they have no competing interests.

Author details

[1]International Monetary Fund, 700 19th St NW, Washington, DC 20431, USA. [2]Inter-American Development Bank, 1300 New York Avenue NW, Washington, DC 20577, USA.

References

1. Aaby P, Coll A, Knudsen K, Samb B, Simondon F, Whittle H. Nonspecific beneficial impact of measles immunisation: analysis of mortality studies from developing countries. Br Med J. 1995;311(7003):481–85.
2. Acemoglu H, Ak M, Akkafa F, Bozkurt A, Ceylan A, Ilcin E, Ozgur S, Ozcirpici B, Palanci Y, Sahinoz S, Sahinoz T, Saka G. Vaccination coverage in the South-East Anatolian Project (SEAP) region and factors influencing low coverage. Public Health. 2006;120(2):145–54.
3. Adler R, Kahane S, Kellam S, Newell K, Reingold A, Smith N, Watt J, Wight S. Immunization levels and risk factors for low immunization coverage among private practices. Pediatrics. 2000;105(6):e73.
4. Akmatov M, Kretzschmar M, Kramer A, Mikolajczyk R. Timeliness of vaccination and its effects on fraction of vaccinated population. Vaccine. 2008;26(31):3805–11.
5. Bakirci N, Torun S. Vaccination coverage and reasons for non-vaccination in a district of Istanbul. BMC Public Health. 2006;6:125.
6. Bardenheier B, Chu S, Rickert D, Rosenthal J, Santoli J, Shefer A, Yusuf H. Factors associated with underimmunization at 3 months of age in four medically underserved areas. Public Health Rep. 2004;119(5):479–85.
7. Barham T, Maluccio J. Eradicating diseases: the effect of conditional cash transfers on vaccination coverage in rural Nicaragua. J Health Econ. 2009; 28(3):611–21.
8. Barker L, Chu S, Luman E, Mokdad A, Strine T, Sutter R. Vaccination coverage of foreign-born children 19-35 months of age: findings from the National Immunization Survey 1999–2000. Pediatrics. 2002;110(2):e15.
9. Berman S, Davis R, Irigoyen M, Kalton G, McCauley M, Rosenthal J, Rodewald L, Sawyer M, Yusuf H. Immunization coverage levels among 19-35 month-old children in four diverse, medically underserved areas of the United States. Pediatrics. 2004;113(4):296–302.
10. Bishar D, Khan M, Koenig M. Health interventions and health equity: the example of measles vaccination in Bangladesh. Popul Dev Rev. 2001;27(2):283–02.
11. Bloom D, Canning D, Weston M. The value of vaccination. World Econ. 2005;6:15–39.
12. Bloom D, Canning D, Seiguer E. The effect of vaccination on children's and cognitive development in the Philippines. Working Paper 69. Program on the Global Demography of Aging. 2011.
13. Bobo J, Gale J, Thapa P, Wassilak S. Risk factors for delayed Immunization in a random sample of 1163 children from Oregon and Washington 35. Pediatrics. 1993;91(2):308–14.
14. Bolton P, Guyer B, Hadpawat A, Holt E, Hughart N, Hussain A. Deficiencies in current childhood immunization indicators. Public Health Rep. 1998;113(6):527–32.
15. Bracamonte P, Ordonez D. El registro de nacimientos: consecuencias en relación al acceso a derechos y servicios sociales y a la implementación de programas de reducción de pobreza en 6 países de Latinoamérica. IDB Project Document. Washington: Inter-American Development Bank; 2006.
16. Breiman R, Phelan M, Rashid M, Streatfield P, Shifa N, Yunus M. Effect of infant immunization on childhood mortality in rural Bangladesh: analysis of health and demographic surveillance data. Lancet. 2004;364(9452):2204–11.
17. Canning D, Driessen J, Razzaque A, Walker D. The effect of childhood measles vaccination on school Enrollment in Matlab, Bangladesh. Working Paper Series 81. Program on the Global Demography of Aging. 2011.
18. Castro L, Rud J. Medición cuantitativa del subregistro de nacimientos e indocumentación. IDB Working Paper 254. Washington: Inter-American Development Bank; 2011.
19. Chaui J, Dayan G, Ellis A, Forlenza R, Kaplan S, Orellana L, Strebel P. Vaccination coverage among children aged 13-59 months in Buenos Aires, Argentina. Rev Panam Salud Publica. 2004;16(3):158–67.
20. Chu S, Luman E, McCauley M, Pickering L, Stokley S. Timeliness of childhood immunizations. Pediatrics. 2002;110(5):935–9.
21. Cody C. Count every child: the right to birth registration. Working Paper. Plan Limited. 2009
22. Corbacho A, Osorio R. Travelling the distance: a GPS-based study of the access to birth registration services in Latin America. IDB Working Paper 307. Washington: Inter-American Development Bank; 2012.
23. Brito S, Corbacho A, Osorio R. Birth registration and the impact on educational attainment. IDB Working Paper IDB-WP-345. Washington: Inter-American Development Bank; 2012.
24. Discover Magazine. Why Does the Vaccine/Autism Controversy Live On? 2009
25. Dombkowski K, Lantz P, Freed G. Risk factors for delay in age-appropriate vaccination. Public Health Rep. 2004;119(2):144–55.
26. Essex C, Geddis D, Smale P. Immunisation status and demographic characteristics of New Zealand infants at 1 year and 2 years of age. N Z Med J. 1995;108(1002):244–6.
27. Fagernas S. The effect of birth registration on child labor and education in early 20th century USA. Working Paper Series 2311, Department of Economics, University of Sussex. 2012.
28. Feilden R, Nielsen O. Immunization and health reform: making reforms work for immunization. A Reference Guide. WHO/V&B/01.44. Geneva: World Health Organization; 2001.
29. Gine X, Yang D. Credit market consequences of improved personal identification: field experimental evidence form Malawi. Am Econ Rev. 2012; 102(6):2923–54.
30. Faustini A, Giorgi R, Perucci C, Spadea T. Choosing immunisation coverage indicators at the local level. Eur J Epidemiol. 2004;19(10):979–85.
31. Harbitz M, Boekle-Giuffrida B. Democratic governance, citizenship, and legal identity. ICF Working Paper. Washington: Inter-American Development Bank; 2009.
32. Harbitz M, Tamargo M. The significance of legal identity in situations of poverty and social exclusion. ICF Technical Note. Washington: Inter-American Development Bank; 2009.
33. Hull B, McIntyre P. Timeliness of childhood immunization in Australia. Vaccine. 2006;24(20):4403–8.
34. Khalegian P. Decentralization and public services: the case of immunization. World Bank Policy Research Working Paper 2989. Washington: World Bank; 2003.
35. Langsten R, Hill K. The accuracy of mother's reports of child vaccinations: evidence from rural Egypt. Soc Sci Med. 1998;46(9):1205–12.
36. Rivers D, Vuong H. Limited information estimators and exogeneity tests for simultaneous probit models. J Econometrics. 1988;39(3):347–66.
37. Schmitt H. Factors influencing vaccine uptake in Germany. Vaccine. 2002;20(1):S2–4.
38. Simpson D, Smith D, Suarez I. Errors and correlates in parental recall of child immunizations: effects on vaccination coverage estimates. Pediatrics. 1997;99(5):e3.
39. UNICEF. The state of the world's children 2012: children in an urban world. New York: UNICEF; 2012.
40. World Health Organization. Economics of immunization: a guide to the literature and other resources. Available: http://apps.who.int/iris/bitstream/10665/68526/1/WHO_V-B_04.02_eng.pdf. Accessed 1 Mar 2017.

11

Patient dumping, outlier payments, and optimal healthcare payment policy under asymmetric information

Tsuyoshi Takahara 🄳

Abstract

We analyze a rationale for official authorization of patient dumping in the prospective payment policy framework. We show that when the insurer designs the healthcare payment policy to let hospitals dump high-cost patients, there is a trade-off between the disutility of dumped patients (changes in hospitals' rent extraction due to low-severity patients) and the shift in the level of cost reduction efforts for high-severity patients. We also clarify the welfare-improving conditions by allowing hospitals to dump high-severity patients. Finally, we show that if the efficiency of the cost reduction efforts varies extensively and the healthcare payment cost is substantial, or if there are many private hospitals, the patient dumping policy can improve social welfare in a wider environment.

Keywords: Patient dumping, Healthcare payment policy, Adverse selection

JEL Classification code: I13, I18, L51

Background

Government agencies in many countries would like to introduce social security systems that decrease healthcare payments while providing high-quality medical services. Two types of healthcare reimbursement policies achieve this end: the retrospective payment system and the prospective payment system.[1] The retrospective payment system is a cost-based system in which insurers pay the entire treatment cost to hospitals. Under the prospective payment system, insurers pay a fixed amount defined by a government agency for each diagnosis per admission. The latter system incentivizes hospitals to reduce treatment costs and may yield socially optimal cost reductions by hospitals.[2] Accordingly, some countries have introduced prospective payments to reduce the cost of social security.[3]

Under the prospective payment system, however, hospitals incur risk when treating extraordinarily expensive patients (also called outlier patients). Hospitals that admit outlier patients incur losses even if they make socially optimal efforts to reduce treatment costs. Subsequently,

an incentive naturally arises for hospitals to refuse treatment to avoid this financial risk, a phenomenon called the dumping problem in the literature.[4] The social cost of patient dumping is obvious. For one thing, it triggers potentially fatal treatment delays. Further, as pointed out by Newhouse [25], the dumping problem stimulates patient convergence on particular hospitals, particularly public hospitals, leading to crowding and longer treatment delays.

Given these social costs associated with the possibility of patient dumping, a clear alternative is to insure hospitals for some fraction of the extra costs incurred to treat each outlier patient.[5] We call this the outlier payment policy for expositional clarity. This policy is precisely what the United States adopted in the 1990s to alleviate the dumping problem. Under this policy, the insurer pays an additional amount equaling some part of the cost exceeding the fixed payment when hospitals admit outlier patients. This additional payment can reduce hospitals' financial risk, thereby contributing to reduced numbers of dumped patients.

The overall welfare effect of the outlier payment policy is not necessarily clear, however, as gains might arise from allowing hospitals to dump patients at their discretion. We argue that adopting the outlier payment policy is

Correspondence: mge012tt@student.econ.osaka-u.ac.jp
Graduate School of Economics, Osaka University, 1-7, Machikaneyama, Toyonaka, Osaka 560-0043, Japan

not always justified, even though hospitals are less likely to dump outlier patients when they are insured against such patients. To substantiate this argument, we consider a canonical model of adverse selection in which there are two hospitals, called private and public for expositional clarity. The sole difference between the two is that the insurer may induce the private hospital to dump its patients whereas it cannot allow the public hospital to do so, perhaps because of legal restrictions. We assume that patients randomly visit one of the hospitals that privately observes the treatment cost for each patient.[6] In this setting, the insurer devises a contract for healthcare payment that is based on the hospital's level of effort. Given the contract, the hospital decides which patients are to be dumped and decides its level of cost reduction efforts accordingly.

To observe the potential welfare consequences of patient dumping, suppose that the insurer chooses not to adopt the outlier payment policy and instead allows the private hospital to dump high-severity patients selectively. Under this patient dumping policy, it is too expensive for the private hospital to treat high-severity patients; consequently, the bulk of them is eventually transferred to the public hospital. Although patient dumping is in itself welfare-reducing, it also endogenously changes the distribution of patients across hospitals and initiates a sorting effect that substantially alleviates information asymmetry regarding patient types. This sorting effect is potentially welfare-improving because it is instrumental in reducing information rent and consequently in realizing more efficient levels of cost reduction for high-severity patients in equilibrium. We show that gains from the sorting effect can outweigh the social cost of patient dumping under some conditions, suggesting that there are situations in which some degree of patient dumping should be tolerated for the betterment of society.

This study yields several findings. First, if the difference in cost reduction efficiency between high- and low-severity patients is large, the patient dumping policy is optimal in a wider environment, even with a high ratio of high-severity patients. Intuitively, under this circumstance, information rent is large, thus making patient dumping an advantageous payment policy. Second, if healthcare payment cost (administrative cost of a healthcare payment system) is large, the outlier payment policy is preferred over patient dumping, [7] because an increase in healthcare payment cost reduces information rent, and therefore, favors outlier payment policy over patient dumping policy. Third, if the number of patients in dumping hospitals (e.g., private hospitals) is large, the patient dumping policy improves welfare to a greater extent. This is because government agencies adopt the patient dumping policy and they need not pay information rent to hospitals that dump high-severity patients, whereas

government agencies pay information rent to all hospitals under the outlier payment policy. As such, we insist that insurers consider the circularity of private hospitals when choosing between outlier payment and patient dumping policies.[8]

The main contribution of this study is showing that patient dumping can be an optimal healthcare payment policy. Numerous studies analyze patient dumping (e.g., Newhouse [25]; Dranove [7]; Eze and Wolfe [14]; Newhouse [26]; Meltzer et al. [23]; Canta [4]. Newhouse [25] shows that patient dumping may occur under the prospective payment system and under competition between hospitals. Dranove [7] notes that the patient dumping policy can be efficient due to specialization among hospitals and concentration of patients. Eze and Wolfe [14] also show the optimality of the patient dumping policy using the example of the United States Veterans Affairs hospital inpatient services. Results of these studies parallel ours. However, efficiencies from patient dumping are "gains from specialization"? in both studies, whereas, in the present study, efficiencies from patient dumping are "gains from information acquisition".

Canta [4] also shows the optimality of the patient dumping policy in a similar environment, considering two types of hospitals. However, our work differs from that of Canta [4] in two points of environment and results. First, Canta [4] does not explicitly analyze the healthcare payment for a public hospital and assumes that a public hospital does not exert a cost reduction effort. In our model, we assume that a public hospital also exerts a cost reduction effort, much like a private hospital, and analyze the effect of the healthcare payment policy on the optimal contract. Through the analysis, we find that the cost reduction effort for high-severity patients and information rent for low-severity patients is greater under the patient dumping policy than under the outlier payment policy. The former effect makes the patient dumping policy advantageous since the distortion is reduced. However, the latter effect makes it disadvantageous since the healthcare payment is increased. Second, Canta [4] assumes that all patients go to the private hospital that can dump high-severity patients and that the public hospital treats only dumped patients. We assume that not all patients go to the private hospital owing to consumer preference or geographical proximity and that a public hospital treats both types of patients. In concrete terms, we assume that a fraction of the patients goes to the private hospital and the remaining go to the public hospital. Although the fraction of patients is given exogenously, in Appendix A. we endogenize the patients' hospital choice. Our assumption is valid in certain countries where patients can choose hospitals freely. As shown in the analysis, the fraction affects the optimal contract under the patient dumping policy.

We assume that insurers offer severity-dependent contracts to hospitals as a healthcare payment policy, and the severity-dependent contract can be interpreted as outlier payment.[9] Allen and Gertler [1] discusses the optimality of this selective payment policy.[10] We assume that hospitals treat patients selectively. This assumption is consistent with the theoretical conclusion of Ellis [10].[11] Keeler et al. [20] shows that outlier payment acts as insurance for hospitals.[12] Previous studies also investigate the optimal scheme under outlier payment (Ma [21]; Ellis and McGuire [12]; Jack [18]; Jack [19]; Mougeot and Naegelen [24]. Ellis and McGuire [12] analyzes a consumer-welfare-maximizing outlier payment scheme. Other works study the optimal ratio of outlier payments. Ma [21] investigates optimal outlier payments under the assumption of two-dimensional efforts (cost reduction and treatment quality) by hospitals. He reveals that insurers should reimburse all treatment costs. Moreover, Mougeot and Naegelen [24] studies optimal outlier payment under asymmetric information between insurers and hospitals, and concludes that insurers should reimburse all treatment costs, even under asymmetric information.

Methods
Environment
We consider a healthcare payment system in which a public insurer offers contracts to a private and a public hospital for treatment of patients with a specific diagnosis. Throughout the analysis, we denote each hospital by j, where $j = pr$ indicates the private hospital and $j = pu$, the public hospital. As stated, the only difference between them is that the insurer may induce the private hospital to dump patients selectively, whereas it cannot allow the public hospital to do so. The reasoning underlying this assumption is that if a public hospital dumps a specific type of patient, he is unlikely to receive any medical attention; in fact, public hospitals in the United States cannot dump any patient. Apart from this distinction, the two hospitals are assumed to have identical technological acumen.

To simplify, we assume that decision making by patients is given exogenously: $\lambda \in (0, 1)$ people select the private hospital, and $(1 - \lambda)$ people select the public hospital.[13] After a patient chooses a hospital, the chosen hospital privately observes patient severity $i \in \{H, L\}$, where $i = H$ denotes a high-severity and $i = L$, a low-severity patient. The insurer knows that any given patient is of the high-severity type with probability $\phi \in (0, 1)$, which is common knowledge.

Hospitals
Each hospital can reduce its treatment cost by exerting effort.[14] The marginal productivity of any cost-reducing effort depends on patient severity, and we assume that

cost reduction is higher for low-severity than high-severity patients for the same level of cost reduction efforts. Cost reduction efforts potentially have adverse consequences for hospitals, such as extended duty hours. For a hospital with patient severity i, total cost $C(i, e)$ can be written as

$$C(i, e) = c - \theta_i e + \frac{1}{2}e^2, \quad i \in \{L, H\}. \tag{1}$$

Here, the cost of treatment, c, is the same for any patient type and is assumed to be sufficiently large. We also assume $\theta_L > \theta_H > 0$, which means that it is easier to reduce the treatment cost for low-severity patients. The last term represents the hospital's disutility from cost reduction efforts. Letting w denote the payment collected from the insurer, the payoff function of a hospital with a type-i patient can be written as[15]

$$\tilde{\pi}(i, w, e) = w - c + \theta_i e - \frac{1}{2}e^2, \quad i \in \{L, H\}. \tag{2}$$

Insurer
The insurer offers each hospital a take-it-or-leave-it contract to each hospital that specifies a healthcare payment and a level of cost reduction effort for each patient severity as reported by the hospital. The contract specifies the payment $w_{\hat{i}}^j$ and the level of cost reduction efforts $e_{\hat{i}}^j$ for a given report $\hat{i}$. Define $\omega_{\hat{i}}^j \equiv (e_{\hat{i}}^j, w_{\hat{i}}^j)$ and $\omega^j \equiv (\omega_H^j, \omega_L^j)$.

The insurer seeks to maximize social welfare, assumed to consist of (i) patients' utility, (ii) the social cost of treatment, and (iii) payment by the insurer. To achieve this, the insurer devises a contract contingent on the hospital's report $\hat{i}$ about patient severity. Given the pair of menu contracts $(\omega^{pr}, \omega^{pu})$, assuming truth-telling, the insurer's payoff is given by

$$
\begin{aligned}
W(\omega^{pr}, \omega^{pu}) = {} & \lambda \left\{ \phi \left\{ \left[1 - C\left(H, e_H^{pr}\right) - \eta w_H^{pr} \right](1 - d) \right. \right. \\
& + \left. \left[\gamma - C\left(H, e_H^{pu}\right) - \eta w_H^{pu} \right] d \right\} + (1 - \phi) \left[1 - C\left(L, e_L^{pr}\right) - \eta w_L^{pr} \right] \right\} \\
& + (1 - \lambda) \left\{ \phi \left[1 - C\left(H, e_H^{pu}\right) - \eta w_H^{pu} \right] + (1 - \phi) \left[1 - C\left(L, e_L^{pu}\right) - \eta w_L^{pu} \right] \right\},
\end{aligned}
\tag{3}
$$

where d is an indicator function that takes $d = 1$ when the private hospital dumps high-severity patients and $d = 0$ otherwise. We normalize patients' utility when they receive immediate medical treatment to 1.[16] In contrast, the utility of dumped patients is given by $\gamma \in (-\infty, 1)$, which captures the ill-effects of patient dumping, such as delayed attention and additional treatment cost.[17] Finally, $\eta \in [1, \infty)$ represents a healthcare payment cost.

Timing
The timing of the game is summarized as follows:

1. the insurer offers contracts to hospitals;

2. a fraction λ of patients select the private hospital, and the remaining fraction $1 - \lambda$ of patients select the public hospital, with no patient being aware of his/her severity;
3. the hospitals observe the severity of the patients;
4. they decide whether or not to dump the patients, and if yes, which patients to dump;
5. they set the level of cost reduction efforts;
6. they report patients' severity to and charge healthcare payments from the insurer, and the contract is implemented.

Results

Optimal healthcare payment under symmetric information

This section characterizes the first-best healthcare payment system as a benchmark. With symmetric information, we suppose that the insurer can observe patient severity and thereby can impose its preferred cost reduction efforts on the hospital without information rent. It is easily seen that the insurer prefers no patient dumping, and the first-best contract must satisfy the following participation constraint for each $i = L, H$ and each $j = pr, pu$:

$$w_i^j - c + \theta_i e_i^j - \frac{1}{2}e_i^{j2} \geq 0. \qquad (PC_i^j)$$

For each $i = L, H$ and each $j = pr, pu$, the insurer's problem is defined as follows:

$$\max_{\omega_i^j} \lambda \left\{ \phi \left[1 - C\left(H, e_H^{pr}\right) - \eta w_H^{pr} \right] + (1 - \phi) \left[1 - C\left(L, e_L^{pr}\right) - \eta w_L^{pr} \right] \right\}$$
$$+ (1 - \lambda) \left\{ \phi \left[1 - C\left(H, e_H^{pu}\right) - \eta w_H^{pu} \right] + (1 - \phi) \left[1 - C(L, e_L^{pu}) - \eta w_L^{pu} \right] \right\}, \qquad (4)$$

subject to $\left(PC_i^j\right)$. All constraints obviously are binding at the optimal solution. Further, there is no reason to treat patients differently as the hospitals are symmetric. This implies that by substituting the participation constraint, the optimization problem for each hospital j can be rewritten as

$$\max_{e_H^j, e_L^j} \phi \left[1 - (1 + \eta) \left(c - \theta_H e_H^j + \frac{1}{2}e_H^{j\,2} \right) \right] \qquad (5)$$
$$+ (1 - \phi) \left[1 - (1 + \eta) \left(c - \theta_L e_L^j + \frac{1}{2}e_L^{j\,2} \right) \right].$$

Solving this optimization problem, we now obtain the first-best allocation. As we assume no disparity in technology, the solution is symmetric between hospitals.

Proposition 1 *In the absence of asymmetric information between the insurer and hospitals, the optimal cost*

reduction efforts and the optimal cost reduction efforts (the first-best contract) are as follows:

$$e_H^{pr^{FB}} = e_H^{pu^{FB}} = \theta_H, \qquad (6)$$

$$e_L^{pr^{FB}} = e_L^{pu^{FB}} = \theta_L, \qquad (7)$$

$$w_H^{pr^{FB}} = w_H^{pu^{FB}} = c - \frac{1}{2}\theta_H^2, \qquad (8)$$

$$w_L^{pr^{FB}} = w_L^{pu^{FB}} = c - \frac{1}{2}\theta_L^2. \qquad (9)$$

Optimal healthcare payment under asymmetric information

Optimal outlier payment policy

In this subsection, we obtain the optimal healthcare payment under outlier payments, or simply the optimal outlier payment policy, under asymmetric information. Formally, any outlier payment policy requires the insurer to devise a contract that satisfies all participation constraints. Furthermore, since the insurer cannot observe patient severity, the optimal contract must satisfy the following incentive compatibility constraint for each $i = L, H$ and each $j = pr, pu$:

$$w_i^j + \theta_i e_i^j - \frac{1}{2}e_i^{j2} \geq w_{\tilde{i}}^j + \theta_i e_{\tilde{i}}^j - \frac{1}{2}e_{\tilde{i}}^{j2}, \; i \neq \tilde{i}. \qquad IC_i^j$$

Because the insurer designs the payment system to bar patient dumping, $d = 0$ in (3), and the insurer's problem can be written as

$$\max_{\omega_i^j} \lambda \left\{ \phi \left[1 - C\left(H, e_H^{pr}\right) - \eta w_H^{pr} \right] + (1 - \phi) \left[1 - C\left(L, e_L^{pr}\right) - \eta w_L^{pr} \right] \right\}$$
$$+ (1 - \lambda) \left\{ \phi \left[1 - C\left(H, e_H^{pu}\right) - \eta w_H^{pu} \right] + (1 - \phi) \left[1 - C\left(L, e_L^{pu}\right) - \eta w_L^{pu} \right] \right\}, \qquad (10)$$

subject to $\left(PC_i^j\right)$ and $\left(IC_i^j\right)$, for each $i = L, H$ and each $j = pr, pu$. The following lemma, which is well known in the literature,[18] is helpful in solving this optimization problem.

Lemma 1 *At the optimal solution, (PC_H^{pr}), (PC_H^{pu}), (IC_L^{pr}), and (IC_L^{pu}) are binding.*

This lemma implies that the following equations must be satisfied:

$$w_H^j = c - \theta_H e_H^j + \frac{1}{2}e_H^{j2}, \qquad (11)$$

$$w_L^j = c - \theta_L e_L^j + \frac{1}{2}e_L^{j2} + e_H^j \Delta\theta, \qquad (12)$$

for $j = pr, pu$, where $\Delta\theta \equiv \theta_L - \theta_H > 0$. Note, also, that the problem faced by one hospital is again independent from and identical to that faced by the other hospital because there is no technology gap in treatment. The optimization problem then can be rewritten as

$$
\max_{e_H^{pr}, e_L^{pr}, e_H^{pu}, e_H^{pu}} \lambda \left\{ \phi \left[1 - (1 + \eta) \left(c - \theta_H e_H^{pr} + \frac{1}{2} e_H^{pr2} \right) \right. \right.
$$
$$
\left. + (1 - \phi) \left[1 - (1 + \eta) \left(c - \theta_L e_L^{pr} + \frac{1}{2} e_L^{pr2} \right) - \eta e_H^{pr} \Delta\theta \right] \right\}
$$
$$
+ (1 - \lambda) \left\{ \phi \left[1 - (1 + \eta) \left(c - \theta_H e_H^{pu} + \frac{1}{2} e_H^{pu2} \right) \right. \right.
$$
$$
\left. \left. + (1 - \phi) \left[1 - (1 + \eta) \left(c - \theta_L e_L^{pu} + \frac{1}{2} e_L^{pu2} \right) - \eta e_H^{pu} \Delta\theta \right] \right] \right\}.
$$

$$(13)$$

Using the above, we obtain the optimal cost reduction effort under the outlier payment policy:

$$
e_H^{pr,O*} = e_H^{pu,O*} = \theta_H - \frac{\eta}{1 + \eta} P \Delta\theta, \tag{14}
$$

$$
e_L^{pr,O*} = e_L^{pu,O*} = \theta_L, \tag{15}
$$

where $P \equiv \frac{1-\phi}{\phi}$. Here, we assume $\theta_H - \frac{\eta}{1+\eta} P \Delta\theta > 0$ to assure the existence of an interior solution.

Next, we obtain the optimal healthcare payment using (11), (12), (14), and (15). It is straightforward to show that

$$
w_H^{pr,O*} = w_H^{pu,O*} = c - \frac{1}{2}\theta_H^2 + \frac{1}{2} \left(\frac{\eta}{1+\eta} P \Delta\theta \right)^2, \tag{16}
$$

$$
w_L^{pr,O*} = w_L^{pu,O*} = c - \frac{1}{2}\theta_L^2 + \left(\theta_H - \frac{\eta}{1+\eta} P \Delta\theta \right) \Delta\theta. \tag{17}
$$

Comparing (6) and (14), we observe that the level of cost reduction efforts for high-severity patients under the outlier payment policy is distorted downward. Since the level of cost reduction efforts under the outlier payment policy is smaller than the first-best level, the total treatment cost and the optimal healthcare payment for high-severity patients are larger (the third term in (16)). In contrast, the optimal cost reduction efforts for low-severity patients under the outlier payment policy is not distorted, and the insurer needs to set a higher healthcare payment (the third term in (17)). This, too, is an effect of information asymmetry. We summarize the optimal contract under the outlier payment policy as follows.

Proposition 2 *When the insurer constructs the healthcare payment system so as not to dump any patient, the optimal healthcare payment compared to the first-best case is such that*

$$
e_H^{pr,O*} = e_H^{pu,O*} < e_H^{prFB} = e_H^{puFB},
$$

$$
e_L^{pr,O*} = e_L^{pu,O*} = e_L^{prFB} = e_L^{puFB},
$$

$$
w_H^{pr,O*} = w_H^{pu,O*} > w_H^{prFB} = w_H^{puFB},
$$

$$
w_L^{pr,O*} = w_L^{pu,O*} > w_L^{prFB} = w_L^{puFB}.
$$

We denote the optimized social welfare in the case of the outlier payment policy as W^{O*}.

Optimal patient dumping policy

We now examine the optimal payment policy when the private hospital is induced to dump high-severity patients. In this case, the insurer sets the healthcare payment for the private hospital with a participation constraint with respect to low-severity patients only. The insurer then obviously offers the first-best contract for low-severity patients. The profit of the private hospital when it admits high-severity patients is given by

$$
\pi(H, e_L^{FB}) = w_L^{FB} - c + \theta_H e_L^{FB} - \frac{1}{2}e_L^{FB} = \theta_L(\theta_H - \theta_L) < 0. \tag{18}
$$

Hence, the private hospital would refuse to treat high-severity patients, which can be observed by the insurer. The insurer's objective function then can be written as

$$
\max_{w_i^j} \lambda \left\{ \phi \left[\gamma - C(H, e_H^{pu}) - \eta w_H^{pu} \right] + (1 - \phi) \left[1 - C(L, e_L^{pr}) - \eta w_L^{pr} \right] \right\}
$$
$$
+ (1 - \lambda) \left\{ \phi \left[1 - C(H, e_H^{pu}) - \eta w_H^{pu} \right] + (1 - \phi) \left[1 - C(L, e_L^{pu}) - \eta w_L^{pu} \right] \right\}, \tag{19}
$$

subject to (PC_L^{pr}), (IC_i^{pu}), and (PC_i^{pu}), for each $i = L, H$ and each $j = pr, pu$. Note that the public hospital still is barred from patient dumping, and thus, the participation constraint for high-severity patients must be satisfied for the public hospital.

To solve this problem, we reapply Lemma 1 and obtain

$$
w_L^{pr} = c - \theta_L e_H^{pr} + \frac{1}{2} e_L^{pr2}, \tag{20}
$$

$$
w_H^{pu} = c - \theta_H e_H^{pu} + \frac{1}{2} e_H^{pu2}, \tag{21}
$$

$$
w_L^{pu} = c - \theta_L e_L^{pu} + \frac{1}{2} e_L^{pu2} + e_H^{pu} \Delta\theta. \tag{22}
$$

Given these, the problem can be rewritten as

$$
\max_{e_L^{pr}, e_H^{pu}, e_L^{pu}} \lambda(1 - \phi) \left[1 - (1 + \eta) \left(c - \theta_L e_L^{pr} + \frac{1}{2} e_L^{pr2} \right) \right]
$$
$$
+ (1 - \lambda)(1 - \phi) \left[1 - (1 + \eta) \left(c - \theta_L e_L^{pu} + \frac{1}{2} e_L^{pu2} \right) - \frac{1}{2} \eta e_H^{pu} \Delta\theta \right]
$$
$$
+ \phi \left[\lambda\gamma + (1 - \lambda) - (1 + \eta) \left(c - \theta_H e_H^{pr} + \frac{1}{2} e_H^{pr2} \right) \right]. \tag{23}
$$

This problem yields the optimal cost reduction efforts under a patient dumping policy:

$$
e_L^{pr,D*} = \theta_L, \tag{24}
$$

$$
e_H^{pu,D*} = \theta_H - (1 - \lambda)\frac{\eta}{1 + \eta} P \Delta\theta, \tag{25}
$$

$$
e_L^{pu,D*} = \theta_L. \tag{26}
$$

Further, the optimal healthcare payment can be obtained by substituting (24), (25), and (26) into (20), (21), and (22):

$$w_L^{pr,D*} = c - \frac{1}{2}\theta_L^2, \tag{27}$$

$$w_H^{pu,D*} = c - \frac{1}{2}\left[\theta_H - (1-\lambda)\frac{\eta}{1+\eta}P\Delta\theta\right]$$
$$\left[\theta_H + (1-\lambda)\frac{\eta}{1+\eta}P\Delta\theta\right], \tag{28}$$

$$w_L^{pu,D*} = c - \frac{1}{2}\theta_H^2 + \left[\theta_H - (1-\lambda)\frac{\eta}{1+\eta}P\Delta\theta\right]\Delta\theta. \tag{29}$$

Unlike previous cases, the optimal contract in this case is asymmetric between hospitals even though we assume no asymmetry in technology. The key is that the insurer need not provide information rent to the private hospital but still pays it to the public hospital. Comparing (17) and (29), we observe that information rent for the public hospital is higher under the patient dumping policy than under the outlier payment policy. In contrast, comparing (14) and (25), we also show that distortion in the level of cost reduction efforts for high-severity patients is smaller under the patient dumping policy than under the outlier payment policy. The optimal healthcare payment system in the case of the patient dumping policy is summarized by the following proposition.

Proposition 3 *The optimal healthcare payment policy under the patient dumping policy is such that*

$$e_L^{pr,D*} = e_L^{pu,D*} = e_L^{pr,O*} = e_L^{pu,O*} = e_L^{pr^{FB}} = e_L^{pu^{FB}},$$
$$e_H^{pu,D*} > e_H^{pu,O*} > e_H^{pu^{FB}},$$
$$w_L^{pr,O*} > w_L^{pr,D*} = w_L^{pr^{FB}},$$
$$w_H^{pu,O*} > w_H^{pu,D*} > w_H^{pu^{FB}},$$
$$w_L^{pu,D*} > w_L^{pu,O*} > w_L^{pu^{FB}}.$$

We denote the optimized social welfare in the case of the patient dumping policy as W^{D*}.

Welfare analysis
Welfare comparison

We thus far have characterized optimal contracts under two distinct regimes: outlier payment and patient dumping. Given the indicated results, we now are ready to compare social welfare between the two policies to illustrate whether a degree of patient dumping should be tolerated and, if so, under what conditions. To this end, we first compute the welfare difference between the two

policies (hereafter, welfare difference) as follows:

$$W^{D*} - W^{O*} = \underbrace{\frac{1}{2}\phi\lambda(1+\eta)\left(\frac{\eta}{1+\eta}P\Delta\theta\right)^2(2-\lambda)}_{\text{Heavy-severity patients}}$$
$$\underbrace{-\phi\lambda(1-\gamma)}_{\text{Patient dumping cost}}$$
$$\underbrace{+\lambda(1-\phi)\eta(\theta_H - \frac{\eta}{1+\eta}P\Delta\theta)\Delta\theta}_{\text{Low-severity patients in the private hospital}}$$
$$\underbrace{-(1-\lambda)(1-\phi)\eta\lambda\frac{\eta}{1+\eta}P\Delta\theta^2}_{\text{Low-severity patients in the public hospital}}. \tag{30}$$

Obviously, the patient dumping policy is preferred over the outlier payment policy when this difference is strictly positive. The first term gives the welfare difference associated with the treatment cost and the payment cost when $i = H$ (which for expositional simplicity we call the welfare difference for high-severity patients). As mentioned, the optimal level of cost reduction efforts for high-severity patients is higher under the patient dumping policy, which always contributes to welfare improvement. The second term gives the welfare difference associated with patients' utility when $i = H$ and $j = pr$ (the welfare difference for high-severity patients in the private hospital). It is always negative because the utility of dumped patients is discounted to γ. The third term gives the welfare difference when $i = L$ and $j = pr$ (the welfare difference for low-severity patients in the private hospital). It is always positive because the insurer need not pay information rent to the private hospital under the patient dumping policy. Finally, the last term reflects the welfare difference when $i = L$ and $j = pu$ (the welfare difference for low-severity patients in the public hospital). It is negative because the insurer must provide a larger information rent in this contingency under the patient dumping policy.

The patient dumping policy clearly is less likely to be optimal when its cost is relatively large (γ is small). We can subsequently conjecture that there is a threshold level $\bar{\gamma}$ such that the outlier payment policy is optimal if and only if $\bar{\gamma} > \gamma$. By rearranging (30), the threshold is computed as

$$\bar{\gamma} = 1 - \underbrace{\frac{1}{2}\frac{\eta^2}{1+\eta}P^2\Delta\theta^2(2-\lambda)}_{\text{High-severity patients}} - \underbrace{\eta P(\theta_H - \frac{\eta}{(1+\eta)}P\Delta\theta)\Delta\theta}_{\text{Low-severity patients in the private hospital}}$$
$$+ \underbrace{(1-\lambda)P^2\frac{\eta^2}{1+\eta}\Delta\theta^2}_{\text{Low-severity patients in the public hospital}}$$
$$= 1 - \eta P\Delta\theta\left(\theta_H - \frac{\eta}{1+\eta}P\Delta\theta\left(1 - \frac{1}{2}\lambda\right)\right). \tag{31}$$

Since $\theta_H - \frac{\eta}{1+\eta}P\Delta\theta > 0$ and $\lambda \in (0,1)$ by assumption, $\theta_H - \frac{\eta}{1+\eta}P\Delta\theta(1 - \frac{1}{2}\lambda) > 0$. We also assume η and $\Delta\theta$ are positive, and by definition P is positive. This implies that $\bar{\gamma} < 1$. We then obtain the following result, which is not surprising by itself but still clarifies that the patient dumping policy can be optimal under some conditions.[19]

Proposition 4 *There is a threshold patient dumping cost $\bar{\gamma}$ that satisfies $\bar{\gamma} \in (-\infty, 1)$.*

The optimal cost reduction efforts and the information rent analysis

We now assess the impact of changes in external conditions on the optimal healthcare payment system via the optimal level of cost reduction efforts and the change in information rent. We particularly focus on changes in the ratios of low-/high-severity patients and public/private hospital patients.

Higher ratio of high-severity patients

We begin with the effect of the ratio of low-/high-severity patients, as captured by P, and examine how a change in P affects the threshold $\bar{\gamma}$. A change in P generally has three effects on differences in social welfare. The first effect is the number effect, that is the effect on the number of patients for which the insurer pays information rent to the hospital. If the number of high-severity patients rises, the number of patients for whom the insurer pays information rent to the hospital declines. The second effect is the distortion effect, which is shown in (14) and (25). It can be seen that the extent of distortion in the level of cost reduction efforts diminishes as the number of high-severity patients rises. The third effect is the information rent effect, which is shown in (17) and (29). The magnitude of the information rent shrinks with an increase (decrease) in the number of high-severity (low-severity) patients.

To evaluate the impact on welfare of a change in P more precisely, it is instructive to decompose welfare differences into three elements as above: the welfare difference for (i) high-severity patients, (ii) low-severity patients in the private hospital, and (iii) low-severity patients in the public hospital. Using algebraic techniques, we obtain

$$-\frac{\partial\bar{\gamma}}{\partial P} = \underbrace{\frac{\eta^2}{1+\eta}P\Delta\theta^2(2-\lambda)}_{\text{High-severity patients}} + \underbrace{\eta[\theta_H - 2\frac{\eta}{1+\eta}\Delta\theta P]\Delta\theta}_{\text{Low-severity patients in the private hospital}}$$

$$\underbrace{-2(1-\lambda)P\frac{\eta^2}{1+\eta}\Delta\theta^2}_{\text{Low-severity patients in the public hospital}}.$$

(32)

1. For high-severity patients, only the distortion effect influences welfare. As seen in (14) and (25), the

distortion effect is larger under the outlier payment policy. As such, if P decreases (i.e., there are many high-severity and few low-severity patients), the gap in welfare under the two cases shrinks, and $\bar{\gamma}$ increases (shown by the first term in (32)).

2. For low-severity patients in the private hospital, the number effect and information rent effect are influential. If there are many high-severity patients, the number of patients for whom the insurer pays information rent to the private hospital is small. This effect moves $\bar{\gamma}$ upward, since it increases social welfare under the outlier payment policy; however, this effect does not affect social welfare under the patient dumping policy. In contrast, the information rent effect moves $\bar{\gamma}$ downward since it is milder under the outlier payment policy. Hence, if the number effect is weaker than the information rent effect, a decrease in P moves $\bar{\gamma}$ downward. When the information rent per patient is smaller (i.e., $\theta_H - \frac{\eta}{1+\eta}P\Delta\theta$ is small), the number effect is weaker (shown by the second term in (32)).

3. For low-severity patients in the public hospital, only the information rent effect is applicable. As seen in (17) and (29), this effect is weaker under the outlier payment policy, which moves $\bar{\gamma}$ downward.

The overall welfare impact of the patient dumping policy is determined by these tradeoffs. In particular, one crucial factor yields the difference in efficiency of cost reduction efforts between the two patient types. We summarize this observation as follows.

Proposition 5 *There exists $\bar{\theta}_H$ such that if $\theta_H > \bar{\theta}_H$, $\frac{\partial\bar{\gamma}}{\partial P} \geq 0$, and if $\theta_H < \bar{\theta}_H$, $\frac{\partial\bar{\gamma}}{\partial P} \leq 0$.*

This result asserts an important policy implication. From Proposition 5, there exists a possibility of welfare improvement by abolishing the outlier payment policy even when the number of high-severity patients is large. If the variance in efficiency of cost reduction efforts is large (i.e., θ_H is small against $\Delta\theta$), the patient dumping policy is preferred over the outlier payment policy for more diseases (i.e., $\bar{\gamma}$ moves downward).

Figure 1 depicts the region in which $\frac{\partial\bar{\gamma}}{\partial P} < 0$ holds. The region tends to shrink as healthcare payment cost η increases. Intuitively, if the healthcare payment cost is large, the optimal information rent is smaller, and the number effect weakens.

Proposition 6 *$\bar{\gamma}$ rises as the healthcare payment cost η increases when P is high.*

Woolhandler and Himmelstein [33] and Woolhandler and Himmelstein [34] empirically investigated per capita

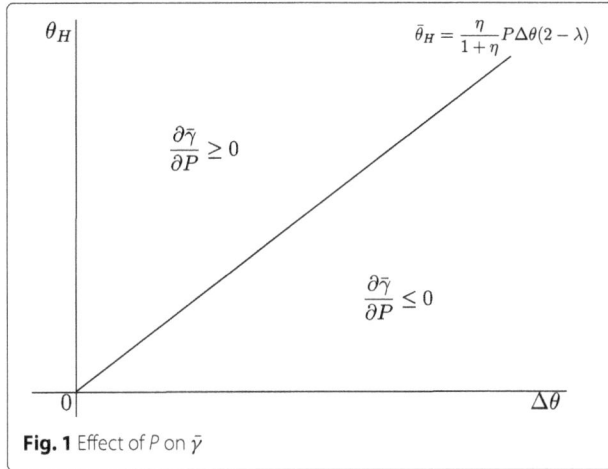

Fig. 1 Effect of P on $\bar{\gamma}$

administrative cost for US and Canadian healthcare payment programs and found that it is higher in the United States than in Canada. As such, our model implies that the patient dumping policy is more advantageous in Canada.

Higher number of patients in the private hospital

We now examine how a change in the proportion of patients who visit the private hospital, as captured by λ, affects the threshold. To this end, it is straightforward to obtain

$$\frac{\partial \bar{\gamma}}{\partial \lambda} = -\frac{1}{2}\frac{\eta^2}{1+\eta}P^2\Delta\theta^2 \leq 0. \tag{33}$$

Note that a change in λ does not affect social welfare under the outlier payment policy since the optimal contract is symmetric between the two hospitals and thus independent of λ. This is not the case under the patient dumping policy, however, as the optimal contract is asymmetric. If the number of patients who select the private hospital increases (i.e., λ increases), the distortion in the cost reduction efforts decreases under the patient dumping policy (25). This moves $\bar{\gamma}$ upward, thereby favoring the patient dumping policy over the outlier payment policy. However, as shown in (28), the optimal information rent increases as λ increases, which yields a countervailing effect and moves λ downward. We can show that this latter effect is generally stronger than the former; hence, an increase in λ always reduces $\bar{\gamma}$ as shown in (33).

Proposition 7 $\bar{\gamma}$ *decreases as* λ *increases.*

It is intuitively clear that patients' initial choice of hospitals, given exogenously in our model, could influence the optimal healthcare payment scheme significantly. According to the proposition, under the assumption that patient dumping is allowed only for private hospitals, social welfare can be improved by abolishing the outlier payment policy against many diseases in areas where more private

hospitals operate. In practice, this implies that a regulatory agency should admit selected regional variations in the healthcare payment scheme as the number of private institutions is expected to be high in urban areas and low in rural areas.

Discussion and conclusions

The main result of this paper is that there are cases in which insurers should not reimburse additional payments to hospitals that admit expensive patients even though doing so may trigger socially expensive patient dumping. A payment scheme that insures against outlier patients exacerbates the extent of information asymmetry between insurers and hospitals and consequently results in less-efficient effort for cost reduction. When this cost is sufficiently significant, insurers should instead allow hospitals to dump expensive patients to specific hospitals as a second-best alternative to the outlier payment policy. We show that such a payment scheme, which tolerates a degree of patient dumping, can ease information asymmetry and improve efficiency under some conditions.

One important limitation of our model is the assumption that patients are allocated randomly to hospitals. However, as we have shown in Appendix A, relaxing this assumption does not alter our main contention in any qualitative way. The analysis would be more complete, though certainly more complicated, if we more explicitly modeled patients' choice of hospitals taking technology difference between hospitals or reputation into consideration. In the future, it might be of interest to explore three-way interactions among insurers, hospitals, and patients.

Endnotes

[1] For instance, see Newhouse [26] for this classification.

[2] Stephan and Berger [32] noted that a patient's pathway (preclinical medical plan) shortens her hospital stay and reduces total treatment cost.

[3] For instance, the United States adopted the prospective payment system in 1983. Some countries, notably Japan, still adopt the retrospective payment system.

[4] This problem was discussed in Ma [21].

[5] If insurers pay all of the treatment cost, hospitals take no risk; such a healthcare payment system is equivalent to the retrospective payment system.

[6] This assumption of asymmetric information is common in the literature. See Chalkley and Malcomson (1998), Sappington and Lewis (1999), Glazer and McGuire [16], Beitia [3], Marchand et al. [22], Chalkley and Khalil [5], Siciliani [30], and, Mougeot and Naegelen [24].

[7] Woolhandler and Himmelstein [33] and Woolhandler and Himmelstein [34] compare the administrative cost of

healthcare programs per capita between the United States and Canada. Skinner et al. [31] investigates the determinants of inefficiency in the Medicare program in the United States.

[8] The Emergency Medical Treatment and Active Labor Act prohibits patient dumping in any region of the United States, and the Centers for Medicare & Medicaid Services, a division of the United States' Department of Health and Human Services, reimburse treatment cost under the Medicare program (this can be considered an outlier payment).

[9] For instance, when insurers define the payment for average-severity patients as the fixed payment under the prospective payment system, the difference of payment for high- and average-severity patients can be interpreted as outlier payment.

[10] Numerous studies examine the optimality of outlier payments: Ellis and McGuire [11], Selden [29], Newhouse [26], Chalkley and Malcomson (1998), Ellis [10], Keeler et al. [20], Glazer and McGuire [16], Glazer and McGuire [17], Meltzer et al. [23], Barros [2], Eggleston [9], Jack [19].

[11] See also Ellis and McGuire [13], Eggleston (2000), Frank et al. [15], and Siciliani [30].

[12] See also Marchand et al. [22].

[13] We assume that each patient does not know his or her severity and chooses a hospital based solely on exogenous factors such as proximity. Of course, we can obtain qualitatively similar results as long as exogenous factors have some effect.

[14] For example, the degree of preventive care by doctors can be interpreted as such a variable.

[15] All propositions hold so long as the hospital's payoff function has the Spence–Mirrlees single crossing property.

[16] In Appendix B. we investigate that the patient dumping policy can be optimal even it has the effect on the treatment quality in the public hospital.

[17] Additional treatment cost includes the social cost indicated by Newhouse [25].

[18] For example, see Salanie [27].

[19] We so far assume that the private/public patient ratio λ is unaffected by the insurer's policy choice. In the Appendix, we show that the following proposition is satisfied even when we patients choice hospital endogenously.

Appendix A: Endogenous hospital choice

In Section 5, we assume that the private/public patient ratio λ is exogenously given and not affected by policy

change since the patients cannot recognize the severity of their condition. However, if the insurer introduces the patient dumping policy and the patients are aware of it, a fraction of patients who select the private hospital under the outlier payment policy may select the public hospital *ab initio* to ensure that they are not dumped and do not to bear the dumping cost even when they do not know the severity of their condition.

Further, in the appendix, we build a Hotelling model that describes the patients' hospital choice. In this model, patients choose a hospital while taking into account the risk of dumping. Lastly, we show that Proposition 4 is satisfied even in this case.

We consider a market where the patients are distributed horizontally and uniformly on the line with length 1. Their location is denoted by x where $x \in [0, 1]$. The private hospital is located on the left end of the line and the public hospital on the right. The utility of a patient located at x and treated at hospital i is given by

$$U(x) = \begin{cases} v - tx & (i = pr) \\ v - t(1 - x) & (i = pu) \end{cases}$$

where v is the benefit of treatment provided by the hospitals under the outlier payment policy and $t(> 0)$ is the marginal transportation cost. Assume that v is large enough and all patients on the line are treated at the hospital. There is no technology gap between the two hospitals, and under the outlier payment policy the value of treatment is the same between the hospitals. The location of the patient who is indifferent between the two hospitals under the outlier payment policy is

$$\bar{x} = \frac{1}{2}.$$

Then, we obtain that the fraction of patients who go to the private hospital is $\bar{\lambda} = \frac{1}{2}$ under the outlier payment policy when we endogenize the patients' hospital choice. Next, we derive the fraction of patients under the patient dumping policy. Under this policy, high-severity patients who go to the private hospital are dumped to the public hospital. Then, the expected utility of patients who go to the private hospital is reduced to v' where $0 < v' < v$. Under the patient dumping policy, the location of the patient who is indifferent between the two hospitals is

$$\tilde{x} = \frac{1}{2} - \frac{v - v'}{2t}.$$

Then, we obtain the fraction of patients who go to the private hospital under the patient dumping policy as $\tilde{\lambda} = \frac{1}{2} - \frac{v-v'}{2t}$. Obviously, $\tilde{\lambda} < \bar{\lambda}$, and we find that the patient dumping policy reduces the number of patients who go to the private hospital.

Increasing the proportion of patients who select the public hospital under the patient dumping policy has three effects.[20] The first is the self-selection effect. Under the outlier payment policy, the expected patient dumping cost is $\phi\lambda\gamma$. However, if the fraction of patients who select the private hospital under the outlier payment policy select the public hospital first, the expected patient dumping policy is reduced to $\phi\tilde{\lambda}\gamma$. Then, the relative superiority of the patient dumping policy becomes substantial. The second is the optimal contract effect. As seen in (25), (26), (28) and (29), the optimal contract for the public hospital depends on λ. As previously demonstrated, in the optimal contract, the cost reduction efforts for high-severity patients and the information rent for low-severity patients are higher under the patient dumping policy than under the outlier payment policy. If λ changes to $\tilde{\lambda}$ under the patient dumping policy, these effects weaken. The third is the number effect. Under the patient dumping policy, the optimal information rent for low-severity patients in the private hospital is reduced to zero. Then, if λ changes to $\tilde{\lambda}$, this information rent-saving effect weakens due to the change in the number of patients, and the superiority of the patient dumping policy diminishes.

Next, we aggregate these effects. We term the optimized social welfare under the patient dumping policy when a fraction of $\tilde{\lambda}$ select the private hospital as $\tilde{W}^{D*}$. We compute the welfare difference between the two policies as follows:

$$
\begin{aligned}
\tilde{W}^{D*} - W^{O*} = &\underbrace{\frac{1}{2}\tilde{\lambda}\frac{\eta^2}{1+\eta}\frac{(1-\phi)^2}{\phi}\Delta\theta^2}_{\text{High-severity patients}} \\
&\underbrace{-\phi\tilde{\lambda}(1-\gamma)}_{\text{Patient dumping cost}} \\
&\underbrace{+(1-\phi)\tilde{\lambda}\eta\left(\theta_H - \frac{\eta}{1+\eta}P\Delta\theta\right)\Delta\theta}_{\text{Low-severity patients in the private hospital}} \\
&\underbrace{-(1-\phi)\eta\Delta\theta\left[(\tilde{\lambda}-\tilde{\lambda})\left(\theta_H - \frac{\eta}{1+\eta}P\Delta\theta\right)+\tilde{\lambda}(1-\tilde{\lambda})\frac{\eta}{1+\eta}P\Delta\theta\right]}_{\text{Low-severity patients in the public hospital}}.
\end{aligned}
$$

$$(34)$$

We denote the threshold γ as $\tilde{\gamma}$ between the two policies when patient movement occurs. By rearranging (34), we obtain

$$
\begin{aligned}
\tilde{\gamma} = 1 &- \left(\frac{1}{2}+\tilde{\lambda}\right)\frac{\eta^2}{1+\eta}P^2\Delta\theta^2 \\
&- \left(\theta_H - \frac{\eta}{1+\eta}P\Delta\theta\right)P\eta\Delta\theta\left(2\frac{\bar{\lambda}}{\tilde{\lambda}}-1\right)
\end{aligned}
$$

$$(35)$$

The second and third terms are negative by assumption. And we obtain that there exists a threshold patient dumping cost $\tilde{\gamma}$ that satisfies $\tilde{\gamma} \in (-\infty, 1)$ even when patient movement occurs.

Appendix B: Congestion effect

In the analysis, we assume that the patients who are treated immediately can obtain constant utility, which is normalized to 1. However, it is conceivable that under the patient dumping policy, a concentration of patients to the public hospital occurs, and the treatment quality provided by the public hospital changes. It will be worse off if the patient concentration imposes a burden on the physicians in the public hospital, where they cannot refuse the treatment for the high-severity patients, considering skilled physicians often shift to private hospitals. However, it will be better if the increase in the number of patients under the patient dumping policy trains the physicians' skill in the public hospital.

In this appendix, we investigate this congestion effect on the welfare and optimal healthcare payment policy under the patient dumping policy. Assume that the utility of a patient treated in the public hospital under the patient dumping policy is reduced by α. That is, the utility of patients who are treated immediately is $1 - \alpha$, and the utility of patients who are dumped by the private hospital is $\gamma - \alpha$. If $\alpha > 0$, the congestion effect improves the treatment quality in the public hospital under the policy, otherwise, $\alpha < 0$. Obviously, when $\alpha > 0$, the patient dumping policy becomes advantageous.

Next, we show the condition under which the patient dumping policy is preferred to the outlier payment policy. We denote the optimized social welfare under the patient dumping policy with the congestion effect as $\hat{W}^{D*}$. The welfare difference between the two policies is as follows.

$$
\begin{aligned}
\hat{W}^{D*} - W^{O*} = &\frac{1}{2}\phi\lambda(1+\eta)\left(\frac{\eta}{1+\eta}P\Delta\theta\right)^2(2-\lambda) - \phi\lambda(1-\gamma) \\
&+ \lambda(1-\phi)\eta\left(\theta_H - \frac{\eta}{1+\eta}P\Delta\theta\right)\Delta\theta \\
&- (1-\lambda)(1-\phi)\eta\lambda\frac{\eta}{1+\eta}P\Delta\theta^2 \\
&- (1-\lambda+\lambda\phi)\alpha
\end{aligned}
$$

$$(36)$$

The last term indicates the welfare loss due to the congestion effect under the patient dumping policy. We term the threshold γ as $\hat{\gamma}$ between the two policies, considering the congestion effect and we obtain

$$
\begin{aligned}
\hat{\gamma} = 1 &- \eta P\Delta\theta\left(\theta_H - \frac{\eta}{1+\eta}P\Delta\theta\left(1-\frac{1}{2}\lambda\right)\right) \\
&+ \frac{(1-\lambda+\lambda\phi)\alpha}{\phi\lambda}.
\end{aligned}
$$

If $\hat{\gamma} < 1$, the following inequality is satisfied.

$$
\frac{\eta P\Delta\theta\left(\theta_H - \frac{\eta}{1+\eta}P\Delta\theta\left(1-\frac{1}{2}\lambda\right)\right)\phi\lambda}{(1-\lambda+\lambda\phi)} > \alpha
$$

If the inequality is satisfied, the patient dumping policy is preferred even when there is the congestion effect under the patient dumping policy. Considering the parameter constraints, the left hand side is negative. Therefore, if the congestion has negative effect on the treatment quality in the public hospital under the patient dumping policy, then the patient dumping policy can be optimal.

Acknowledgements
During the course of this study, I talked to many people whose knowledge and ideas contributed significantly to the analysis in this paper. In particular, I thank Junichiro Ishida, Shingo Ishiguro, and Noriaki Matsushima for their comments and the helpful discussions I had with them. I also thank Akifumi Ishihara, Hiroshi Kitamura, Akira Miyaoka, Keizo Mizuno, Ryo Ogawa, Wataru Tamura, and participants at the Applied Microeconomic Theory Workshop, the Japan Association for Applied Economics 2012 spring meeting, the Japanese Economic Association 2012 spring meeting, the Contract Theory Workshop Summer Camp 2012 in Shinshu, the Applied Economic Theory Workshop for Alumni, the Workshop in Macroeconomics for Young Economists, the 13th International Meeting of the Association for Public Economic Theory(PET13), the Lunchtime Workshop at Kyoto University, and Kwansei Gakuin Industrial Organization Workshop for their constructive comments.

Competing interests
The author declares that he/she has no competing interests.

References
1. Allen R, Gertler P. Regulation and the provision of quality to heterogeneous consumers: The case of prospective pricing of medical services. J Regul Econ. 1991;3(4):361–75.
2. Barros PP. Cream-skimming, incentives for efficiency and payment system. J Health Econ. 2003;22(3):491–43.
3. Beitia A. Hospital quality choice and market structure in a regulated duopoly. J Health Econ. 2003;22(6):1011–36.
4. Canta C. Efficiency, access, and the mixed delivery of health care services. mimeo. 2012. https://chiaracanta.files.wordpress.com/2009/11/canta_151020122.pdf.
5. Chalkley M, Khalil F. Third party purchasing of health services: Patient choice and agency. J Health Econ. 2005;24(6):1132–53.
6. Chalkley M, Malcomson JM. Contracting for health services when patient demand does not reflect quality. J Health Econ. 1998;17(1):1–19.
7. Dranove, D. Rate-setting by diagnosis related groups and hospital specialization. RAND J Econ. 1987;18(3):417–27.
8. Eggleston, K. Risk selection and optimal health insurance-provider payment systems. J Risk Insur. 2000;67(2):173–96.
9. Eggleston, K. Multitasking and mixed systems for provider payment. J Health Econ. 2005;24(1):211–23.
10. Ellis RP. Creaming, skimping and dumping: provider competition on the intensive and extensive margins. J Health Econ. 1998;17(5):537–55.
11. Ellis RP, McGuire TG. Provider behavior under prospective: reimbursement: Cost sharing and supply. J Health Econ. 1986;5(2):129–51.
12. Ellis RP, McGuire TG. Optimal payment system for health services. J Health Econ. 1990;9(4):375–96.
13. Ellis RP, McGuire TG. Hospital response to prospective payment: Moral hazard, selection, and practice style effects. J Health Econ. 1996;15(3):257–77.
14. Eze P, Wolfe B. Is dumping socially inefficient? An analysis of the effect on Medicare's prospective payment system on the utilization of veterans affairs inpatient services. J Public Econ. 1993;52(3):329–44.
15. Frank RG, Glazer J, McGuire TG. Measuring adverse selection in managed health care. J Health Econ. 2000;19(6):829–54.
16. Glazer J, McGuire TG. Optimal risk adjustment in markets with adverse selection: an application to managed care. Amer Econ Rev. 2000;90(4):1055–71.
17. Glazer J, McGuire TG. Setting health plan premiums to ensure efficient quality in health care: minimum variance optimal risk adjustment. J Public Econ. 2002;84(2):153–73.
18. Jack, W. Purchasing health care services from providers with unknown altruism. J Health Econ. 2005;24(1):73–93.
19. Jack, W. Optimal risk adjustment with adverse selection and spatial competition. J Health Econ. 2006;25(5):908–26.
20. Keeler EB, Carter G, Newhouse JP. A model of the impact of reimbursement schemes on health plan choice. J Health Econ. 1998;17(3):297–320.
21. Ma CA. Health care payment system: cost and quality incentives. J Econ Manage Strat. 1994;3(1):93–112.
22. Marchand M, Sato M, Schokkaert E. Prior health expenditures and risk sharing with insures competition quality. RAND J Econ. 2003;34(4):647–69.
23. Meltzer D, Chung J, Basu A. Does competition under Medicare prospective payment selectively reduce expenditures on high-cost patients? RAND J Econ. 2002;33(3):447–68.
24. Mougeot M, Naegelen F. Supply-side risk adjustment and outlier payment policy. J Health Econ. 2008;27(5):1196–200.
25. Newhouse JP. Two prospective difficulties with prospective payment of hospitals, or, it's better to be a resident than a patient with an complex problem. J Health Econ. 1983;2(3):269–74.
26. Newhouse JP. Reimbursing health plans and health providers: Efficiency in production versus selection. J Econ Lit. 1996;34(3):1236–63.
27. Salanie B. A economics of contracts: primer. Cambridge: The MIT Press; 2005.
28. Sappington DEM, Lewis TR. Using subjective risk adjusting to prevent patient dumping in the health care industry. J Econ Manag Strat. 1999;8(3):351–82.
29. Selden TM. A model of capitation. J Health Econ. 1990;8(3):397–409.
30. Siciliani L. Selection of treatment under prospective payment system in the hospital sector. J Health Econ. 2006;25(3):479–99.
31. Skinner JS, Elliott S, Fischer, Wennberg J. The efficiency of Medicare In: Wise DA, editor. Analysis in the Economics of Aging, NBER Book Series - The Economics of Aging. Chapter 6. Chicago: University of Chicago Press; 2005. p. 129–60.
32. Stephan AE, Berger DL. Shortened length of stay and hospital cost reduction with implementation of an accelerated clinical care pathway after elective colon resection. Surgery. 2003;133(3):277–83.
33. Woolhandler S, Himmelstein DU. The Deteriorating administrative efficiency of the U.S. health care system. N Engl J Med. 1991;324(18):1253–8.
34. Woolhandler S, Himmelstein DU. Costs of health care administration in the United States and Canada. N Engl J Med. 2003;349(8):768–75.

12

Worldwide assessment of healthcare personnel dealing with lymphoedema

Henrike Schulze[1]*, Marisa Nacke[2], Christoph Gutenbrunner[1] and Catarina Hadamitzky[3]

Abstract

Background: Lymphoedema is a pandemic with about 250 million people suffering from this condition worldwide. Lymphatic diseases have considerable public health significance, but yet few professionals are specialised in their management causing a substantial burden on health resources.

Aims and objectives: This study aims to give an overview of the approximate number of medical professionals, professional societies, institutions and companies dealing with lymphoedema in various countries. Concepts of improvement for current human resources are considered.

Methods: An online database analysis (Google search engine and PubMed) was carried out for each country of the world. Additionally, relevant congress participant lists as well as member lists of significant medical societies and reports of the World Health Organisation were analysed.

Results: Overall distribution of tertiary level professionals specialised in this field is heterogenous. A decrescent gradient of professionals can be seen between developed and developing countries and between urban and rural areas. Countries in general do not seem to have yet met the current demand for specialists at tertiary level in this field.

Conclusions: This study intends to draw attention to the current medical coverage gaps due to a low number of lymphoedema specialists at tertiary level. It wishes to start a discussion about structured reimbursement and certification of knowledge and skills that are essential incentives for experts to act as multiplicators and change the lack of care in the mid-term. Current fail prescriptions and evitable disability and sick certificates represent a high financial burden that could be reinvested in a correct management. Policy makers must focus in the two above mentioned essential measures. Medical training and the consequent development of the industry will then naturally take place, as it was the case for other professional groups in the past.

Keywords: Lymphology, Lymphoedema, Lymphatic diseases, Medical healthcare resources, Medical education

Background

Lymphoedema, also known as elephantiasis, is a chronic disease characterised by massive swelling of limbs or tissues. The disease affects about 250 million patients worldwide [1]. It occurs through accumulation of fluid and other tissue elements that would normally be drained by the lymphatic system. The origin can be genetic or, more commonly, secondary to injuries.

Secondary causes of lymphoedema vary according to geographic distribution [2]. In developing countries, it is often a corollary of parasitic infections through Filaria or Loa Loa or caused by Podoconiosis and has massive global public health significance [3].

In developed countries, secondary lymphoedema mainly occurs after cancer therapy [4]. It is strongly associated with prevalent cancer types, e.g. breast or prostate cancers [5]. Depending on the type and extent of treatment, the anatomic location, the heterogeneity of assessment methods, and the follow-up, the reported incidence of cancer-related lymphoedema varies [6, 7]. Because lymphatic swelling can occur decades after cancer treatment, cancer patients undergoing lymph node dissection should be considered at lifetime risk.

---

* Correspondence: henrikeschulze@hotmail.de
[1]Clinic of Rehabilitation Medicine, Hannover Medical School, Carl-Neuberg-Straße 1, 30625 Hannover, Germany
Full list of author information is available at the end of the article

Despite its epidemiological relevance, only few professionals are specialised in the management of lymphatic diseases [8–10]. Lymphology is a mostly overlooked field in medical schools and exposure of medical professionals to this field varies greatly [10, 11]. The lack of professional knowledge especially at the level of general practitioners, as first medical contacts, is considered to be a problem that impacts early detection, leads to misdiagnosis and inappropriate treatment and results in poor management of health resources [9, 10, 12–17]. Natural exacerbation of the swelling causes increased demand on healthcare resources but can also lead to life threatening infections as well as psychosocial exclusion followed by a diminished quality of life or even depression [18–21].

Appropriate management of lymphoedema, including surgical procedures, can cure the condition in 30–40% of the cases [22] but also conservative therapy with manual lymphatic drainage and compression leads to an improvement of patients' quality of life and increases their presence at work [23, 24]. Although the number of healthcare professionals specialised in lympho-vascular diseases seems to be insufficient, this phaenomenon has been left unquantified until now. In the literature of the last decade only a single publication [13] directly addresses the discrepancy between offered and demanded services in this field of healthcare. Nevertheless, medical professionals could improve the current healthcare situation through their multiplication characteristics by influencing the interdisciplinary work with nurses and/or physiotherapists regarding the chosen therapy and by spreading rare knowledge in universities, hence promoting research. Empowerment of future generations could create a stronger relationship between the local health services and lymphoedema patients in the future [25].

The objective of this study was to gain an overview of the approximate number of medical physicians and researchers currently dealing with lymphoedema. Another aim was to assess the ratio between healthcare professionals and general population in vast geographical areas, and this despite low numbers of specialised healthcare professionals with tertiary level of training to be found in this field of rare knowledge. Additionally, professional societies and companies associated with lymphoedema were counted in order to understand possible concepts of improvement for current human resources, as professional training and certification allow further development in this important field. Furthermore, potential policy implications such as structured reimbursement or higher public research funding were included in the discussion of this study.

Methods

In order to map medical professionals, societies, institutions and industrial companies dedicated to lymphoedema, research was performed exclusively online for each single country of the world in three independent phases. The targeted professional groups were physicians and researchers. The search included published data from 2005 to 2015 and was restricted to six languages, namely English, German, French, Spanish, Portuguese and Italian.

In the first phase, a data collection was performed with the Google search engine. For each single *country name*, the word *lympho*edema* was introduced, and the top ten listed websites were analysed. Then, these terms were successively combined with the following words: *physician* or *medical doctor, researcher, chronic o*edema, lymphatic filariasis, podoconiosis, elephantiasis* and *cancer* (Fig. 1). It also allowed retrieving information on professional societies and industrial companies.

In the second phase, the search was conducted with the same keywords in the PubMed database. Relevant studies from the database were identified by their titles and abstracts. In case of uncertainties, the full text was retrieved and authors and participating institutions were listed in the corresponding countries.

In the third phase, duplicates were removed. Cross analysis on congress participants listed in scientific meetings dealing with the topic of lymphatic diseases was performed and relevant reports from the WHO were analysed. If available, member lists of medical societies for lymphatic diseases were included in the analysis. The quantifications of specialised professionals were not performed on numeric data, but on the personal data available online for each expert, including affiliation, address, and fields of interest.

Data extraction and analysis

A data extraction form was developed in Excel. Individual physicians and researchers were assigned to one of the following categories depending on their main focus: *surgery, conservative therapy, research, filariasis, podoconiosis* and *medical imaging*. Their professional affiliations were recorded along with the postal and digital address. When the information was originated in research papers, experts were grouped by geographic distribution, not by paper. International research groups had their members therefore grouped separately according to their country of residence. Experts were counterchecked individually for their qualifications (medical doctors or e.g. biologists) and a Google search for data under their name was performed to assign them to a main focus as stated above. Medical societies and institutions were also sorted by country as well as main focus and likewise pharmaceutical companies (Fig. 1). The

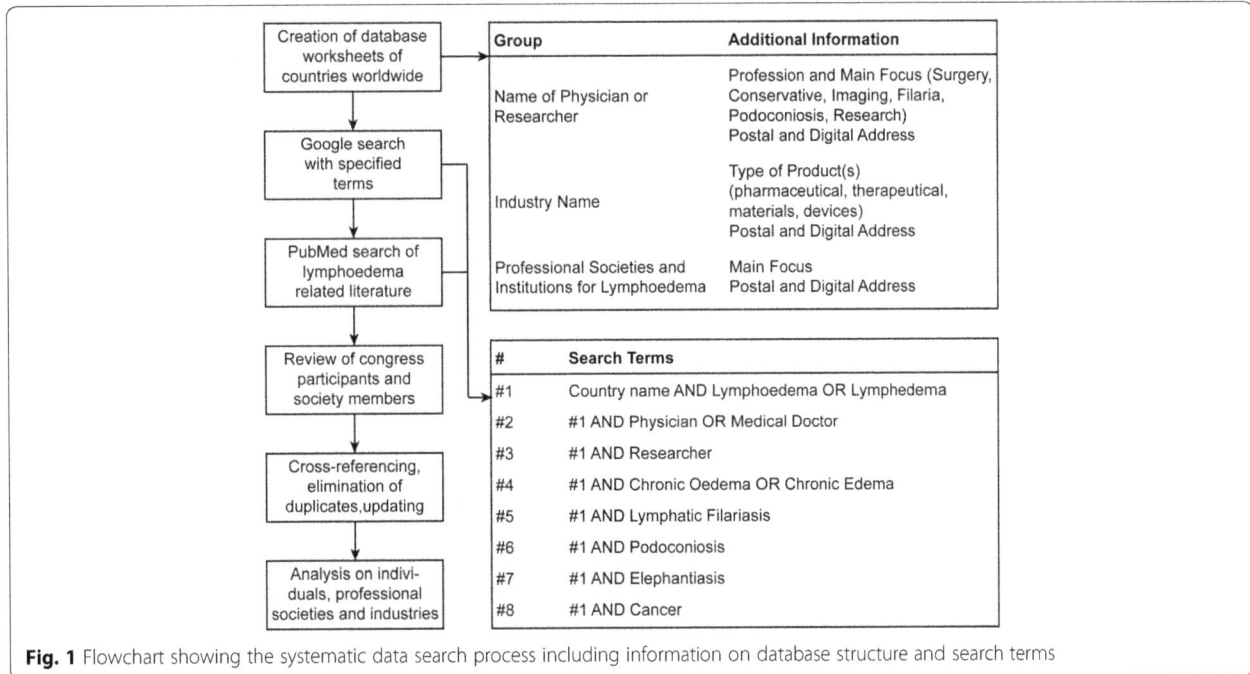

Fig. 1 Flowchart showing the systematic data search process including information on database structure and search terms

main findings were analysed narratively as statistical pooling was not adequate for this scoping study.

Ethics approval was not required for this study, as online information is publicly accessible and there is no reasonable expectation of privacy.

Results

The conducted research included 208 countries on six continents. Of the entirety of countries in the world, 123 countries provided online information on at least one of the researched topics (59% of the total sample).

Activities could be mapped in twelve out of 23 countries in North and Central America; 13 out of 17 in South America; 27 out of 49 countries in Europe; 14 out of 20 countries in Oceania; 25 out of 48 Asian countries and 32 out of 51 countries in Africa.

First, the exact numbers of tertiary level professionals dedicated to lymphatic diseases were analysed (Fig. 2). As expected, their distribution is very heterogeneous, e. g. Pakistan, with a population of more than double than Germany, has only four listed professionals, the latter having 432. A high absolute number of professionals

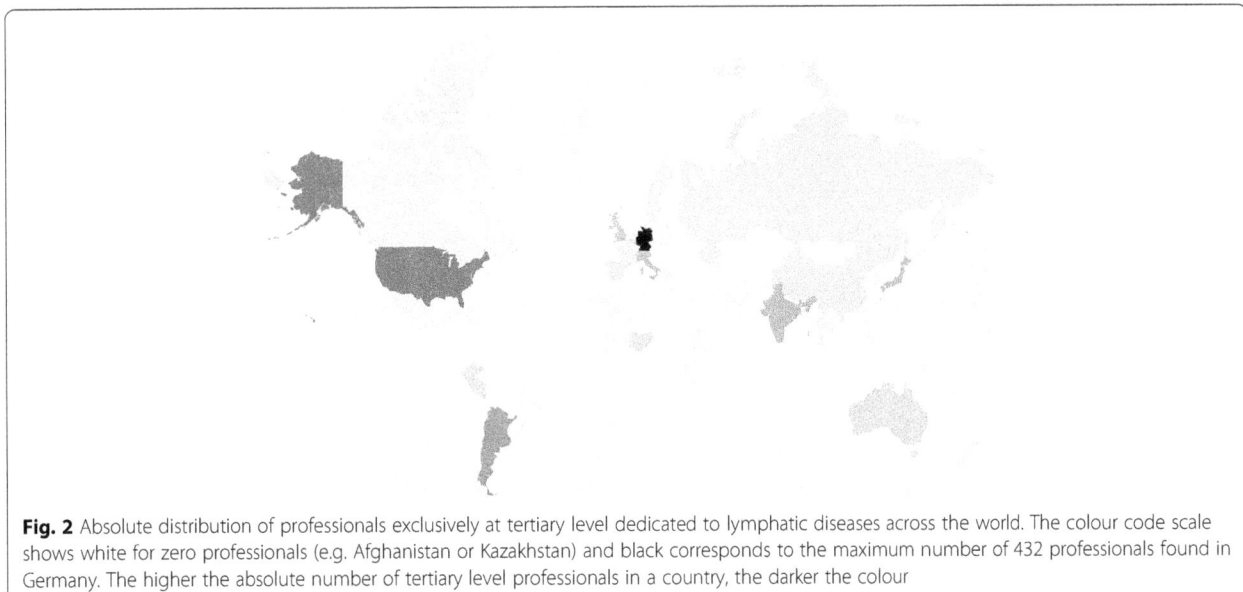

Fig. 2 Absolute distribution of professionals exclusively at tertiary level dedicated to lymphatic diseases across the world. The colour code scale shows white for zero professionals (e.g. Afghanistan or Kazakhstan) and black corresponds to the maximum number of 432 professionals found in Germany. The higher the absolute number of tertiary level professionals in a country, the darker the colour

could be tracked in Europe ($n = 1310$) (Fig. 3a; Table 1). Whilst being the continent with the lowest absolute number of tertiary level professionals currently working in the field of lymphology, Oceania has the highest ratio of professionals per capita (165 professionals per 38.5 million people) (Fig. 3a and b, Table 1). Europe, on the contrary, displays only an average level of coverage of its population of half a billion notwithstanding the high absolute numbers of professionals. Asia, on the lower

extreme, has a coverage ratio of tertiary level professionals per million inhabitants below one (Fig. 3b, Table 1).

Additionally, we split the focus of the tertiary level professionals into clinical activity and research (Fig. 3b; Table 1). Professionals with both foci were included in both statistics. When considering only clinically active physicians per million inhabitants, e.g. Europe had high ratios (0.89 ppm), whereas Africa, with a total of 26 clinically active physicians, has according to our research criteria practically inexistent medical coverage in this field. Similar coverage exists for researchers in most continents excluding Oceania. Oceania has a high ratio of researchers per million inhabitants (3.5 ppm).

Also, in Europe inequality is such, that some countries presented very poor medical coverage of lymphoedema despite belonging to the European continent. Differences can already be seen comparing five European countries (Fig. 3c). Interestingly, countries with a large population such as Japan do not seem to reach the higher ratios of less populated countries like Switzerland (Table 2). The uneven distribution of tertiary level physicians was not only present at a global level, but also within single countries. Spain, with a total of 34 active physicians, can be considered a paradigm of depletion in rural areas with most physicians to be found in Madrid ($n = 5$), Valencia ($n = 17$) or Barcelona ($n = 6$) (Fig. 4).

Data regarding the specialty of physicians (Table 3) showed that most are focused on the conservative management of the disease ($n = 641$), most of them being located in Europe ($n = 535$). Concerning the operative therapy of lymphoedema, our online search was able to identify the highest number of surgeons in Europe ($n = 295$), followed by Asia ($n = 139$). Surprisingly, very few physicians are specialised in imaging procedures of lymphatic vessels ($n = 64$) despite the overlap with imaging methods used in cancer management. Concerning filarial lymphoedema, only 40 specialists could be mapped. Our search led to just two medical specialists dedicated to podoconiosis. In Asia ($n = 163$) and Oceania ($n = 21$) most physicians additionally are researchers, showing a strong potential for innovation in these continents. This is also true for North America.

Our search regarding professional societies and institutions dedicated to this field of medicine showed that the leading single country is the U.S. with 161 societies (Table 4). European countries altogether have 598 societies mentioning lymphoedema as one of their points of interest, all specialties included, but oftentimes the professionals involved in these societies or institutions are the same at regional, national and international level. Additionally, some Asian countries as India are well organised in this field with a total online track of 96 Indian societies. Table 4 also shows where industrial companies dedicated to lymphoedema products are located.

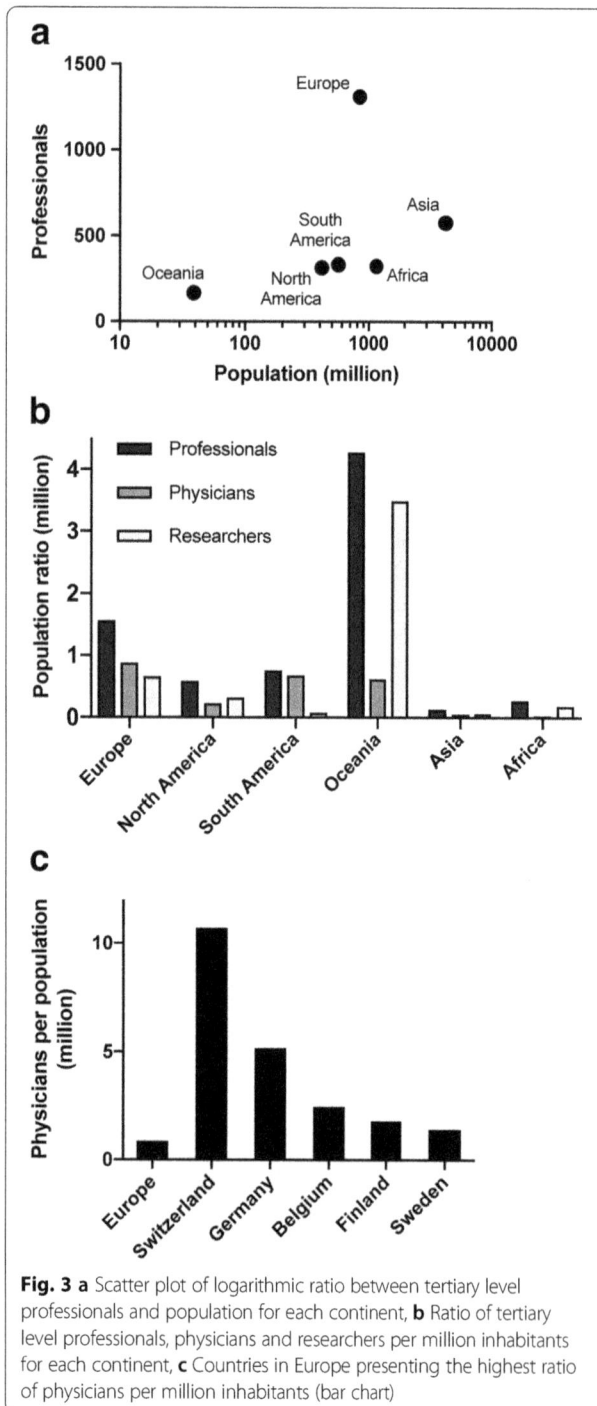

Fig. 3 a Scatter plot of logarithmic ratio between tertiary level professionals and population for each continent, **b** Ratio of tertiary level professionals, physicians and researchers per million inhabitants for each continent, **c** Countries in Europe presenting the highest ratio of physicians per million inhabitants (bar chart)

Table 1 Data for each continent for Fig. 2

Continent	Professionals[a]	Physicians	Researchers	Population (in million)	Professionals/population (per million)	Physicians/population (per million)	Researchers/population (per million)
Europe	1310	739	550	833.9	1.57	0.89	0.66
North America	332	128	182	562.6	0.59	0.23	0.32
South America	314	281	33	414.1	0.76	0.68	0.08
Oceania	165	24	135	38.5	4.28	0.62	3.50
Asia	577	253	298	4222.9	0.14	0.06	0.07
Africa	323	26	221	1159.8	0.27	0.02	0.19

[a]Professionals are regarded as physicians, researchers and also other persons involved in the topic of lymphoedema such as stakeholders at the World Bank who provide money for lymphoedema research and education

Leading countries are the U.K. ($n = 33$) and the U.S. ($n = 42$). Respectively, most companies can be found in Europe ($n = 90$) and North America ($n = 49$). Developing countries are virtually depleted of industrial companies in this field, forcing them to import needed products or simply failing to provide them.

Discussion

The social burden of the lymphoedema pandemic is inversely proportional to the low number of medical professionals dedicated to its management or research. It is translated in inadequate prescriptions, poor management of health resources, as well as time of work absenteeism, social exclusion and stigma of patients [12, 18, 19, 25–27]. The conducted study aimed at a semi-quantification of the problem by showing where medical professionals can be found, and where their coverage must be expanded.

Aspects of online search methods

One possible limitation of our study resulted from restricting our search to the internet. Certainly, local offers of lymphoedema management exist that were not visible online. About 67% of the world's population does not have access to the internet [28]. Especially in developing regions patients still seek advice from traditional healers [29–35]. This is supported by reports from the Caribbean, showing that most patients only seek care from university-trained but more expensive healthcare providers when traditional treatment has shown to be ineffective [26, 27]. If patients and their communities are taught about their disease, it has been shown that a loco-cultural understanding of the disease can coexist with the biomedical one [36]. Therefore, additional low-cost programs should be established, as they improve lymphoedema outcomes, even leading to an important economic benefit as patients are able to work again or work more [24]. Examples of low-cost interventions are training of communities on hygiene measures of the lymphoedema limb as well as demonstrations for the application of topic antibiotics on secondary wound

infections and bandaging. When comparing the yearly costs per patient in hygiene and/or bandaging materials including antibiotic ointments (direct healthcare costs) with the gain in working days/salary since program implementation (indirect workforce costs), Stillwaggon et al. [24] could calculate per-person savings of more than 130 times the per-person costs of their program. This demonstrates the importance of understanding the cultural background when planning health resources in these societies [37]. The online selection bias might nevertheless have the advantage of listing only professionals that have reached a certain degree of impact, at least at regional level. This study therefore mimics the barriers encountered by lymphoedema patients seeking healthcare providers with the support of online search engines but might not be exact concerning the current local healthcare measures provided by the communities.

Language bias

Considering the language barrier, the analysis was limited to six languages spoken by the main authors. Regions of the world not using the latin alphabet were impermeable to our search thus creating false negatives mainly in the data on Asia and North Africa. Therefore, although our search was thoroughly performed with the name of every single country in the world, the fact that we were using western languages in our search reduced our scope of investigation extensively, especially considering that Asia is an extremely populated region of the world. Retrospectively, most countries failing to provide any online information were small in size and population. Additionally, some of these countries use specific local terms to name lymphoedema. Common synonyms are "big foot" in Haiti [29] or "mossy foot" in Ethiopia [38] (Table 5). These alternative terms might have led to incomplete listing of involved professionals in the respective regions of Africa, Central America and Asia.

Importance of developing adequate training offers

General analysis of the absolute number of professionals qualified at tertiary level in this field reveals a great need

Table 2 Overview of the leading countries and ratios per continent of professionals, physicians, researchers and societies

	Professionals	Physicians	Researchers	Professionals/population (per million)	Physicians/population (per million)	Researchers/population (per million)	Societies/Population (per million)
Europe	Germany	Germany	UK	Switzerland	Switzerland	Belgium	Switzerland
Highest quantity / ratio	432	421	79	13.80	10.74	5.70	6.22
Population (in million)	80.9	80.9	64.5	8.2	8.2	11.2	8.2
North America	USA	USA	USA	Grenada	Grenada	Grenada	Grenada
Highest quantity / ratio	241	75	148	47.01	18.81	28.21	9.40
Population (in million)	318.9	318.9	318.9	0.1	0.1	0.1	0.1
South America	Argentina	Argentina	Brazil	Argentina	Argentina	Guiana	Bermuda
Highest quantity / ratio	181	168	15	4.21	3.91	2.62	15.34
Population (in million)	43.0	43.0	206.0	43.0	42.0	0.7	0.1
Oceania	Australia	Australia	Australia	Amer. Samoa	Amer. Samoa	Amer. Samoa	Tuvalu
Highest quantity / ratio	80	10	70	162.36	18.04	144.32	101.08
Population (in million)	23.5	23.5	23.5	0.1	0.1	0.1	< 0.1
Asia	Japan	India	Japan	Micronesia	Japan	Micronesia	Micronesia
Highest quantity / ratio	138	102	78	9.61	0.47	9.61	9.61
Population (in million)	127.1	1295.3	127.1	0.1	127.1	0.1	0.1
Africa	Nigeria	Cameroon	Nigeria	Sao Tome	Comoros	Sao Tome	Sao Tome
Highest quantity / ratio	76	3	72	21.47	2.60	21.47	10.73
Population (in million)	177.5	22.8	177.5	0.2	0.8	0.2	0.2

for Asian, North American and European countries to organise training offers. In the reminiscent regions, countries do not seem to possess enough professionals to offer the whole spectrum of medical training on lymphatic diseases (Fig. 2; Table 3). Therefore, it is paramount that healthcare providers in Asia, North America and Europe embrace this challenge, take responsibility and promote training offers to improve global geographical coverage. Lymphology should already be taught in undergraduate medical school in order to close the knowledge gap [11]. Analysing general medical care in most countries of Africa shows that although this continent is responsible for 24% of the burden of diseases worldwide, it is only disserved by 3% of the total healthcare providers [39]. One could postulate that if financial resources invested in humanitarian treatment of disease in developing countries in the past had instead been used for medical training, the present situation might not be as unbalanced. In these countries, in spite of an established prevalence of 40 million patients affected with lymphoedema as a consequence of lymphatic filariasis, few are able to receive proper medical support and treatment [9, 10, 40], especially as the patients are more likely to get the disease if they have a low or medium socioeconomic status and might therefore not be able to afford treatments [41, 42]. On the other hand, the treatment of filariasis constitutes one of the success stories of mass drug administration (Global Programme to

Eliminate Lymphatic Filariasis - GPELF) with decreased primary infections following the global programs of eradication [43]. Community healthcare workers carried out the pharmacologically driven programs. Nevertheless, healthcare workers were not specifically informed about lymphoedema and lacked the clinical expertise of tertiary level professionals to diagnose this condition as a possible corollary of filaria infection. This constituted a lost opportunity of broad geographic impact perpetuating inadequate management, poor treatment and failure to meet the specific needs of patients with lymphoedema after filarial infection [26, 27, 31, 44, 45]. But, even so, substantial health and economic benefits have risen from the program, especially in what concerns lymphoedema prevention by treating the causal worm [42]. National strategies are often followed by new investments. The government of Ethiopia just recently invested in the fight against neglected tropical diseases (including lymphoedema/podoconiosis) in order to achieve the goal of eliminating these until 2020 according to a set up national plan [45]. An important addition to national strategies would be to collect statistical data on the current prevalence of the disease and apply epidemiologic information in the creation of medical support where help is needed [46, 47].

The heterogeneity of medical training is not restricted to developing countries. A lack of specialised physicians especially exists in poorer, more rural and remote areas

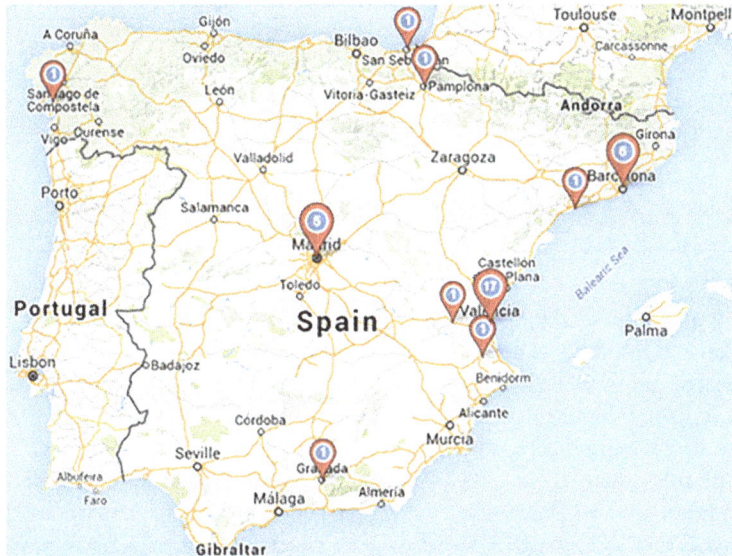

Fig. 4 Geographical distribution of physicians in Spain in absolute numbers

as described for Australia [48] and similar findings were postulated even across the U.K. [8]. In the case of Spain, most mapped physicians were located in cities. Lymphoedema consultation services are mostly based in hospitals and for public insurance patients the access is restricted, making it more difficult to seek qualified treatment [8]. With the exception of some regions of Germany and Switzerland, professionals specialised in lymphatic diseases were very seldom general practitioners, rendering this distributary problem a characteristic of most countries worldwide.

Lymphoedema researchers

Regarding the data on the number of researchers dedicated to lymphoedema, one of our main difficulties during our search was to identify if these professionals were physicians, or belonged to other professional branches e. g. biologists. Nevertheless, this academic distinction has little influence on the capacity of researching solutions for a disease, as this plurality might be beneficiary for innovation. Most researchers originate from continents

with developed countries such as Oceania or Europe. Awareness and public funding of research are still low on upcoming continents such as South Asia although things have started to change [49]. Young researchers are less attracted to investigate a field they have never heard about as most of their universities have failed to include lymphatic diseases in the university curricula. An important milestone of a global strategy to address the problem of medical care of lympho-vascular diseases should also include measures to break the vicious circle of the lack of research. This has to be achieved outside of the laboratories at sub graduate level through innovative training offers.

Professional societies including lymphatic diseases in their topics of interest

Patients trying to find qualified medical healthcare professionals online, will be confronted with similar limitations encountered in this study. Nevertheless, patients express a deep need for guidance and information [50]. A medical doctor with expertise in lymphatic diseases

Table 3 Distribution of physicians' specialties in the field of lymphology according to continent

	Surgery	Conservative Therapy	Medical Imaging	Filaria	Podoconiosis	Research
Africa	8	3	0	4	0	**16**
Asia	139	28	27	21	0	**163**
Oceania	6	5	0	5	0	**21**
Europe	295	**535**	25	5	1	234
North America	**68**	36	10	4	0	**68**
South America	**61**	34	2	1	1	5
Total	577	641	64	40	2	507

The highest numbers of physicians' specialists of each continent are marked bold

Table 4 Overview of societies, institutions and industry specialised in lymphatic diseases per continent including leading countries

	Europe	North America	South Amercia	Africa	Asia	Oceania
Professional societies and institutions	598	218	54	138	319	75
Leading country	*Germany: 88*	*USA: 161*	*Argentina: 33*	*Ethiopia: 16*	*India: 96*	*Australia: 31*
Industry	90	49	none	3	6	2
Leading country	*UK: 33*	*USA: 42*	*none*	*Kenya, Tanzania, South Africa: 1*	*Taiwan: 3*	*Australia: 2*

that cannot be found by patients searching online is equivalent to a very localised resource. Therefore, we also analysed the number of professional societies, as they play a paramount role in providing information on the spectrum of expertise of their members. Physicians were easily found in South America as the Pan-American Society for Lymphology and Phlebology published a list of physicians. Other examples of societies providing well-structured information are to be found in Germany and Switzerland. There was no clear correlation between the number of professionals specialised in lymphology in a region or country, and the number of professional societies active in this field. But most problematic was the complete lack of independent societies for lymphatic diseases in most countries of the world that could contribute to high level postgraduate education and facilitate discussions about diagnosis and treatment guidelines.

Industrial activities in lymphology

In our analysis of the distribution of industrial activity connected to lymphoedema, North America and Europe were the leading continents. The associated industry is currently not pharmaceutical but mainly biotechnological focussing on measurement devices, surgery microscopes and compression garments. Similarly to pharmaceutical companies, biotechnology companies show less interest in e.g. Africa or South America most likely due to poor distribution networks and low profit margins.

Additional policies for palliation of current deficits

It is somewhat striking to see this disparity of numbers of specialised physicians in developed countries. We believe the reasons for their relatively high number in some countries as e.g. Belgium or Germany to be historical. The first lymphoedema clinic was founded in Germany and already in the late seventies, German healthcare insurances started reimbursing lymphoedema therapy modalities. Although many physiotherapists in Germany are trained in manual lymphatic drainage, only medical doctors are entitled to prescribe it. Therefore, there is a positive peer pressure between both professional groups. This leads to some degree of medical training in this field [51], mostly of general physicians as well as doctors in physical and rehabilitation medicine [52]. Why do other developed countries with a similar number of lymphedema patients still lack specialised human health resources? Improving the quality of management of this disease in Germany and the Benelux was not solely due to medical professionals in itself but

Table 5 Overview of local dialect terms and their medical translation for symptoms of lymphatic diseases

Local term	General term	Country
Gwo pye (Creol dialect) or *big foot*	Elephantiasis	Haiti [29]
Maklouklou or *gwo gren*	Hydrocele	Haiti [29]
Dicipela	Erysipela	Dominican Republic [26, 32]
Seca	Large boil in the groin or upper thigh	Dominican Republic [26, 32]
Mossy foot	Podoconiosis	Ethiopia [38]
Biaye or *edoa*	Inguinal lymphadenitis	Ghana [30]
Ahu par or *esam*	Fever with chills and rigors accompanied by swollen groin glands and legs	Ghana [30]
Gyepim, dubah (both in Ahanta and Nzema dialect) or *large leg*	Elephantiasis	Ghana [30]
Etow (Ahanta), *wheba* (Ahanta), *tuekeh* (Nzema) or *edoma holokpoo*	Hydrocele	Ghana [30]
Yanaikkal	Lymphoedema or elephantiasis of the lower leg	India [56]
Veraveekkam or *veravadam*	Hydrocele	India [56]

mostly to the professional group of the physiotherapists. Here, reimbursement of lymphoedema treatment was adequate, but only allowed to those physiotherapists having undergone validated specialised training. This motivating restriction never happened in the medical profession. The medical chamber of doctors in Germany failed until now to recognise a medical subspecialty in lymphatic diseases, although reiterated proposals have been delivered by professional societies since the nineties. Until today, all physicians are entitled to manage lymphoedema patients. Also, the reimbursement for this medical act is very low and calculated for periods of three months regardless of the number of times the patient has to be seen in that time interval, leading to low motivation to treat this chronic disease. Paradoxically, European policy makers do not seem to be aware of the costs of fail prescriptions and poor management.

In the U.S. severe reimbursement barriers still exist for lymphatic diseases [18, 53]. Here, not only direct costs, but also travel costs and loss of earning prohibit patients to seek proper medical treatment [25, 54].

Interestingly, in the U.K., where the number of medical doctors specialised in this field is also below demand, nurses established a culture of lymphoedema treatment based on patient self-management and training of family members to provide lymphatic drainage. Showing patients how to manage their lymphoedema reduces exacerbations and improves their quality of life [24, 55]. Therefore, it is not neutral to decide which professionals will become key players in this field. It is not sufficient to limit the reimbursement to certified professionals, but special incentives for patient training and empowerment should also be promoted. They eventually increase the patients' independence from the same providers of care that are so scarce in most health systems.

Conclusions

Lymphoedema patients oftentimes experience a chaotic journey from diagnosis to treatment due to scarce support by the medical system. The time prior to diagnosis and thereafter prior to health reimbursement must be shortened. Interventions in this health sector would ideally be based on the knowledge of the extent of the problem. The present study represents a first attempt to quantify a group of professionals characterised by a deficiency of data. Not only the medical expertise in lymphology is not officially recognised as a subspecialty (except for the Netherlands and the United Kingdom) and experts are therefore not listed as such in the corresponding professional chambers, but also the number of professionals specifically offering health services in this field is globally very limited. With the right policies, as certification and homologation of knowledge at tertiary level, restriction of patient care solely to specialised

healthcare providers, structured reimbursement and sufficient research funding, the current situation can be improved. Targeted incentives for medical professionals trained in this field would then ameliorate the management of these diseases, optimise the use of already available financial resources, promote the passage of knowledge and skills in universities, promote research, empower patients and influence interdisciplinary work. These professionals can potentially become the true motors of a worldwide solution. The authors of the study strongly support the use of their database for further research according to the principles of share of good practice.

Abbreviations
ppm: Parts per Million; WHO: World Health Organization

Acknowledgements
We would like to thank David Beverungen for his support in technical issues.

Funding
This work was supported by the European Union [527658 – LLP-1-2012-1-DE-ERASMUS-ESMO]. Henrike Schulze, Marisa Nacke and Catarina Hadamitzky were co-financed by this institution. This study presents the work of independent scientists and does not necessarily reflect the views of the European Commission or its services.

Authors' contributions
HS carried out the data gathering and analysis and wrote the manuscript. MN contributed to the design of figures and tables and provided comments on all drafts. CG provided comments on the draft. CH supervised the study, substantially contributed to data analysis and interpretation and revised all drafts. All authors read and approved the final manuscript.

Competing interests
We confirm that this manuscript describes original work and has neither been published elsewhere nor is under consideration by any other journal. All authors have approved the manuscript and agree with its submission to Health Economics Review. The study authors have no competing interests.

Author details
[1]Clinic of Rehabilitation Medicine, Hannover Medical School, Carl-Neuberg-Straße 1, 30625 Hannover, Germany. [2]Cancer Research UK, Beatson Institute, Glasgow, UK. [3]Practice for Lympho-Vascular Diseases, Bahnhofstraße 12, Hannover, Germany.

References
1. Földi M, Földi E. Földi's textbook of lymphology for physicians and Lymphoedema therapists. 3rd rev ed. München: Urban & Fischer; 2012.
2. Cano J, Rebollo MP, Golding N, Pullan RL, Crellen T, Soler A, et al. The global distribution and transmission limits of lymphatic filariasis: past and present. Parasit Vectors. 2014;7:466.

3.   Wynd S, Melrose WD, Durrheim DN, Carron J, Gyapong M. Understanding the community impact of lymphatic filariasis: a review of the sociocultural literature. Bull World Health Organ. 2007;85:493–8.

4.   Szuba A, Rockson SG. Lymphedema: classification, diagnosis and therapy. Vasc Med. 1998;3:145–56.

5.   Cormier JN, Askew RL, Mungovan KS, Xing Y, Ross MI, Armer JM. Lymphedema beyond breast cancer: a systematic review and meta-analysis of cancer-related secondary lymphedema. Cancer. 2010;116:5138–49.

6.   Ozaslan C, Kuru B. Lymphedema after treatment of breast cancer. Am J Surg. 2004;187:69–72.

7.   Lawton G, Rasque H, Ariyan S. Preservation of muscle fascia to decrease lymphedema after complete axillary and ilioinguinofemoral lymphadenectomy for melanoma. J Am Coll Surg. 2002;195:339–51.

8.   Moffatt CJ, Franks PJ, Doherty DC, Williams AF, Badger C, Jeffs E, et al. Lymphoedema: an underestimated health problem. QJM - Mon J Assoc Phys. 2003;96:731–8.

9.   Yahathugoda TC, Wickramasinghe D, Weerasooriya MV, Samarawickrema WA. Lymphoedema and its management in cases of lymphatic filariasis: the current situation in three suburbs of Matara, Sri Lanka, before the introduction of a morbidity-control programme. Ann Trop Med Parasitol. 2005;99:501–10.

10. Stout NL, Brantus P, Moffatt C. Lymphoedema management: an international intersect between developed and developing countries. Similarities, differences and challenges. Glob Public Health. 2012;7:107–23.

11. Vuong D, Nguyen M, Piller N. Medical education: a deficiency or a disgrace. J Lymphoedema. 2011;6:44–9.

12. Morgan PA, Murray S, Moffatt CJ, Honnor A. The challenges of managing complex lymphoedema/chronic oedema in the UK and Canada. Int Wound J. 2012;9:54–69.

13. Davies R, Fitzpatrick B, Neill AO, Sneddon M. Lymphoedema education needs of clinicians: a national study. J Lymphoedema. 2012;7:14–24.

14. Bogan LK, Powell JM, Dudgeon BJ. Experiences of living with non-cancer-related lymphedema: implications for clinical practice. Qual Health Res. 2007;17:213–24.

15. Williams AF, Moffatt CJ, Franks PJ. A phenomenological study of the lived experiences of people with lymphoedema. Int J Palliat Nurs. 2004;10:279–86.

16. Leard T, Barrett C. Successful Management of Severe Unilateral Lower Extremity Lymphedema in an outpatient setting. Phys Ther. 2015;95:1295–306.

17. Wang W, Keast DH. Prevalence and characteristics of lymphoedema at a wound-care clinic. J Wound Care. 2016;25:S11–2, S14-5.

18. Armer J, Feldman J, Fu M, Stout N, Lasinski B, Tuppo C, et al. ALFP: identifying issues in lymphoedema in the US. J Lymphoedema. 2009;4:3–9.

19. Suma TK, Shenoy RK, Kumaraswami V. A qualitative study of the perceptions, practices and socio-psychological suffering related to chronic brugian filariasis in Kerala, southern India. Ann Trop Med Parasitol. 2003;97:839–45.

20. Bartlett J, Deribe K, Tamiru A, Amberbir T, Medhin G, Malik M, et al. Depression and disability in people with podoconiosis: a comparative cross-sectional study in rural northern Ethiopia. Int Health. 2016;8:124–31.

21. Penha TR, Botter B, Heuts EM, Voogd AC, von Meyenfeldt MF, van der Hulst. Quality of life in patients with breast Cancer-related lymphedema and reconstructive breast surgery. J Reconstr Microsurg. 2016;32:484–90.

22. Becker C, Assouad J, Riquet M, Hidden G. Postmastectomy lymphedema: long-term results following microsurgical lymph node transplantation. Ann Surg. 2006;243:313–5.

23. Morgan PA, Franks PJ, Moffatt CJ. Health-related quality of life with lymphoedema: a review of the literature. Int Wound J. 2005;2:47–62.

24. Stillwaggon E, Sawers L, Rout J, Addiss D, Fox L. Economic costs and benefits of a community-based lymphedema management program for lymphatic Filariasis in Odisha state, India. Am J Trop Med Hyg. 2016;95:877–84.

25. Stanton MC, Best A, Cliffe M, Kelly-hope L, Biritwum NK, Batsa L, et al. Situational analysis of lymphatic filariasis morbidity in Ahanta West District of Ghana. Tropical Med Int Health. 2016;21:236–44.

26. Person B, Addiss D, Bartholomew LK, Meijer C, Pou V, Gonzálvez G, et al. A qualitative study of the psychosocial and health consequences associated with lymphedema among women in the Dominican Republic. Acta Trop. 2007;103:90–7.

27. Rath K, Swain BK, Mishra S, Patasahani T, Kerketta AS, Babu BV. Peripheral health workers' knowledge and practices related to filarial lymphedema

care: a study in an endemic district of Orissa, India. Am J Trop Med Hyg. 2005;72:430–3.

28. Pushter J, Stewart R. Smartphone ownership and internet usage continues to climb in emerging economies. Pew Research Center. 2016. http://www.pewglobal.org/2016/02/22/internet-access-growing-worldwide-but-remains-higher-in-advanced-economies/ Accessed 23 Feb 2018.

29. Coreil J, Mayard G, Louis-Charles J, Addiss D. Filarial elephantiasis among Haitian women: social context and behavioural factors in treatment. Tropical Med Int Health. 1998;3:467–73.

30. Ahorlu CK, Dunyo SK, Koram KA, Nkrumah FK, Aagaard-Hansen J, Simonsen PE. Lymphatic filariasis related perceptions and practices on the coast of Ghana: implications for prevention and control. Acta Trop. 1999;73:251–61.

31. Richard SA, Mathieu E, Addiss DG, Sodahlon YK. A survey of treatment practices and burden of lymphoedema in Togo. Trans R Soc Trop Med Hyg. 2007;101:391–7.

32. Person B, Addiss DG, Bartholomew LK, Meijer C, Pou V, van den Borne B. Health-seeking behaviors and self-care practices of Dominican women with lymphoedema of the leg: implications for lymphoedema management programs. Filaria J. 2006;5:13.

33. Babington LM, Kelley BR, Patsdaughter CA, Soderberg RM, Kelley JE. From recipes to recetas: health beliefs and health care encounters in the rural Dominican Republic. J Cult Divers. 1999;6:20–5.

34. Aarons DE. Medicine and its alternatives. Health care priorities in the Caribbean. Hast Cent Rep. 1999;29:23–7.

35. Bandyopadhyay L. Lymphatic filariasis and the women of India. Soc Sci Med. 1996;42(10):1401.

36. Cassidy T, Worrell CM, Little K, Prakash A, Patra I, Rout J, et al. Experiences of a community-based lymphedema management program for lymphatic Filariasis in Odisha state, India: an analysis of focus group discussions with patients, families, community members and program volunteers. PLoS Negl Trop Dis. 2016;10:e0004424.

37. Pachter LM. Culture and Clinical care. Folk illness beliefs and behaviors and their implications for health care delivery. JAMA. 1994;271:690–4.

38. Davey G, Burridge E. Community-based control of a neglected tropical disease: the mossy foot treatment and prevention association. PLoS Negl Trop Dis. 2009;3:e424.

39. International Finance Corporation WBG. The business of health in Africa partnering with the private sector to improve People's lives. Washington DC 2008.

40. Addiss DG, Brady MA. Morbidity management in the global Programme to eliminate lymphatic Filariasis: a review of the scientific literature. Filaria J. 2007;6:2.

41. Mutheneni SR, Upadhyayula SM, Kumaraswamy S, Kadiri MR, Nagalla B. Influence of socioeconomic aspects on lymphatic filariasis: a case-control study in Andhra Pradesh, India. J Vector Borne Dis. 2016;53:272–8.

42. Turner HC, Bettis AA, Chu BK, McFarland DA, Hooper PJ, Ottesen EA, et al. The health and economic benefits of the global programme to eliminate lymphatic filariasis (2000-2014). Infect Dis Pov. 2016;5:54.

43. Omura S, Crump A. The life and times of ivermectin - a success story. Nat Rev Microbiol. 2004;2:984–9.

44. Schellekens SM, Ananthakrishnan S, Stolk WA, Habbema JDF, Ravi R. Physicians' management of filarial lymphoedema and hydrocele in Pondicherry, India. Trans R Soc Trop Med Hyg. 2005;99:75–7.

45. Mengitsu B, Shafi O, Kebede B, Kebede F, Worku DT, Herero M. Ethiopia and its steps to mobilize resources to achieve 2020 elimination and control goals for neglected tropical diseases webs joined can tie a lion. Int Health. 2016;8(Suppl 1):i34–52.

46. Cooper G, Bagnall A. Prevalence of lymphoedema in the UK: focus on the southwest and West Midlands. Br J Commun Nurs. 2016;Suppl:S6–14.

47. Yimer M, Hailu T, Mulu W, Abera B. Epidemiology of elephantiasis with special emphasis on podoconiosis in Ethiopia: a literature review. J Vector Borne Dis. 2015;52:111–5.

48. Wakerman J, Humphreys JS, Wells R, Kuipers P, Entwistle P, Jones J. Primary health care delivery models in rural and remote Australia: a systematic review. BMC Health Serv Res. 2008;8:276.

49. Sadana R, D'Souza C, Hyder AA, Chowdhury AMR. Importance of health research in South Asia. BMJ. 2004;328:826–30.

50. Bulley C. Making a case for funding for lymphoedema services. J Lymphoedema. 2007;2:22–9.

51. Ärztekammer Westfalen-Lippe. Curriculäre Fortbildung Lymphologie für Ärzte/innen". https://www.aekwl.de/index.php?id=5557. Accessed 23 Feb 2018.

52. Fialka-Moser V, Korpan M, Varela E, Ward A, Gutenbrunner C, Casillas JM, et al. The role of physical and rehabilitation medicine specialist in lymphoedema. Ann Phys Rehabil Med. 2013;56:396–410.

53. Shaitelman SF, Cromwell KD, Rasmussen JC, Stout NL, Armer JM, Lasinski BB, et al. Recent progress in the treatment and prevention of cancer-related lymphedema. CA Cancer J Clin. 2015;65:55–81.

54. Ramaiah KD, Radhamani MP, John KR, Evans DB, Guyatt H, Joseph A. The impact of lymphatic filariasis on labour inputs in southern India: results of a multi-site study. Ann Trop Med Parasitol. 2000;94:353–64.

55. Lu S-R, Hong R-B, Chou W, Hsiao P-C. Role of physiotherapy and patient education in lymphedema control following breast cancer surgery. Ther Clin Risk Manag. 2015;11:319–27.

56. Ramaiah KD, Kumar KN, Ramu K. Knowledge and beliefs about transmission, prevention and control of lymphatic filariasis in rural areas of South India. Tropical Med Int Health. 1996;1:433–8.

13

Variation in the relationship between birth weight and subsequent obesity by household income

Jonas Minet Kinge[1,2]

Abstract

There is evidence to suggest that high birth weight increases subsequent BMI. However, little attention has been paid to variations in this impact between population groups. This study investigates the relationship between high birth weight and subsequent obesity, and whether or not this relationship varies by household income. Data was taken from fourteen rounds of the Health Survey for England (between 2000–2014; $N = 31,043$) for children aged 2–16. We regressed obesity in childhood against birth weight, accounting for interactions between birth weight and household income, using sibling-fixed effects models. High birth weight was associated with increased risk of subsequent obesity. This association was significantly more pronounced in children from low-income families, compared with children from high-income families. A 1 kg increase in birth weight increased the probability of obesity by 7% in the lowest income tertile and 4% in the highest income tertile. This suggests that early socioeconomic deprivation compound the effect of high birth weight on obesity.

Keywords: Birth weight, Obesity, Body mass index, Socioeconomic status, Sibling fixed-effects

Background

The well-known fetal origins hypothesis stresses the importance of fetal development in links between measures of fetal and infant health and later-life health outcomes [1, 2]. In relation to this, it has been suggested that intrauterine growth rate is closely linked to the fetal development of tissues and organs that in postnatal life control eating patterns, physical activity, and metabolism, such as the hypothalamus, pancreatic b-cells, fat tissue, and muscles [3–6]. Hence, a question of interest is whether the prenatal period affects later risk of overweight and obesity. A vast number of studies, including a systematic review and a meta-analysis, have found an association between high birth weight and the risk of overweight in children, adolescents, and adults [7, 8]. The interpretation of these associations may be difficult, however, because many of the studies compared persons who were born to different mothers and brought up in different families. Hence, several researchers have examined the within-family association between birth weight and later body mass index (BMI) in siblings, using sibling-fixed effects designs, and found significant associations [6, 9–11].

While the association between birth weight and subsequent obesity is established, little attention has been paid to variation in this effect between population groups. Such considerations are pertinent given that theory and evidence suggests that parents allocate their investments unequally among their children, and by this reinforce or compensate for initial differences [12]. A growing number of studies also suggests that investment responses vary by family socioeconomic status (SES).

Parental investment responses to a high birth weight may vary by a family's SES because expectations for children's BMI, parenting knowledge about diet and exercise, and the availability of resources to respond to childhood obesity. It has been suggested that parental resources may affect (a) preferences for equity in their

Correspondence: Jonas.Minet.Kinge@fhi.no
[1]Norwegian Institute of Public Health, Pb 4404 Nydalen, 0403 Oslo, Norway
[2]Department of Health Management and Health Economics, University of Oslo, Oslo, Norway

children's outcomes, (b) the productivity of investments in obese children, and (c) knowledge about potential ways to compensate for a high BMI, leading some parents to reinforce and others to compensate [13, 14].

This means that the relationship between birth weight (BW) and later BMI might vary by socioeconomic factors. The framework in Fig. 1 show that household environment, which captures parental behavior for individual i (Z_i), may affect subsequent obesity (Y_i) in three ways. It affects obesity indirectly via its effect on birth weight (B_i), which in turn affects subsequent obesity (arrow 1); it affects obesity directly (arrow 2); and, it affects obesity by modifying the relationship between birth weight and obesity (arrow 3).

The aim of the following study is to measure the third effect (arrow 3), i.e., whether or not the relationship between BW and later BMI varies by household environment, which in this study is measured by SES. A small but growing literature has examined whether a family's SES mitigates the effects of poor child endowments on child outcomes [15–20]. These studies find that poorly endowed children achieve worse outcomes and that the negative impacts of a poor endowment are often larger for children born in disadvantaged families. For example, Almond, Edlund [15] examine the effect of pollution from the Chernobyl disaster on the Swedish cohort that was in utero at the time of the disaster. Those who suffered the greatest radiation exposure were less likely to qualify for high school, and had lower math grades. However, the damage was much larger among those children whose parents were less educated. We have not found any studies that have looked at whether or not the impact of high birth weight on obesity varies by the family SES.

To investigate whether or not the relationship between birth weight and subsequent obesity varies by SES we used data from the Health Survey for England (HSE). The HSE contains measures of children's anthropometrics, household characteristics (like SES) and other individual characteristics. The survey is representative for English children and includes the BW of children aged 2–16 years. This dataset provides us with a unique opportunity to examine the effects of high BW on obesity by SES.

Interactions between SES and high BW

There are a number of theories suggesting that health issues may have consequences that are more negative in children from low SES families, compared with high SES families. Currie and Hyson [21] offers three hypotheses predictive of an interactive effect between SES and BW on later life health outcomes. These hypotheses refer to the model of parental investments in children's human capital. In this model, parents who are assumed to care about their children's outcomes, maximize their own utility subject to a production function for outcomes and a budget constraint. Although Currie and Hyson [21] discuss the impact of low BW on health and human capital, their discussion has been modified to the case for high BW and later life obesity.

The first hypotheses regarding interactive effects relate to the production function for child health. The idea is that the efficiency with which inputs can be transformed into outcomes may be permanently altered by the fact of the children's BW. If low-SES children with high BW suffer from a higher incidence of "obesity increasing environmental influences", than high BW children from high-SES families, this theory predicts that they will have a higher prevalence of obesity.

Currie and Hyson [21] secondly discuss hypotheses that focus on differences in taste between high-SES and low-SES groups. Suppose for example, that BW reflects unmeasured maternal behaviors that continue to affect the outcomes of the child after birth. Such behaviors could be related to exercise and diet as both pre-pregnant body mass index and maternal

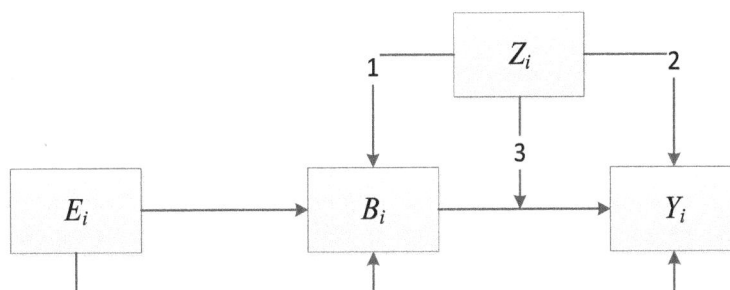

Fig. 1 The impact of birth weight on subsequent obesity. E = genetic endowments; B = birth weight; Z = socioeconomic status; Y = obesity; i = indexes individuals

weight change has an impact on offspring birthweight [22, 23]. A mother that is unwilling to take actions necessary to improve the health of the newborn (e.g. exercise and diet during pregnancy), may also be less likely to make costly investments after the child is born (e.g. help the child with achieving a healthy weight). That is, BW can be influenced by investment in the prenatal period, and this investment could continue after birth. If the propensity to invest in children correlates with social class, then we will observe that high BW has a more pronounced effect on obesity in low-SES children.

Finally, Currie and Hyson [21] discuss hypotheses that focus on the constraints facing parents. For example, the poor face credit constraints, which prevent them from making worthwhile investments in their children. E.g., investments could be in a lifestyle intervention or participation in costly children's sports. Related to this Conley [24] proposed a theory that resource-allocation decisions vary by social class. When resources are limited, concentrating resources on higher-ability children may be the least risky strategy to ensure success of at least one child. Hence, low SES families may be forced to concentrate limited resources on the ablest child to maximize positive returns for their investments. Conversely, socially advantaged families have more options. They have the means to ensure that high-ability children obtain the minimal level of investments to secure success while directing a higher share of resources toward lower-ability children in an effort to compensate for initial endowment differences. This theory is largely supported by findings from Hsin [14], who used time diaries to investigate maternal time investment in response to birth weight.

The theories and empirical findings above are based on studies of low birth weight and subsequent outcomes. Whether or not it is likely that similar mechanisms apply in terms of high birth weight and subsequent obesity can be explored empirically.

Data and variables
Data source
The analysis was based on data from fourteen rounds (2000–2014) of the *Health Survey for England* (HSE) [25]; 2014 is the most recent year of data available. We excluded 2003 as no information on BW is available that year. The HSE is a repeated cross-sectional survey, which draws a different sample of nationally representative individuals living in England each year. To maximize the sample size we included the children boost samples when available.

All adults (16+) within the household (up to a maximum of 10) are eligible for interview, plus up to two children (0-15). The interviewer randomly selects the children to interview in a household with more than two children. For children aged 0–12, parents answer on behalf of the child, but the child is present.

The dependent variable
We used BMI from measured height and weight values measured by the interviewer. One useful feature of the HSE is that the BMI values are not based on self-reported height and weight, which reduces the likelihood of measurement error. We measured obesity as a binary variable taking the value one if a child was obese and zero otherwise. The obesity cut-off values were based on BMI and are age- and gender-specific, defined according to WHO guidelines for children aged 5–19 years [26] and 2–5 years [27]. This means that the definition of obesity varied by age and gender.

Birth weight (BW)
BW was recorded for all children under the age of 16. This was done by the interviewer asking the parent or legal guardian about the BW of the children taking part in the survey. As we have relied on parents' recall of BW, this may be inaccurate. However, prior studies have shown good agreement between maternal recall and medical records of their pregnancy and child's birth outcomes [28–30]. In fact, Lederman and Paxton [31] stated, "Maternal recall is a satisfactory substitute for clinical data, being consistent with the record, and more complete, yet easier to obtain for clinical studies."

We treated the BW variable as a continuous variable. However, as the relationship between BW and subsequent obesity might be nonlinear we have repeated the analyses with a categorical BW variable. More details and the results of this analysis is in Appendix 1.

Household income
We used household income as our measure of SES. This measure is available for both the boost and the core samples, while parents' education or occupation is only available for the core sample, if we used these it would reduce our sample size substantially. Following Case, Lubotsky [32], Currie, Shields [33], the main measure of income that we used was current total pretax annual household income, which is provided in 31 bands in the data, ranging from less than £520 to more than £150,000. We took midpoints of these bands. Since the data were collected over a period of 14 years we deflated them (to 2005 prices) using the consumer price index for the UK. Hence, we have a

pseudocontinuous measure for total family income, which was then equivalised using McClements household score provided in the HSE to account for household size and composition. Finally we converted the equivalised household income into natural logarithms for use in the analyses.

Covariates

We included the following covariates in the regressions: age; sex; interactions between age and sex; ethnicity (white/non-white); Government Office Region (GOR) of residence (nine categories); survey year (fourteen categories). In addition, we included a dummy variable for being the oldest sibling, as birth order has a known effect on health [34]. We also control for maternal age at delivery (five categories <20, 20-30, 30-40, 40+, missing maternal age (2.5% of the children)) as both high and low maternal age is associated with reduced health in the child [35]; and a dummy variable for whether or not the child was born prematurely.

Rather than stratifying by sex, we controlled for it in the analysis. Two recent reviews did not reveal a different association between birth weight and overweight/obesity by sex [7, 8]. In addition, we tried to include interactions between BW and sex in our models below and they were not significant ($p = 0.23$).

Methods

We modelled childhood obesity for individual i as:

$$Y_i = c_0 + c_1 B_i + c_2 Z_i + X_i \gamma + u_i \qquad (1)$$

where Y is a binary measure of obesity for individual i; B is a measure of BW; Z is a measure of household income; and X is a vector of individual, maternal and household characteristics. u is an error term and c and γ are coefficients to be estimated. To allow for the effect of birthweight to vary by income we ran a second model including an interaction between BW and income:

$$Y_i = c_0 + c_1 B_i + c_2 Z_i + c_3 Z_i x B_i + X_i \gamma + u_i \qquad (2)$$

were the ZxB is an interaction between household income and BW. If the Eq. [2] has a better fit than Eq. [1] it suggests that the impact of BW varies significantly by household income. We tested this by a likelihood ratio test.

We cannot rule out that omitted variables bias the relationship between BW and obesity. As children are brought up in different families both early life conditions and parental background factors can affect BW and obesity. To mitigate this we ran the following model using sibling-fixed effects specifications:

$$Y_{ij} = c_0 + c_1 B_{ij} + X_{ij} \gamma + \varepsilon_j + u_{ij} \qquad (3)$$

$$Y_{ij} = c_0 + c_1 B_{ij} + c_3 Z_j x B_{ij} + X_i \gamma + \varepsilon_j + u_{ij} \qquad (4)$$

where ij denotes individual i in family j, and ε represents a family fixed effect. This means that we compared only siblings within each family, and X is a vector of control variables that are not shared between siblings. These are: birth order; maternal age at delivery; whether or not the child was born prematurely; and, the child's age interacted with gender. Household income does not vary across siblings, which means that we cannot include household income in itself in the models. However, the interaction between household income and BW (ZxB) might still be unique for each sibling and is included in Eq. 4.

Our outcome of interest is a limited dependent variable and our primary models are linear probability models (LPM) with heteroscedasticity robust standards errors. This will yield the best least squares approximation of the true conditional expectation function and we can interpret the coefficients as marginal effects. There are two reasons for choosing LPM over, e.g., logit or probit models. Firstly, the interpretation of interactions in non-linear models is less clear as the coefficients are multiplicative [36]. Secondly, non-linear fixed effects models has been shown to provide biased results [37], [Greene W, Han C, Schmidt P. The bias of the fixed effects estimator in nonlinear models. Unpublished Manuscript, Stern School of Business, NYU. 2002;29]. However, we re-ran part of our regressions with logit models and calculated marginal effects for interactions according to Ai and Norton [36]. The conclusions did not change.

We apply survey weights reported in the HSE to each observation. The individual survey weights were generated separately for adults and children. For children (aged 0 to 15), the weights were generated from the household weights and the child selection weights – the selection weights corrected for only including a maximum of two children in a household. The combined household and child selection weights were adjusted to ensure that the weighted age/sex distribution matched that of all children in co-operating households. The survey weights were not used in the regressions with sibling-fixed effects.

It is possible that observations are independent across households, but not within households. We therefore also controlled for clustered sampling within household using unique household identifiers that produced Huber/White/sandwich robust variance estimators that allowed for within-household dependence [38].

Results

Roughly, two thirds of the full sample was also included in the sibling analyses (Table 1). Although the sociodemographic characteristics were comparable, the obesity prevalence was higher in the full sample (11.2%), than in the sibling sample (10.5%).

Predicted smoothed values of subsequent obesity by BW are in Fig. 2. The predictions are based on locally weighted regressions, with a bandwidth of 0.8. They show that obesity prevalence increased with BW. This pattern was found both in the children with a household income above and below the median. However, the figures suggest that the obesity prevalence increased relatively more in the children with a household income below median, compared with the children in families with an income above median. The findings in the full sample and in the sibling sample were similar, though the differences by household income appear to be more pronounced in the sibling sample.

Table 1 Summary statistics of the estimation samples

	Full	Sibling
Total (N)	31,043	19,460
Male (N)	15,718	9,806
Female (N)	15,325	9,654
Birth weight (mean)	3.34	3.35
Obese (%)	11.2	10.5
Age (mean)	9.0	9.1
Maternal age at birth (mean)	28.9	28.7
Preterm birth (%)	5.0	5.6
LN household income (mean)	9.8	9.8
Survey year (%)		
2000	1.09	1.10
2001	7.70	7.79
2002	16.93	17.80
2004	3.16	3.19
2005	6.13	6.20
2006	0.32	0.37
2007	15.86	15.78
2008	15.41	15.36
2009	8.37	8.24
2010	11.17	10.86
2011	3.29	3.06
2012	3.40	3.53
2013	3.73	3.43
2014	3.46	3.29

Linear BW was associated with increased risk of obesity, while the log of household income was associated with reduced risk of obesity in regressions with covariates (Table 2). The interaction between BW and income was significant and the LR-test suggests a significantly better fit in the model with the interaction. These results were found in the full sample and the sibling sample. The BW-coefficient was significant in the sibling fixed effects specification. In addition, the interactions between income and BW remained significant in the sibling fixed effects models. This suggests that the impact of BW on subsequent obesity varies significantly with household income. The effect of BW was larger in children from low-income families.

When we stratified the children into tertiles by income, we also observe a more pronounced effect of BW on obesity, in the lowest income tertile (Table 3). Similar findings were done in the sibling fixed effects analysis, where the effect of BW, on obesity, was 0.067 in the lowest income tertile while it was 0.036 in the highest income tertile.

As shown in Fig. 2, the effect of BW on subsequent obesity might not be linear. Hence, we reran the analysis with a categorical BW variable. The findings, which are presented in Appendix 1, supports the results, presented in Tables 2 and 3 using linear BW. In low-income children, the association between high BW and obesity was significantly more pronounced, compared with high-income children.

Discussion

The aims of this study were to investigate the relationship between birth weight and subsequent obesity, and whether or not this relationship varies by household income. Our main findings were that of a significant correlation between high birth weight and subsequent obesity, and that the correlation varied significantly by household income. The effect of BW on subsequent obesity was more pronounced in children from low-income households compared with children from high-income households.

We provide evidence to show that children born with high birth weight had significantly higher obesity prevalence, than those of normal birth weight. Variables shared between siblings did not explain our findings, according to the sibling fixed effects models. These results are qualitatively similar to those in other studies, which have also shown that high birth weight is associated with increased risk of subsequent overweight and obesity [7, 8]. Our findings also support earlier studies that have used sibling fixed effects and found a significant impact of birth weight on obesity [6, 11]. However, direct comparisons of the

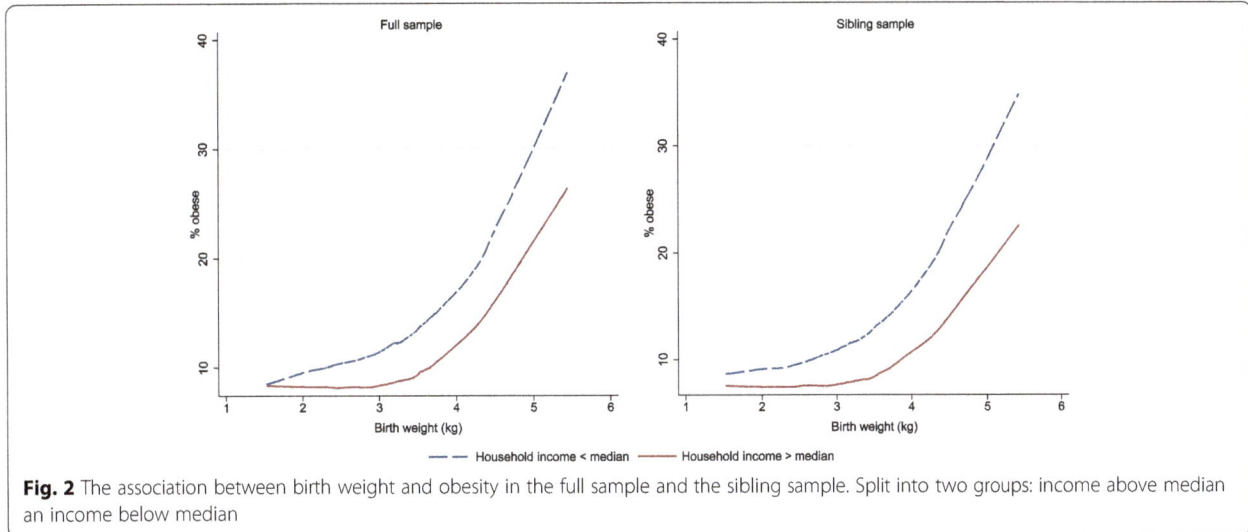

Fig. 2 The association between birth weight and obesity in the full sample and the sibling sample. Split into two groups: income above median an income below median

coefficients are difficult as most other studies report their findings in odds ratios, while we reported marginal effects. A few studies have shown an association between birth weight and subsequent obesity using UK data [39, 40]. However, this study is, to our awareness, the first study using UK data and a sibling fixed effects design.

Our main finding is however, that the association between birth weight and subsequent obesity varied

significantly by household income; the association was more pronounced in children from lower income households. Children born with high birth weight in low-income households were more likely to be obese than those of normal birth weight in low-income household, and were more likely to be obese than those in higher income households who was born with the same birth weight. This trend was also observed after controlling for individual and household characteristics and in

Table 2 OLS of the effect of birth weight in kilos (continuous) and income on obesity in the full sample and the sibling sample

| | No interactions (Eq. 1/Eq. 3) | | With interactions (Eq. 2/Eq. 4) | |
	Coef.	t	Coef.	t
Full sample*				
Birth weight	0.0403	9.81	0.1273	3.04
Log of household income	-0.0220	-8.11	0.0078	0.56
Birth weight X income			-0.0089	-2.13
LR test of basic model vs. model with interaction			*p = 0.01*	
Sibling sample*				
Birth weight	0.0353	6.77	0.1503	2.76
Log of household income	-0.0227	-6.51	0.0170	0.94
Birth weight X income			-0.0118	-2.17
LR test of basic model vs. model with interaction			*p = 0.01*	
Sibling fixed effects**				
Birth weight	0.0434	5.64	0.1874	2.34
Log of household income	*[equal across siblings]*		*[equal across siblings]*	
Birth weight X income			-0.0148	-1.8
LR test of basic model vs. model with interaction			*p < 0.01*	

* Covariates: age; sex; interactions between age and sex; ethnicity; Government Office Region (GOR) of residence; survey year; birth order; maternal age at delivery; and, whether or not the child was born prematurely
** Covariates: birth order; maternal age at delivery; whether or not the child was born prematurely; and, the child's age interacted with gender

Table 3 The effect of the birth weight (continuous) on the probability of obesity. Stratified by household income. Results for the full sample and for sibling fixed effects analysis

	Full sample		Sibling fixed effects	
	Coef.	*t*	*Coef.*	*t*
All	0.0375	10.58	0.0434	5.64
Low income	0.0521	7.59	0.0670	4.5
Medium income	0.0329	5.28	0.0310	2.37
High income	0.0354	6.52	0.0356	2.92

Covariates: birth order; maternal age at delivery; whether or not the child was born prematurely; and, the child's age interacted with gender

sibling fixed effects models. While a number of studies have investigated the impact of birth weight on subsequent obesity controlling for socioeconomic variables in multivariate analyses, we are not aware of any published studies that have stratified their analyses by socioeconomic status to investigate whether or not the association between birth weight on obesity varies by socioeconomic status.

Our findings are consistent with the theories proposed in the introduction. For example, the theory on strategic investment propose that parental allocation decisions largely are driven by conscious investments strategies of the parents [24]. This results in low-income families concentrating their limited resources on the higher-ability children, to maximize their human capital returns. While high-income parents adopt compensatory strategies because they can afford this, i.e. they devote more resources to the less endowed children, while still ensuring enough resources to their other children to maximize their probability of success.

An alternative explanation might be that low income parents might be more likely to lack the psychological and material resources to handle high need children [14]. Caring for high birth weight children might be more burdensome, not only are they at increased risk for being obese, they are also more likely to suffer from a number of chronic illnesses [41, 42] and have worse academic outcomes [43, 44]. Successful obesity interventions does not only demand a persistent effort from the child, they are also more likely to be successful if the parents are involved [45]. In this case, our results would not be a result of conscious investments, but from immediate responses to the current situation. Although our study cannot separate out one of these alternative explanations, it offers a strong empirical finding: the impact of birth weight on subsequent obesity varies by household income.

There are a number of implications of these findings. The fetal origins literature emphasizes fetal development and its consequences for later life health outcomes [1, 2]. However, this study finds that environmental and social factors may alter the biological effect of high BW on later life obesity. This suggests that the conditions in utero is less important for the development of obesity than the epidemiological literature has suggested as the home environment may—depending on whose home it is—promote or prevent the development of subsequent obesity in those being born with a high birth weight. If this is true, studies that do not account for heterogeneity in the effect of high BW on obesity may, on the one hand, overestimate the effect in lower SES families, but, on the other hand, underestimate the effect for children born into high SES families. Our findings also suggest that socioeconomic inequalities in obesity might be related to conditions in utero.

The present study has limitations. First, our measure of obesity was BMI, which has been criticized, e.g., because it does not incorporate body fat, which is an independent predictor of ill health [46]. In addition, earlier studies have suggested that birth weight is positively associated with both lean body mass and fat in adults [47]. Although we used age and gender specific cut-off values for obesity, caution is necessary when BMI is used as children and adolescents can experience growth in height and weight during brief periods [48]. Second, the children, in the sibling fixed effects models, were members of families with more children and were less obese than were the children in the total study population. Thus, the results of the sibling comparisons may not be fully representative for the total population of English children.

Conclusion

Our study has shown that, as in previous studies, high BW was associated with increased risk of subsequent obesity. In addition, we have shown that the association between BW and obesity was more pronounced in children from lower income households. High household income buffers the effect of birth weight on subsequent obesity.

Appendix 1
Treating birth weight as a categorical variable

In the following BW is grouped into three categories. "Low BW" defined as a BW < 2.5 kg; "normal BW" defined as a BW between 2.5 and 4.5 kg; and, "High BW" defined as BW > 4.5 kg.

When BW was included as a categorical variable we found a significant and positive effect of high BW, compared with normal BW, on obesity (Table 4 in Appendix 1). The LR-tests also suggest that the models that included interactions between BW and income had a significantly better fit. I.e. the effect of high BW on subsequent obesity was higher in children from low income families.

Table 4 OLS of the effect of birth weight (categorical variable) and income on obesity in the full sample and the sibling sample

	No interactions (Eq. 1/Eq. 3)		With interactions (Eq. 2/Eq. 4)	
	Coef.	t	Coef.	t
Full sample*				
High birth weight	0.0516	7.81	0.2025	2.35
Low birth weight	-0.0263	-2.26	-0.0743	-0.91
Log of household income	-0.0212	-7.85	-0.0197	-6.72
High birth weight X income			-0.0153	-1.78
Low birth weight X income			0.0051	0.61
LR test of basic model vs. model with interaction			p = 0.06	
Sibling sample**				
High birth weight	0.0458	5.69	0.2293	2.14
Low birth weight	-0.0222	-1.48	-0.0807	-0.8
Log of household income	-0.0218	-6.26	-0.0199	-5.25
High birth weight X income			-0.0187	-1.75
Low birth weight X income			0.0062	0.6
LR test of basic model vs. model with interaction[a]			p = 0.05	

* Covariates: age; sex; interactions between age and sex; ethnicity; Government Office Region (GOR) of residence; survey year; birth order; maternal age at delivery; and, whether or not the child was born prematurely
** Covariates: birth order; maternal age at delivery; whether or not the child was born prematurely; and, the child's age interacted with gender

Table 5 The effect of the birth weight (categorical variable) on the probability of obesity. Stratified by household income. Results for the full sample and for sibling fixed effects analysis

	Full sample		Sibling fixed effects	
	Coef.	t	Coef.	t
All				
High birth weight	0.0525	9.58	0.0358	3.63
Low birth weight	-0.0127	-1.02	-0.0316	-1.39
Low income				
High birth weight	0.0709	6.03	0.0556	2.7
Low birth weight	-0.0246	-1.17	-0.0203	-0.56
Medium income				
High birth weight	0.0507	5.33	0.0411	2.4
Low birth weight	-0.0159	-0.69	0.0027	0.06
High income				
High birth weight	0.0454	5.78	0.0177	1.23
Low birth weight	-0.0051	-0.24	-0.0750	-1.94

Covariates: birth order; maternal age at delivery; whether or not the child was born prematurely; and, the child's age interacted with gender

When we stratified the children into tertiles by income we also observe that the effect of BW was more pronounced in the lowest income tertile (Table 5 in Appendix 1). Similar findings were done in the sibling fixed effects analysis.

Abbreviations
BMI: Body mass index; BW: Birth weight; HSE: Health survey for England; LPM: Linear probability models; SES: Socioeconomic status

Acknowledgements
I would like acknowledge the project « The burden of obesity in Norway: morbidity, mortality, health service use and productivity loss» funded by the Norwegian Research Council through grant 250335/F20. The funding source had no involvement in the in study design; in the collection, analysis and interpretation of data; in the writing of the articles; and in the decision to submit it for publication. I thank Øystein Kravdal, Jane Greve and seminar participants at NHESG for helpful comments.

Competing interests
The author declares that he/she has no competing interests.

References

1. Barker DJ. The fetal and infant origins of adult disease. Br Med J. 1990; 301(6761):1111.
2. Currie J, Almond D. Human capital development before age five. Handb labor econ. 2011;4:1315–486.
3. Catalano PM, Hauguel-De MS. Is it time to revisit the Pedersen hypothesis in the face of the obesity epidemic? Am J Obstet Gynecol. 2011;204(6):479–87.
4. Martin-Gronert M, Ozanne S. Metabolic programming of insulin action and secretion. Diabetes Obes Metab. 2012;14(s3):29–39.
5. Simmons R, editor Perinatal programming of obesity. Seminars in perinatology; 2008: Elsevier.
6. Eriksen W, Sundet JM, Tambs K. Birth weight and the risk of overweight in young men born at term. Am J Hum Biol. 2015;27(4):564–9.
7. Schellong K, Schulz S, Harder T, Plagemann A. Birth weight and long-term overweight risk: systematic review and a meta-analysis including 643,902 persons from 66 studies and 26 countries globally. PLoS One. 2012;7(10): e47776.
8. Zhao Y, Wang S-F, Mu M, Sheng J. Birth weight and overweight/obesity in adults: a meta-analysis. Eur J Pediatr. 2012;171(12):1737–46.
9. Johansson M, Rasmussen F. Birthweight and body mass index in young adulthood: the Swedish young male twins study. Twin Res. 2001;4(5):400–5.
10. Pietilainen KH, Rissanen A, Laamanen M, Lindholm AK, Markkula H, Yki-Jarvinen H, et al. Growth patterns in young adult monozygotic twin pairs discordant and concordant for obesity. Twin Res. 2004;7(5):421–9.
11. The NS, Adair LS, Gordon-Larsen P. A Study of the Birth Weight–Obesity Relation Using a Longitudinal Cohort and Sibling and Twin Pairs. Am J Epidem. 2010.
12. Grätz M, Torche F. Compensation or Reinforcement? The Stratification of Parental Responses to Children's Early Ability. Demography. 2016;53(6): 1883–904.
13. Restrepo BJ. Parental investment responses to a low birth weight outcome: who compensates and who reinforces? J Popul Econ. 2016;29(4):969–89.
14. Hsin A. Is biology destiny? Birth weight and differential parental treatment. Demography. 2012;49(4):1385–405.
15. Almond D, Edlund L, Palme M. Chernobyl's Subclinical Legacy: Prenatal Exposure to Radioactive Fallout and School Outcomes in Sweden*. Q J Econ. 2009;124(4):1729–72.
16. Lin M-J, Liu J-T, Chou S-Y. As low birth weight babies grow, can well-educated parents buffer this adverse factor? A research note. Demography. 2007;44(2):335–43.
17. Zvara BJ, Schoppe-Sullivan SJ. Does parent education moderate relations between low birth weight and child cognitive development outcomes? Fam Sci. 2010;1(3-4):212–21.
18. Halla M, Zweimüller M. Parental response to early human capital shocks: evidence from the Chernobyl accident. 2014.
19. Beach B, Saavedra M. Mitigating the Effects of Low Birth Weight: Evidence from Randomly Assigned Adoptees. American J Health Econ. 2015;1(3):275–96.
20. Cheadle JE, Goosby BJ. Birth weight, cognitive development, and life chances: A comparison of siblings from childhood into early adulthood. Soc Sci Res. 2010;39(4):570–84.
21. Currie J, Hyson R. Is the Impact of Health Shocks Cushioned by Socioeconomic Status? The Case of Low Birthweight. Am Econ Rev. 1999; 89(2):245–50.
22. Stamnes Koepp UM, Frost Andersen L, Dahl-Joergensen K, Stigum H, Nass O, Nystad W. Maternal pre-pregnant body mass index, maternal weight change and offspring birthweight. Acta Obstet Gynecol Scand. 2012;91(2):243–9.
23. Yan J. Maternal pre-pregnancy BMI, gestational weight gain, and infant birth weight: A within-family analysis in the United States. Econ Hum Biol. 2015; 18:1–12.
24. Conley D. Bringing sibling differences in: Enlarging our understanding of the transmission of advantage in families. Social class: How does it work. 2008:179-200.
25. National Centre for Social Research and Department of Epidemiology and Public Health University College London (UCL). Health Survey for England. Colchester: UK Data Archive 1997 - 2013.
26. World Health Organization. Growth reference 5-19 years: BMI-for-age (5-19 years). Geneva: WHO. Available online at: http://www.who.int/growthref/who2007_bmi_for_age/en/. Accessed 12 2011.
27. 27. WHO Child Growth Standards: Length/height-for-age, weight-for-age, weight-for-length, weight-for-height and body mass index-for-age: Methods and development. [Internet]. World Health Organization; 2006. Available from: http://www.who.int/childgrowth/standards/technical_report/en/.
28. Tomeo CA, Rich-Edwards JW, Michels KB, Berkey CS, Hunter DJ, Frazier AL, et al. Reproducibility and validity of maternal recall of pregnancy-related events. Epidemiology. 1999;10(6):774–6.
29. Tate AR, Dezateux C, Cole TJ, Davidson L, Group MCSCH. Factors affecting a mother's recall of her baby's birth weight. Int J Epidemiol. 2005;34(3):688–95.
30. O'Sullivan JJ, Pearce MS, Parker L. Parental recall of birth weight: how accurate is it? Arch Dis Child. 2000;82(3):202–3.
31. Lederman SA, Paxton A. Maternal reporting of prepregnancy weight and birth outcome: consistency and completeness compared with the clinical record. Matern Child Health J. 1998;2(2):123–6.
32. Case A, Lubotsky D, Paxson C. Economic Status and Health in Childhood: The Origins of the Gradient. Am Econ Rev. 2002;92(5):1308–34.
33. Currie A, Shields MA, Price SW. The child health/family income gradient: Evidence from England. J Health Econ. 2007;26(2):213–32.
34. Donovan SJ, Susser E. Commentary: advent of sibling designs. Int J Epidemiol. 2011;40(2):345–9.
35. Fall CHD, Sachdev HS, Osmond C, Restrepo-Mendez MC, Victora C, Martorell R, et al. Association between maternal age at childbirth and child and adult outcomes in the offspring: a prospective study in five low-income and middle-income countries (COHORTS collaboration). Lancet Glob Health. 2015;3(7):e366–e77.
36. Ai C, Norton EC. Interaction terms in logit and probit models. Econ Lett. 2003;80(1):123–9.
37. Greene W. The behaviour of the maximum likelihood estimator of limited dependent variable models in the presence of fixed effects. Econ J. 2004; 7(1):98–119.
38. Kish L, Frankel MR. Inference from complex samples. J Royal Stat Soc Series B (Methodological). 1974:1-37.
39. Phillips DI, Young JB. Birth weight, climate at birth and the risk of obesity in adult life. Int J Obes Relat Metab Disord. 2000;24(3):281–7.
40. Reilly JJ, Armstrong J, Dorosty AR, Emmett PM, Ness A, Rogers I, et al. Early life risk factors for obesity in childhood: cohort study. BMJ. 2005;330(7504):1357.
41. Flaherman V, Rutherford GW. A meta-analysis of the effect of high weight on asthma. Arch Dis Child. 2006;91(4):334–9.
42. Yeazel MW, Ross JA, Buckley JD, Woods WG, Ruccione K, Robison LL. High birth weight and risk of specific childhood cancers: A report from the Children's Cancer Group. J Pediatr. 1997;131(5):671–7.
43. Cesur R, Kelly IR, editors. From cradle to classroom: high birth weight and cognitive outcomes. Forum for Health Economics & Policy; 2010: De Gruyter.
44. Kirkegaard I, Obel C, Hedegaard M, Henriksen TB. Gestational age and birth weight in relation to school performance of 10-year-old children: a follow-up study of children born after 32 completed weeks. Pediatrics. 2006;118(4):1600–6.
45. Young KM, Northern JJ, Lister KM, Drummond JA, O'Brien WH. A meta-analysis of family-behavioral weight-loss treatments for children. Clin Psychol Rev. 2007;27(2):240–9.
46. Burkhauser RV, Cawley J. Beyond BMI: the value of more accurate measures of fatness and obesity in social science research. J Health Econ. 2008;27(2):519–29.
47. Skidmore PM, Cassidy A, Swaminathan R, Richards JB, Mangino M, Spector TD, et al. An obesogenic postnatal environment is more important than the fetal environment for the development of adult adiposity: a study of female twins. Am J Clin Nutr. 2009;90(2):401–6.
48. Troiano RP, Flegal KM. Overweight children and adolescents: description, epidemiology, and demographics. Pediatrics. 1998; 101(Supplement 2):497–504.

14

Standardised mortality rate for cerebrovascular diseases in the Slovak Republic from 1996 to 2013 in the context of income inequalities and its international comparison

Beáta Gavurová* ⓘ, Viliam Kováč and Tatiana Vagašová

Abstract

Non-communicable diseases represent one of the greatest challenges for health policymakers. The main objective of this study is to analyse the development of standardised mortality rates for cerebrovascular disease, which is one of the most common causes of deaths, in relation to income inequality in individual regions of the Slovak Republic. Direct standardisation was applied using data from the Slovak mortality database, covering the time period from 1996 to 2013. The standardised mortality rate declined by 4.23% in the Slovak Republic. However, since 1996, the rate has been higher by almost 33% in men than in women. Standardised mortality rates were lower in the northern part of the Slovak Republic than in the southern part. The regression models demonstrated an impact of the observed income-related dimensions on these rates. The income quintile ratio and Gini coefficient appeared to be the most influencing variables. The results of the analysis highlight valuable baseline information for creating new support programmes aimed at eliminating health inequalities in relation to health and social policy.

Keywords: Standardised mortality rate, Cerebrovascular diseases, Income inequality, Regional disparities, the Slovak Republic

Background

The health status of a country's population is the result of a complex interplay of genetic features, socio-economic situations, and environmental, nutritional, and lifestyle factors, as well as of the general availability of health care including preventive programmes [1]. The data on mortality are common indicators used to measure and compare a country's health status at the local, national, and international level, as these data are regularly and widely collected. Understanding the health status of a population should form the baseline for establishing effective health policies, allocation of funds, and prioritisation of health care in the country [2–4]. The Slovak Republic has currently developed proposals for reforms in the health

sector, and these changes should be based on relevant analyses concerning the health status of a population and demographic indicators. In terms of mortality, it is desirable to examine the leading causes of death because these conditions require increased attention from health policymakers in the Slovak Republic.

The most common causes of death include cardiovascular diseases, which cause approximately 45% of all deaths in the Slovak Republic. In particular, ischaemic heart diseases and cerebrovascular diseases are the leading causes of mortality in the Slovak Republic [5].

The World Health Organization defines cerebrovascular diseases as rapidly developing clinical signs of focal cerebral dysfunction that last for more than 24 hours or lead to death without the presence of an apparent cause other than cerebrovascular malformations. Ischaemic stroke is defined as blockage of the blood vessels affecting tissue

*Correspondence: beata.gavurova@tuke.sk
Technical University of Košice, Němcovej 32, Košice, Slovakia

in the central nervous system. Unlike transient ischaemic attack, ischaemic infarction may be symptomatic or asymptomatic. Cerebrovascular diseases are a predominant cause of death in developed countries [6]. They present long-term and significant socio-economic issues worldwide [7–9]. The incidence of transient ischaemic attacks in Europe and in the United States is estimated to range from 0.37 to 1.1 per 1,000 inhabitants per year, which exponentially increases with age regardless of race and gender from 6 to 16 per 1,000 inhabitants aged 85 years and older per year [10]. Its prevalence is estimated to range from 0.4% to 4.1%. In 2002, experts had already examined the development of the mortality rate due to cerebrovascular diseases in Europe, the United States, and in Japan [11, 12]. Their studies confirmed that the worst results at that time occurred in eastern European countries. With the increasing life expectancy as well as the number of elderly, a rise in the prevalence of cerebrovascular diseases can be expected in many developed countries.

Despite the advanced multidisciplinary research on cerebrovascular disease in many countries, respective analyses are absent for the Slovak Republic. The available partial analyses of medical fields assess the country's population health issues separately, in the context of outputs from various casuistries. They do not provide comprehensive or relevant baselines for health and social policy, because they lack a contextual link with demographic processes such as the ageing of the population and correlations with socioeconomic characteristics and regional disparities in health. Knowledge of these determinants, the causal relations, and their quantification should be incorporated into targeted research studies and would provide important information for many policymakers as well as for the creation of targeted metrics representing the health status of the Slovak population within the strategic framework of the healthcare system. A systemic problem that occurs with prevention programmes is that if they are not properly targeted or are implemented with inappropriate tools, they lose their primary effect, and thus efforts to increase the effectiveness of the health system do not achieve the desired countrywide results.

The situation outside of the Slovak Republic is far more positive. Multidimensional analyses of mortality and its determinants have long been at the heart of many disciplines, including the medical, economic, social sciences. This is clearly evidenced by the quality of the available epidemiological scientific research studies [13, 14] as well as the further development of similar fields [15–20]. In addition to scientific research institutions, the issue of morbidity and mortality is also explored by international institutions – for instance, the World Health Organization, Eurostat, and the Organisation for Economic Co-operation and Development [6].

The aim of this study is to identify the most vulnerable groups of people in the past 17 years and to find the regions of the Slovak Republic with the highest cerebrovascular disease mortality rate while considering the income inequality between regions.

The main objectives of this study are as follows:

- To analyse the progression of mortality rate due to cerebrovascular diseases in the Slovak Republic in comparison with selected European countries;
- To reveal regional differences, both in the level and progression of the cerebrovascular disease mortality rate, in the Slovak Republic;
- To quantify the relationship between the mortality rate and income indicators in the individual regions of the Slovak Republic.

The main contribution of this study is the identification of regional discrepancies in the mortality rate of cerebrovascular diseases in the Slovak Republic and the analysis of their reasons in relation to each region's income indicators. When examining the relationship between mortality and income indicators, we expected to observe a positive linear relationship between mortality and the explored indicators – unemployment rate, poverty, Gini coefficient, social benefits, and income quintile ratio. On the contrary, a negative linear relationship was expected for disposable income.

Methods

The data and methodology section offers an overview of the applied dataset and methodology.

Data

The mortality rate was computed from data on the number of deaths due to cerebrovascular diseases – marked as codes I60 to I69 – according to sex, five-year age groups and individual regions of the Slovak Republic from 1996 to 2013. Under the conditions of their contract, the National Health Information Centre (Národné centrum zdravotníckych informàcií) of the Slovak Republic provides a primary source of data on national health statistics.

Mid-year population data by sex, age group and individual region for all explored years were obtained from the Statistical Office of the Slovak Republic (Štatistický úrad Slovenskej Republiky). Mortality rate was age-standardised to the revised European standard population by the age groups adopted by Eurostat in the last revision in 2012. For international comparisons, countries with extreme cerebrovascular disease mortality rates were selected, as were countries of the Visegrad Group – the Czech Republic, Hungary, Poland, and the Slovak Republic, which show similarities due to their shared post-socialist development. The data were available from 2004 to 2012.

In particular regions of the Slovak Republic, we tested the relationship between the standardised mortality rate and the following socio-economic indicators:

- Unemployment rate – expressed as the share of unemployed inhabitants of the number of economically active inhabitants in the previous year;
- Disposable income of a household – the mean equivalised net income per household – expressed in EUR per month;
- Poverty – the share of the population with an income lower than the at-risk-of-poverty threshold compared to the whole population;
- Gini coefficient;
- Income quintile ratio – $S80/S20$ ratio;
- Social benefits – the amount of all social benefits received by an individual – expressed in EUR per month.

The data on unemployment rate were obtained from the Statistical Office of the Slovak Republic, and the other indicators were downloaded from the European Union Statistics on Income and Living Conditions, which is the most extensive statistical survey on income, living conditions and poverty indicators in the European Union from 2004 to 2013.

There are a few notes to consider regarding the definition of the chosen income indicators. The unemployment rate indicates the ratio of the number of unemployed inhabitants out of the number of economically active inhabitants in the previous year. The mean equivalised net income per household represents the household disposable income divided by the equivalent household size. Individual household members are assigned weights – 1 for the first adult household member, 0.5 per each additional adult member, 0.5 per each adolescent 14 years of age and over and 0.3 per each child younger than 14 years of age. The at-risk-of-poverty threshold is set at 60% of the national median of individual equivalised disposable income. It expresses the percentage of inhabitants with an equivalent disposable income below a set boundary.

The Gini coefficient is an indicator of monetary poverty that represents inequality in income distribution and is defined as the relationship of cumulative shares of the population arranged according to the level of equivalised disposable income compared to the cumulative share of the equivalised total disposable income they receive. It ranges in value from 0, meaning absolute income equality – everyone has the same income – to 1, signalling absolute income inequality – one person has the entire income and all others have none. The income quintile ratio – $S80/S20$ ratio – is a measure of the income distribution inequality. It is calculated as the proportion of the total income of 20% of the richest people in society – located in the top quintile – relative to the total income of the 20% poorest

people – located in the lowest quintile. Social benefits include all types of monetary social help targeted for poor, disabled, or otherwise handicapped people.

Methodology

To examine the relationships between these variables, we applied correlation and regression analyses. Through the regression, we quantified the effect of individual income indicators functioning as independent variables on the standardised mortality rate as the dependent variable at a certain significance level.

The general equation used in regression analysis is as follows:

$$Y = \beta_0 + \sum_{i=1}^{v} (\beta_i X_i) + \epsilon \tag{1}$$

- Y – explained variable;
- β_0 – constant;
- v – number of explanatory variables;
- β_i – fitted coefficient of the ith explanatory variable, whilst $i \in \mathbb{N}$;
- X_i – the ith explanatory variable;
- ϵ – residual.

In our analysis, we implemented a modelling process with an outcome in the form of regression models. We applied the linear regression method. To determine the statistical significance of the regression models, four methods were employed – the coefficient of determination and its adjusted version, the bayesian information criterion, and the Akaike information criterion.

The standardised mortality rate SMR serves as an explanatory variable. It was constructed for cerebrovascular diseases in particular. The explanatory variables mentioned in the regression analysis are as follows:

- UR – unemployment rate;
- I – mean net disposable income of a household – expressed in EUR per month;
- P – share of population with an income lower than the at-risk-of-poverty threshold in relation to the whole population;
- GC – Gini coefficient;
- IQR – income quintile ratio;
- SB – amount of all social benefits of an individual – expressed in EUR per month.

Mortality rate was expressed as the standardised mortality rate, which is defined as the number of total deaths per 100,000 inhabitants. We applied the method of direct standardisation to eliminate variances resulting from differences in the age structure of the populations across regions and over time, ensuring the necessary conditions for comparing regions of the Slovak Republic.

The standardised cerebrovascular disease mortality rate by sex was calculated for the individual regions of the Slovak Republic during the period from 1996 to 2013 in Microsoft Access using Structured Query Language, and contingency analysis was conducted in Microsoft Excel. Regression analysis was performed in statistical software R. The dataset was in the form of time series panel data combined with cross-sections.

To study the population statistics, we applied descriptive statistical methods, in particular measures of central tendency – minimum, maximum, mean, median and mode – and measures of variability – interquartile range, standard deviation and coefficient of variation.

Results
Development of standardised mortality rates for cerebrovascular diseases in the selected European Union members

Cerebrovascular diseases are a leading cause of death in almost all European Union countries, representing approximately 11% of all deaths in these countries [21]. The comparability of the data over time and across different countries was ensured by Eurostat's Working Group on Public Health Statistics. In contrast to the 2004 to 2010 data, the 2011 to 2012 data were collected with a legal basis [22, 23], however, the comparability of the data was checked before dissemination.

Figure 1 depicts the progression in the cerebrovascular disease mortality rate of the European Union countries with the most extreme values throughout the time period from 2004 to 2012. The trend in standardised mortality rate was identified as slightly decreasing, with the exception of the trend in Bulgaria. The highest percentage declines were recorded in countries such as Estonia, where it reached 63.13%, and the Czech Republic with a 39.74% decline. However, a slight increase at a level of 0.69% was revealed in Bulgaria, while the standardised

mortality rates were on average 3.2 times higher than the average of the entire European Union. The smallest decline in standardised mortality rate occurred in the Slovak Republic, at a level of 4.23%. While the standardised mortality rate of all the observed countries decreased from 2006 to 2008, the Slovak Republic recorded a very sharp increase of 42.7%. The average of the entire European Union was characterised by a relatively high decline in the standardised mortality rate for cerebrovascular diseases, reaching 31.5%. The Slovak Republic significantly lagged behind the other countries in improvements in the mortality rate within a given time span. In the last year with available statistics, the Visegrad Group members showed standardised mortality rates above the average of the entire European Union. The Slovak Republic had the worst standardised mortality rate at 160 per 100,000 inhabitants, followed by Hungary at 158 per 100,000 inhabitants, the Czech Republic at 142 per 100,000 inhabitants and finally Poland at 132 per 100,000 inhabitants.

Development of the standardised mortality rate for cerebrovascular diseases in the Slovak Republic

The focus of further analyses was on the standardised mortality rate for cerebrovascular diseases in the Slovak Republic. In the long term, during the period from 1996 to 2013, the trend in standardised mortality rate was cyclical and slightly decreasing.

The standardised mortality rate for men recorded a 24.99% decrease from 211.92 per 100,000 inhabitants in 1996 to 158.96 per 100,000 inhabitants in 2013, compared to a 24.09% drop from 165.64 per 100,000 inhabitants in 1996 to 125.73 per 100,000 inhabitants in 2013 for women. Throughout the period from 1996 to 2013, the standardised mortality rate for men was higher by 33% compared to the rate among women. A maximum gender gap was observed in 2007 at a level of 37%, while a minimum difference of 26% was found in 2013, as seen in Fig. 2.

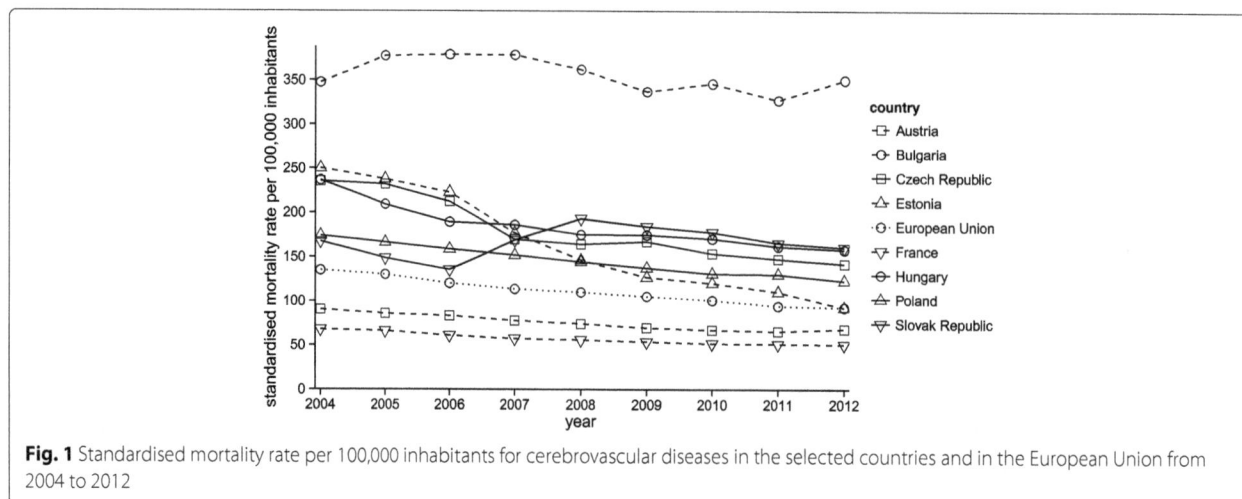

Fig. 1 Standardised mortality rate per 100,000 inhabitants for cerebrovascular diseases in the selected countries and in the European Union from 2004 to 2012

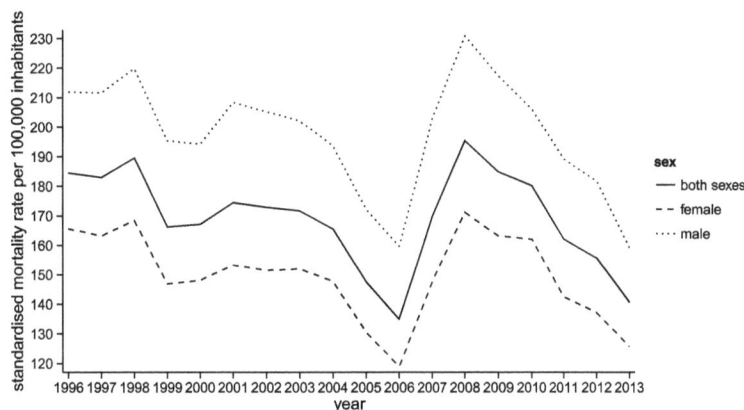

Fig. 2 Standardised mortality rate per 100,000 inhabitants for cerebrovascular diseases according to the sexes in the Slovak Republic from 1996 to 2013

Age plays an important role in the analysis of mortality because it is a significant predictor and an indicator of at-risk age groups. To eliminate fluctuations in the number of deaths, the observed period from 1996 to 2013 was divided into the three periods. Each phase covers 6 years. The first period begins in 1996 and ends in 2001, the second period lasts from 2002 to 2007, and the third period runs from 2008 to 2013 [24]. The number of deaths according to age group, represented by the histogram displayed in Fig. 3, reflects the observations for the three different time periods to detect the age group with the most number of deaths. It shows an exponential growth in the number of deaths up to the group of 75-year-old to 79-year-old people for the first time period and up to the group of 80-year-old to 84-year-old people for the second and also the third period. Regarding old age mortality, negative linear trends in frequencies are demonstrated.

The median standardised mortality rate was set at the 75-year-old to 79-year-old age group, representing 50% of deaths above this age group. In relation to the advanced age of death, it can be supposed that the background or origin of cerebrovascular diseases is chronic in many cases of death. The interquartile range lies between the 65-year-old to 69-year-old and 80-year-old to 84-year-old age groups, representing the age characteristics of half of the deaths in the period from 1996 to 2001. From 2002 to 2013, the first quartile transitioned to the 70-year-old to 74-year-old age group and the third quartile did not change, and thus a 50% share of deaths was narrowed down to the age group of 70-year-old to 84-year-old people.

The results reveal a decreased level of premature mortality for cerebrovascular diseases, which was typically represented by deaths up to the 75th year of age [25]. This finding may be partly related to the ageing of the Slovak population as well as to an increase in life expectancy at birth from 77.5 years in 2000 to 79.9 years in 2012. Therefore, in the following analysis, the values of the

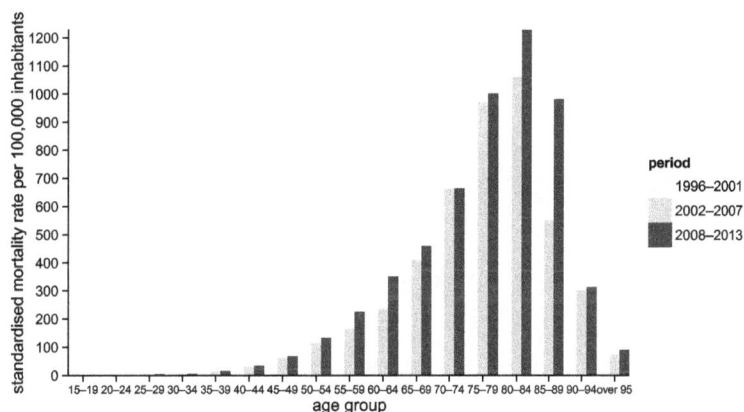

Fig. 3 Standardised mortality rate per 100,000 inhabitants for cerebrovascular diseases according to the age groups and the time period in the Slovak Republic from 1996 to 2013

standardised mortality rate are considered to eliminate bias. For a deeper analysis of the mortality caused by cerebrovascular diseases in the Slovak Republic, it was desirable to examine regional differences based on sex and using a long-term approach.

Regional differences in the development of standardised mortality rate for cerebrovascular diseases in the Slovak Republic

Based on the Nomenclature of Units for Territorial Statistics geocode standard, the Slovak Republic is divided into 8 geographic regions: the Banská Bystrica Region, the Bratislava Region, the Košice Region, the Nitra Region, the Prešov Region, the Trencín Region, the Trnava Region, and the Žilina Region.

As seen in Table 1, in terms of the individual regions of the Slovak Republic for men, the standardised mortality rates range from 143.42 per 100,000 inhabitants in the Prešov Region to 288.73 per 100,000 inhabitants in the Banská Bystrica Region between 1996 and 2001; they further vary from 108.57 per 100,000 inhabitants in the Bratislava Region to 237.10 per 100,000 inhabitants in the Nitra Region in the period from 2002 to 2007, and finally from 113.05 per 100,000 inhabitants in the Žilina Region to 241.8 per 100,000 inhabitants in the Nitra Region during the last period from 2008 to 2013.

Table 2 reflects the descriptive statistics of standardised mortality rate in each time period. Throughout the entire explored time span, the median standardised mortality rate for men increased from 197.70 per 100,000 inhabitants to 205.15 per 100,000 inhabitants, representing a deterioration in mortality accompanied by considerable period-over-period increases in the Prešov Region, at levels of 5.39% and 33.84%; in the Košice Region, at levels of 11.18% and 0.82%; and in the Nitra Region, at levels

Table 2 Descriptive statistics of standardised mortality rates for cerebrovascular diseases for men in the Slovak Republic

Indicator	1996–2001	2002–2007	2008–2013
Minimum	143.42	108.57	113.05
Maximum	288.73	237.10	241.80
Median	197.70	199.71	205.15
Mean	206.24	188.82	197.54
Standard deviation	45.47	41.71	37.43
Coefficient of variation	22.05	22.09	18.95

Source: based on own elaboration by the authors

of 0.20% and 1.98% between each two successive periods, respectively, as seen in Table 1. In all three time periods, the Banská Bystrica Region, the Nitra Region, and the Trnava Region had a standardised mortality rate above the median for men, while the Bratislava Region and the Žilina Region consistently showed values lower than the median. Although the standardised mortality rate attained in the Banská Bystrica Region was high, this region also showed the greatest progress in improving mortality results. The reduced variability in standardised mortality rate for cerebrovascular diseases was confirmed by the values of standard deviation as well as the coefficient of variation, which recorded a downward trend throughout the entire time span, as displayed in Table 2. As for the variability of each region, the highest value was achieved in the Bratislava Region, at a level of 26.21. The lowest value, 14.90, was observed in the Žilina Region. Although the Bratislava Region could be considered the best in terms of mortality, the variability results showed quite high volatility in positive results in this region.

The standardised mortality rate was an average of 33% lower for women than for men. During the period

Table 1 Standardised mortality rate per 100,000 inhabitants for cerebrovascular diseases for men in the regions of the Slovak Republic according to the time periods

Region	1996–2001		2002–2007			2008–2013			Coefficient of variation
	SMR	Rank	SMR	Rank	Change	SMR	Rank	Change	
BC	288.73	8th	218.83	7th	−24.21%	208.01	5th	−4.94%	20.58
BL	170.40	2nd	108.57	1st	−36.29%	113.05	1st	4.13%	26.21
KI	187.03	4th	207.93	5th	11.18%	209.64	6th	0.82%	22.71
NI	236.62	7th	237.10	8th	0.20%	241.80	8th	1.98%	15.90
PV	143.42	1st	151.15	2nd	5.39%	202.30	4th	33.84%	24.99
TA	231.51	6th	214.40	6th	−7.39%	217.46	7th	1.43%	15.30
TC	208.38	5th	191.49	4th	−8.10%	192.04	2nd	0.29%	16.50
ZI	183.84	3rd	181.14	3rd	−1.47%	196.01	3rd	8.21%	14.90

Legend: *SMR* standardised mortality rate, *BC* the Banská Bystrica Region, *BL* the Bratislava Region, *KI* the Košice Region, *NI* the Nitra Region, *PV* the Prešov Region, *TA* the Trnava Region, *TC* the Trencín Region, *ZI* the Žilina Region
Note: Change is computed as period-over-period change
Source: based on own elaboration by the authors

from 1996 to 2001, its values for women range from 110.44 per 100,000 inhabitants in the Prešov Region to 227.15 per 100,000 inhabitants in the Banská Bystrica Region. From 2002 to 2007, the minimum value increased only to 83.79 per 100,000 inhabitants in the Bratislava Region. Conversely, the maximum value peaks at a level of 183.33 per 100,000 inhabitants in the Nitra Region. In the period from 2008 to 2013, the Bratislava Region with a value of 89.78 per 100,000 inhabitants remained the best, compared with the Nitra Region at a level of 183.33 per 100,000 inhabitants, representing the worst mortality rate of all regions. According to Table 3, the percentage changes in the standardised mortality rate for women expose relatively large differences between the regions. In the period from 2002 to 2007, a majority of the regions recorded a decline in percentage compared with the period from 1996 to 2001. The highest percentage decreases were recorded in the Bratislava Region, at a value of 34.64%; in the Banská Bystrica Region, with a value of 29.94%; and in the Trencín Region, with a value of 17.44%.

Similarly as seen in Table 4, the median standardised mortality rate falls from 153.41 per 100,000 inhabitants to 142.90 per 100,000 inhabitants. In the last time period, the median increases to 151.63 per 100,000 inhabitants. This trend was accompanied by an increase in the growth rate of standardised mortality rate in all regions except for the Košice and Nitra Regions. However, the most growth occurred in the Prešov Region, at a level of 34.10%. The Nitra Region showed no change in growth rate, although it increased during the entire examined time span in the Košice Region as well as in the Prešov Region. The Banská Bystrica Region, Nitra Region, and Trnava Region had a standardised mortality rate above the median, while the Bratislava Region and the Žilina Region consistently

Table 4 Descriptive statistics of standardised mortality rates for cerebrovascular diseases for women in the Slovak Republic

Indicator	1996–2001	2002–2007	2008–2013
Minimum	110.44	83.79	89.78
Maximum	227.15	183.33	183.33
Median	153.41	142.90	151.63
Mean	156.25	140.17	150.36
Standard deviation	36.07	30.93	28.16
Coefficient of variation	23.08	22.07	18.73

Source: based on own elaboration by the authors

showed values lower than the median throughout the whole time span. The standard deviation as well as the coefficient of variation showed a downward trend. As for women, the rates of variability gained the highest values in the Prešov Region, at a level of 25.87, and in the Bratislava Region, at a level of 25.69. On the contrary, the lowest values are found in the Trnava Region, at a value of 14.12, and in the Žilina Region, reaching a value of 15.33.

To clearly show the regional disparities, Figs. 4 and 5 represent the status of the Slovak regions in terms of their average standardised mortality rates for cerebrovascular diseases during the whole time span, both for men and women. The worst values were observed in the southern regions – namely, the Nitra Region and the Banská Bystrica Region. In contrast, better results were associated with northern Slovakia – the Žilina Region and the Prešov Region – and the most favourable standardised mortality rate for cerebrovascular diseases occurred in the Bratislava Region. It is remarkable to observe the northern regions with lower standardised mortality rates and the southern regions with higher standardised mortality rates. These differences likely relate to the risk factors, the

Table 3 Standardised mortality rate per 100,000 inhabitants for cerebrovascular diseases for women in the regions of the Slovak Republic according to the time periods

Region	1996–2001		2002–2007			2008–2013			Coefficient of variation
	SMR	Rank	SMR	Rank	Change	SMR	Rank	Change	
BC	227.15	8th	159.14	6th	−29.94%	167.45	6th	5.22%	21.38
BL	128.20	2nd	83.79	1st	−34.64%	89.78	1st	7,16%	25.69
KI	141.56	4th	149.35	5th	5.51%	150.54	4th	0.79%	22.05
NI	171.61	7th	183.33	8th	6.83%	183.33	8th	0%	17.91
PV	110.44	1st	113.88	2nd	3.11%	152.71	5th	34.10%	25.87
TA	170.73	6th	161.75	7th	−5.26%	170.67	7nd	5.51%	14.12
TC	165.27	5th	136.44	4th	−17.44%	146.02	3th	7.02%	16.69
ZI	135.01	3rd	133.69	3rd	−0.98%	142.38	2rd	6.50%	15.33

Legend: *SMR* standardised mortality rate, *BC* the Banská Bystrica Region, *BL* the Bratislava Region, *KI* the Košice Region, *NI* the Nitra Region, *PV* the Prešov Region, *TA* the Trnava Region, *TC* the Trencín Region, *ZI* the Žilina Region
Note: Change is computed as period-over-period change
Source: based on own elaboration by the authors

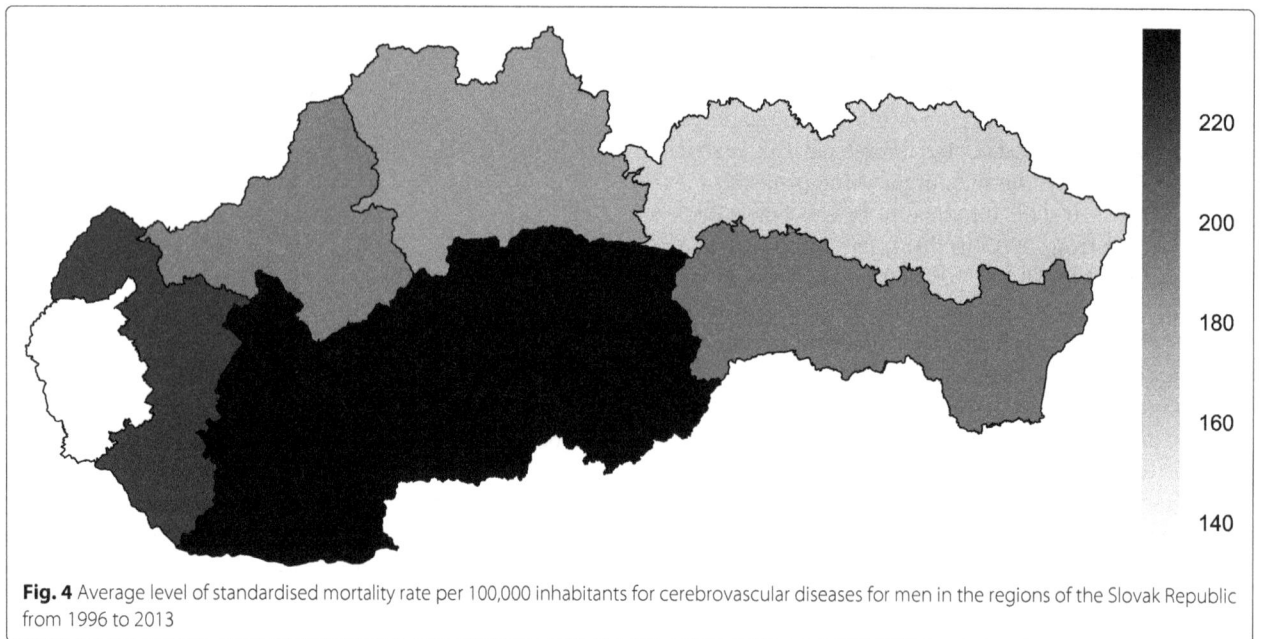

Fig. 4 Average level of standardised mortality rate per 100,000 inhabitants for cerebrovascular diseases for men in the regions of the Slovak Republic from 1996 to 2013

socio-economic indicators and the environmental factors influencing cerebrovascular diseases in these individual regions.

Regression analysis

The examined models are presented in Table 5. Fitted coefficients and p-values are displayed for each variable involved in the particular model.

The following Table 6 demonstrates the quantified standardised beta coefficients for the explanatory variables of the regression models.

The subsequent Table 7 visualises significance of the quantified variables involved in the regression models in form of p-value.

The first model series represents a model set expressing the standardised mortality rate by all the variables except for the constant value. The first two models – M_1 and M_2 – were part of this series. In the first step, the poverty indicator was deleted from the modelling process as the variable with the worst p-value. The best model in this series was represented by the second model, M_2.

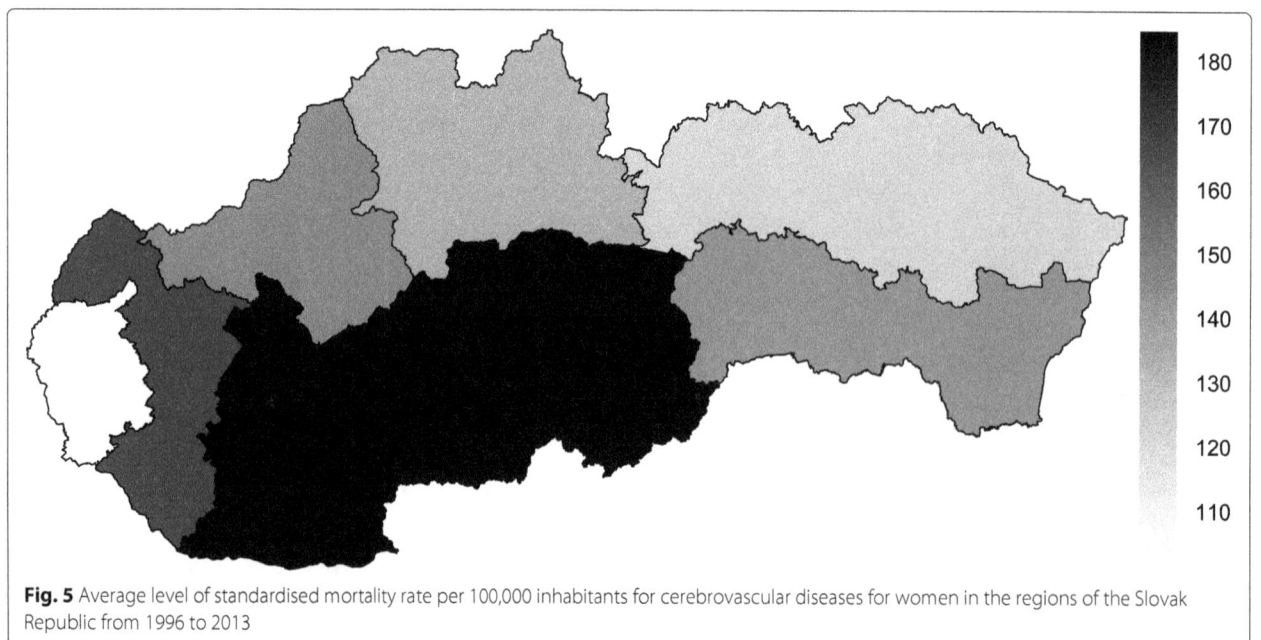

Fig. 5 Average level of standardised mortality rate per 100,000 inhabitants for cerebrovascular diseases for women in the regions of the Slovak Republic from 1996 to 2013

Table 5 Beta coefficients

Coefficient	M_1	M_2	M_3	M_4
β_0			−410.606	−594.3626
UR	0.0659	0.0587	0.2213	0.0551
I	0.0819	0.0134	0.8793	
P	0.2529		0.68	0.0279
GC	0.0206	0.0042	0.3616	0.0315
IQR	0.0113	0.0034	0.4439	0.0269
SB	0.0784	0.0659	0.2365	0.0654

Source: based on own elaboration by the authors

Table 7 Significance of variables

Variable	M_1	M_2	M_3	M_4
β_0			0.7488	0.072
UR	0.0659	0.0587	0.2213	0.0551
I	0.0819	0.0134	0.8793	
P	0.2529		0.68	0.0279
GC	0.0206	0.0042	0.3616	0.0315
IQR	0.0113	0.0034	0.4439	0.0269
SB	0.0784	0.0659	0.2365	0.0654

Source: based on own elaboration by the authors

The M_2 model explained the standardised mortality rate as follows:

$$M_2 = -1.9361UR - 3.8777I + 6.5488GC - 5.5587IQR + 1.3006SB$$

(2)

The coefficient of determination of this model reached a value of 0.9557, and although the adjusted coefficient of determination declined to 0.3584, the dataset can be considered well fitted by the model M_2. The model's p-value for F statistics was 0.0311. The choice of the second model M_2 was also confirmed by the bayesian information criterion, which reached −5.10 in the model M_2, whereas the corresponding value for the first model M_1 was −2.97. The Akaike information criterion further confirmed this situation, as its value for the first model M_1 was 297.13 and was 240.41 for the second model M_2. Moreover, all the included variables fulfilled at least the ten-percent significance level with only two dimensions – unemployment rate and social benefits – slightly overstepping the five-percent significance level. The Gini coefficient had the largest impact on mortality rate, with a beta coefficient reaching 6.5488. The income quintile share ratio had the next largest effect, with a value of −5.5587, followed by income with a value of 3.8777, unemployment rate with a value of −1.9361 and finally social benefits with a value of 1.3006.

Table 6 Standardised beta coeffcients

Variable	M_1	M_2	M_3	M_4
β_0			2.2240×10^{-15}	2.6543×10^{-15}
UR	−2.1068	−1.9361	−2.1068	−2.1489
I	−1.0149	−3.8777	−1.0149	
P	1.7317		1.7317	2.3268
GC	9.8444	6.5488	9.8444	10.927
IQR	−10.1619	−5.5587	−10.162	−11.709
SB	1.3940	1.3006	1.3940	1.4170

Source: based on own elaboration by the authors

The second model series was based on the previous one with only one alternation – a constant value in the form of the intercept was added. In the first step, income was removed from the modelling process because its p-value was the highest of all the involved variables. The second model of the series was again the best, although it cannot be taken into consideration, because only the correct constant value would remain in the successive step of the modelling process.

$$M_4 = 2.6543 \times 10^{-15} - 2.1489UR + 2.3268P + 10.927GC - 11.709IQR + 1.4170SB$$

(3)

Model M_4 fits the dataset well; this was confirmed by the coefficient of determination, which reached a value of 0.9824, and its adjusted version, showing a value of 0.2456. The model itself fulfilled the five-percent significance level, with a p-value for F statistics of 0.0433. Therefore, continuing this modelling process was pointless. The bayesian information criterion expressed the same result – the value for the third model M_3 was −0.55, whereas it was −2.97 for the fourth model M_4. The Akaike information criterion further confirmed this situation – the third model M_3 had a value of 231.50 and the fourth model M_4 a value of 231.00.

Discussion

The variability of the standardised mortality rate gradually declined during the given time periods. The worst standardised mortality rates were recorded in the Banská Bystrica Region as well as in the Nitra Region, and the best value was recorded in the Bratislava Region throughout the explored time span. The standardised mortality rate values were lower in the northern part of the Slovak Republic compared with the southern part of the country. However, the Bratislava Region and also the Prešov Region showed the highest variability in standardised mortality rate. In contrast, the lowest variability was typical for the Žilina Region and the Trnava Region. Although the Bratislava Region was considered the best in terms of mortality rate, the variability results in this region demonstrated high volatility in positive results. However, the Žilina Region showed a high level of stability of positive results regarding mortality rate. As for men, only the Banská Bystrica Region showed a permanent percentage drop in standardised mortality rate between the observed time periods, while the opposite tendency was indicated in the Košice Region, the Nitra Region, and in the Prešov Region. The other regions demonstrated a volatile development rate. As for women, a permanent percent increase in standardised mortality rate was observed in the Košice Region and Prešov Region.

The regression analysis revealed several dimensions that had an impact on standardised mortality rate. Of all the examined variables, unemployment rate, household disposable income and income quintile ratio had a negative impact, helping to reduce the mortality rate. However, at-risk-of-poverty status, Gini coefficient and social benefits positively influenced mortality rate. All these dimensions appeared statistically significant and reliably described the standardised mortality rate.

From the perspective of the indicators examined in this study, mortality rate can be described by unemployment rate, household disposable income, share of at-risk-of-poverty population, Gini coefficient, income quintile ratio, and social benefits. This finding was statistically confirmed. The factor with the largest influence was income quintile ratio, which had the highest beta coefficient in the model M_4 that can be regarded as being the most meaningful model than others, since the second model series - the models M_3 and M_4 - contains the intercept β_0. Based on this finding, we suggest considering income quintile ratio within the Slovak population when arranging out-of-pocket payments to ensure that low-income groups are not at risk due to high payments for delivered health care.

Slovak men recorded higher values of standardised mortality rate by nearly 33% compared with women. However, an average decline of 24% in standardised mortality rate was observed for both sexes from 1996 to 2013. The reason for the sharp increase in mortality from 2006 to 2008 is described in a study by Hlavatý and Liptáková [26]. They revealed that in 2005 and 2006, the absolute number of deaths for cerebrovascular diseases, marked as $I60$ to $I69$ according to the World Health Organization's International Statistical Classification of Diseases, was undervalued by 50% in favour of deaths for hypertension, which were marked as $I10$ to $I15$, due to an incorrect coding of the causes of death in statistical processing. After 2006, the National Health Information Centre conducted a revision of the coding, leading to a sharp increase in deaths from cerebrovascular diseases. Since

2007, all causes of deaths have been coded according to international recommendations by Eurostat and the World Health Organization documented in the Manual on the certification of causes of death in Europe [27]. The greatest difference between men and women occurred in 2007, while the smallest gap was revealed in 2013. The incidence of mortality for cerebrovascular diseases has shifted to higher ages over the years. People at the highest risk were in the age group of 70 to 84 years from 1996 to 2001 and from 75 to 84 years from 2002 to 2013.

A limitation of this study is the lack of availability of data on individual income level in the mortality database, and thus summary measures for income indicators in each region were applied.

The variability in mortality rate development in each year shows that the development of mortality should also be examined in terms of regional disparities to reflect the factors strongly contributing to the development in mortality rate in individual regions [28, 29]. By mapping regional disparities, prevention programmes and other interventions that could regulate mortality in individual regions can be effectively established. By implementing active prevention programmes targeted to selected population groups as well as to particular regions, mortality and morbidity can be actively controlled, and these programs also contribute to increase the effectiveness of the health system [30, 31].

Many educational activities devoted to prevention programmes for cerebrovascular disease risk factors are clearly priorities of the health policy in the Slovak Republic, namely the Monika project [32], the Cindi project [33], the National Programme of Prevention Heart Conditions in Adults [34], and the National Action Plan for the prevention of obesity for the years 2015–2025 [35]. Their aim is to ensure effective long-term education of the population at all societal levels.

As for international comparisons, the standardised mortality rate for cerebrovascular diseases in the Slovak population showed alarming values in comparison with the entire European Union average. Many studies [36–38] have shown that there is a diversity of health policy approaches to reducing the incidence of risk factors affecting cerebrovascular diseases, such as unhealthy lifestyles, smoking, and obesity as well as lower access to health care associated with the population's socio-economic status.

Carefully prepared mortality analyses can provide a valuable platform for developing the methodology of avoidable mortality, which currently is solely dependent on the health systems of interest to its creators [24, 39, 40]. The results of the available methodologies of avoidable mortality [41] warrant caution in their interpretation because each one has a specific methodology and inclusion or exclusion diagnoses. According to many authors

[8, 42, 43], mortality provides a reliable picture of public health and is also the most objective way of measuring health.

Conclusion

To conclude, at the present time, the mortality rate for cerebrovascular diseases has decreased in many European Union countries as well as in Slovakia.

Mortality is characterised by a relatively large amount of inertia in its development, and therefore, it is not expected that the described differences between the Slovak Republic population and that of the other European countries will be diminished in the next few years. In our study, we present an evaluation of the development of mortality rates for cerebrovascular diseases in the Slovak Republic. In addition, our objective was to quantify the regional disparities and to analyse the development of the mortality rate in relation to income inequalities in the individual regions of the Slovak Republic. Income quintile ratio appears to be the most influencing dimension in these models of standardised mortality rate. Considering the process of demographic ageing as well as the increase in the number of older people in the European Union and worldwide, responsibility for health should be prioritised.

Acknowledgements

This paper was created within the project supported by the Scientific Grant Agency of the Ministry of Education, Science, Research and Sport of the Slovak Republic 1/0986/15 Proposal of the dimensional models of the management effectiveness of ICT and information systems in health facilities in Slovakia and the economic-financial quantification of their effects on the health system in Slovakia.
Our thanks go out to the National Health Information Centre of the Slovak Republic for providing access to the central mortality database for the explored period as well as the other studied data along with the Statistical Office of the Slovak Republic.
Our acknowledgments also belong to the Ministry of Health of the Slovak Republic for its cooperation in creation of the new conceptions and methodologies and for its support of our research activities.

Authors' contributions

BG participated in the sequence alignment and drafted the manuscript. VK participated in the design of the study and performed the statistical analysis. TV participated in the statistical analysis and carried out the epidemiology overview. All authors read and approved the final manuscript.

Competing interests

The authors declare that they have no competing interests.

References

1. Dahlgren G, Whitehead M. Policies and strategies to promote social equity in health. Arbetsrapport – Institutet för Framtidsstudier. 2007;14:1–69. http://www.iffs.se/en/publications/working-papers/policies-and-strategies-to-promote-social-equity-in-health/.

2. Carreras M, García-Goni M, Ibern P, Coderch J, Vall-Llosera L, Inoriza JM. Estimates of patient costs related with population morbidity: can indirect costs affect the results? Eur J Health Econ. 2011;12(4):289–95. doi:10.1007/s10198-010-0227-5.

3. Šimrová J, Barták M, Vojtíšek R, Rogalewicz V. The costs and reimbursements for lung cancer treatment among selected health care providers in the Czech Republic. E+M Ekonomie a Manage. 2014;17(3):74–86. doi:10.15240/tul/001/2014-3-007.

4. Mohelska H, Maresova P, Valis M, Kuca K. Alzheimer's disease and its treatment costs: case study in the Czech Republic. Neuropsychiatr Dis Treat. 2015;11:2349–54. doi:10.2147/NDT.S87503.

5. Health Statistics Yearbook of the Slovak Republic 2013. Bratislava: National Health Information Center; 2015. http://www.nczisk.sk/Documents/rocenky/rocenka_2013.pdf.

6. Truelsen T, Begg S, Mathers C. The global burden of cerebrovascular disease 2000. Cerebrovascular disease 21-06-06. http://www.who.int/healthinfo/statistics/bod_cerebrovasculardiseasestroke.pdf.

7. Clarke P, Latham K. Life course health and socioeconomic profiles of Americans aging with disability. Disabil Health J. 2014;7(1):15–23. doi:10.1016/j.dhjo.2013.08.008.

8. Kinge JM, Morris S. Variation in the relationship between BMI and survival by socioeconomic status in Great Britain. Econ Hum Biol. 2014;12:67–82. doi:10.1016/j.ehb.2013.05.006.

9. Page A, Lane A, Taylor R, Dobson A. Trends in socioeconomic inequalities in mortality from ischaemic heart disease and stroke in Australia, 1979–2006. Eur J Prev Cardiol. 2012;19(6):1281–9. doi:10.1177/1741826711427505.

10. Easton JD, Saver JL, Albers GW, Alberts MJ, Chaturvedi S, Feldmann E, Hatsukami TS, Higashida RT, Johnston SC, Kidwell CS, Lutsep HL, Miller E, Sacco RL. Definition and evaluation of transient ischemic attack: a scientific statement for healthcare professionals from the American Heart Association/American Stroke Association Stroke Council; Council on Cardiovascular Surgery and Anesthesia; Council on Cardiovascular Radiology and Intervention; Council on Cardiovascular Nursing; and the Interdisciplinary Council on Peripheral Vascular Disease, The American Academy of Neurology affirms the value of this statement as an educational tool for neurologists. Stroke. 2009;40(6):2276–93. doi:10.1161/STROKEAHA.108.192218.

11. Levi F, Lucchini F, Negri E, Vecchia CL. Trends in mortality from cardiovascular and cerebrovascular diseases in Europe and other areas of the world. Heart. 2002;88(2):119–24.

12. Bella SD, Sarti S, Lucchini M, Bordogna MT. A comparative analysis of inequality in health across Europe. Sociol Res Online. 2011;16(4). doi:10.5153/sro.2492.

13. Palmer JR, Boggs DA, Wise LA, Adams-Campbell LL, Rosenberg L. Individual and neighborhood socioeconomic status in relation to breast cancer incidence in African-American women. Eur J Prev Cardiol. 2012;176(12):1141–6. doi:10.1093/aje/kws211.

14. Morgan SD, Redman S, D'Este C, Rogers K. Knowledge, satisfaction with information, decisional conflict and psychological morbidity amongst women diagnosed with ductal carcinoma in situ (DCIS). Patient Educ Couns. 2011;84(1):62–8. doi:10.1016/j.pec.2010.07.002.

15. Soltes M, Radonak J. A risk score to predict the difficulty of elective laparoscopic cholecystectomy. Videosurgery Miniinvasive Tech. 2014;9(4):608–12. doi:10.5114/wiitm.2014.47642.

16. Buzink S, Soltes M, Radonak J, Fingerhut A, Hanna G, Jakimowicz J. Laparoscopic surgical skills programme: preliminary evaluation of grade i level 1 courses by trainees. Videosurgery Miniinvasive Tech. 2012;7(3):188–92. doi:10.5114/wiitm.2011.28895.

17. Poelman MM, van den Heuvel B, Deelder JD, Abis GSA, Beudeker N, Bittner RR, Campanelli G, van Dam D, Dwars BJ, Eker HH, Fingerhut A, Khatkov I, Koeckerling F, Kukleta JF, Miserez M, Montgomery A, Brands RMM, Conde SM, Muysoms FE, Soltes M, Tromp W, Yavuz Y, Bonjer HJ. Eaes consensus development conference on endoscopic repair of groin hernias. Surg Endosc Interv Tech. 2013;27(10):3505–19. doi:10.1007/s00464-013-3001-9.

18. Zavadil M, Rogalewicz V, Kotlanova S. PHP325 – development of hospital-based HTA unit processes in the Czech hospital environment. Value Health. 2015;18(7):570. doi:10.1016/j.jval.2015.09.1879.

19. Škampová V, Rogalewicz V, Celedová L, Cevela R. Ambulatory geriatrics in the Czech Republic: A survey of geriatricians' opinions. Kontakt. 2014;16(2):119–31. doi:10.1016/j.kontakt.2014.04.002.

20. Maresova P, Mohelska H, Dolejs J, Kuca K. Socio-economic aspects of alzheimer's disease. Curr Alzheimer Res. 2015;12(9):903–11.

21. Organisation for Economic Co-operation and Development. Health at a glance: Europe 2014. 2014. doi:10.1787/23056088.

22. Regulation (EC) No 1338/2008 of the European Parliament and of the Council of 16 December 2008 on Community statistics on public health and health and safety at work (Text with EEA relevance). OJ. 2008;L 354: 70–81. http://eur-lex.europa.eu/legal-content/EN/TXT/PDF/?uri=CELEX: 32008R1338&from=EN.

23. Commission Regulation (EU) No 328/2011 of 5 April 2011 implementing Regulation (EC) No 1338/2008 of the European Parliament and of the Council on Community statistics on public health and health and safety at work, as regards statistics on causes of death (Text with EEA relevance). OJ. 2011;L 90:22–24. http://eur-lex.europa.eu/legal-content/EN/TXT/PDF/?uri=CELEX:32011R0328&from=EN.

24. Mészáros J, Burcin B. Vývoj odvrátitelnej úmrtnosti na Slovensku. Slovenská štatistika a demografia. 2008;18(2–3):24–39.

25. Gay JG, Paris V, Devaux M, de Looper M. Mortality amenable to health care in 31 OECD countries estimates and methodological issues. Organisation Econ Co-operation Development Health Working Papers. 2011;55:1–39.

26. Hlavatý T, Liptáková A. Správa o stave zdravotníctva na Slovensku. Bratislava: Ministry of Health of the Slovak Republic; 2011. http://www.health.gov.sk/Clanok?sprava-o-stave-zdravotnictva-na-slovensku.

27. Project "Preparation of an EU training package on certification of causes of Death" EUROSTAT - ISTAT Contract N° 200235100007, Manual on certification of causes of death in Europe. Rome: Italian National Institute of Statistics; 2003. http://www.moh.gov.cy/MOH/MOH.nsf/0/9CE89CE81E91903EC22579C600266A75/$file/Manual%20on%20certification%20of%20causes%20of%20death%20in%20Europe.pdf.

28. Turrell G, Hewitt B, Haynes M, Nathan A, Corti BG. Change in walking for transport: a longitudinal study of the influence of neighbourhood disadvantage and individual-level socioeconomic position in mid-aged adults. Int J Behav Nutr Phys Act. 2014;11(151). doi:10.1186/s12966-014-0151-7.

29. Šoltés V, Gavurová B. The functionality comparison of the health care systems by the analytical hierarchy process method. E+M Ekonomie a Manag. 2014;17(3):100–17. doi:10.15240/tul/001/2014-3-009.

30. Šoltés V, Gavurová B. The possibilities of day surgery system development within the health policy in Slovakia. Health Econ Rev. 2014;4:1–12. doi:10.1186/s13561-014-0035-1.

31. Šoltés M, Gavurová B. Identification of the functionality level of day surgery in Slovakia. Ekonomický Casopis. 2014;62(10):1031–51.

32. Baráková A, Avdičová M, Čorňák V, Hraška V. Vybrané informácie zo zdravotníckej štatistiky o vývoji ochorení obehovej sústavy v SR. Projekt MONIKA. Bratislava: Public Health Office of the Slovak Republic, National Health Information Center; 1999.

33. Avdičová M, Egnerová A, Hrubá F. Prevalence of risk factors of cardiovascular diseases: results of the CINDI screening. Banská Bystrica: State Institute of Public Health of the Slovak Republic; 2000.

34. Kamenský G, Murín J. Kardiovaskulárne ochorenia – najväčšia hrozba. Bratislava: AEPress; 2009.

35. Národný akčný plán v prevencii obezity na roky 2015–2025. Bratislava: Public Health Authority of the Slovak Republic; 2015. http://www.uvzsr.sk/docs/info/podpora/NAPPO_2015-2025.pdf.

36. Dragano N, Bobak M, Wege N, Peasey A, Verde PE, Kubinova R, Weyers S, Moebus S, Möhlenkamp S, Stang A, Erbel R, Jöckel KH, Siegrist J, Pikhart H. Neighbourhood socioeconomic status and cardiovascular risk factors: a multilevel analysis of nine cities in the Czech Republic and Germany. BMC Publ Health. 2007;7:255. doi:10.1186/1471-2458-7-255.

37. Behanova M, Katreniakova Z, Nagyova I, van Ameijden EJC, Dijkshoorn H, van Dijk JP, Reijneveld SA. The effect of neighbourhood unemployment on health-risk behaviours in elderly differs between Slovak and Dutch cities. Eur J Public Health. 2015;25(1):108–14. doi:10.1093/eurpub/cku116.

38. Wojtyniak B, Jankowski K, Zdrojewski T, Opolski G. Regional differences in determining cardiovascular diseases as the cause of death in Poland: time for change. Kardiologia Polska. 2012;70(7):695–701.

39. Newey C, Nolte E, McKee M, Mossialos E. Avoidable mortality in the enlarged European Union. 2004. https://www.researchgate.net/publication/228988065_Avoidable_Mortality_in_the_Enlarged_European_Union.

40. Davila-Cervantes CA, Agudelo-Botero M. Avoidable mortality in Mexico and its contribution to years of life lost. Analysis by degree of state marginalization. Papeles de Poblacion. 2014;20(82):267–86.

41. Gavurová B, Vagašová T. Meranie efektívnosti zdravotnej starostlivosti v krajinách EÚ konceptom liecitelnej úmrtnosti. eXclusive J. 2014;2(3):50–62.

42. Kalwij A. An empirical analysis of the importance of controlling for unobserved heterogeneity when estimating the income-mortality gradient. Demograph Res. 2014;31(30):913–39. doi:10.4054/DemRes.2014.31.30.

43. Niu G, Melenberg B. Trends in mortality decrease and economic growth. Demography. 2014;51:1755–73. doi:10.1007/s13524-014-0328-3.

15

Convergence and determinants of health expenditures in OECD countries

Son Hong Nghiem[1]* ⓘ and Luke Brian Connelly[2]

Abstract

This study examines the trend and determinants of health expenditures in OECD countries over the 1975-2004 period. Based on recent developments in the economic growth literature we propose and test the hypothesis that health care expenditures in countries of similar economic development level may converge. We hypothesise that the main drivers for growth in health care costs include: aging population, technological progress and health insurance. The results reveal no evidence that health expenditures among OECD countries converge. Nevertheless, there is evidence of convergence among three sub-groups of countries. We found that the main driver of health expenditure is technological progress. Our results also suggest that health care is a (national) necessity, not a luxury good as some other studies in this field have found.

Keywords: Health expenditure, Convergence, OECD countries

Background

Rising real per capita incomes, technological innovation and ubiquitous insurance against medical treatment and the ageing of the population are generally considered to exert important influences on the growth of health expenditures. The causal inter-relationships between these factors, though, are complex. Despite common perceptions, the bulk of health expenditure growth is not due to population ageing *per se* [19, 49], but the growth in demand for new medical technologies (MTs) that improve and/or extend life as real per capita incomes grow [15, 20, 49, 71, 73]. Yet the foregoing statement—while true—is also deceptively simplistic. First, since shares of GDP not only reflect expenditures but income, it is true not only to say that national income drives health expenditures, but also that health expenditures drive national income growth. The link between health *per se* and growth and health and productivity has been explored by a number of

authors (Narayan et al. [45] provide an overview; also see Pradhan [59]). Second, the distinction between age-related and technology-related sources of health expenditure growth is likely to be—at least in part—a false distinction. The demand for technological innovation in the health sector will increase not only with income, but also with needs, many of which are correlated with ageing. Finally, there is also some recent and somewhat contradictory evidence from the US [7] that the health sector suffers from Baumol's [9] "cost disease". Specifically, this empirical work suggests that the health sector is a "non-progressive" sector of the economy, being characterised as labour-intensive and relatively devoid of innovations that enhance labour productivity. The latter results are curious and probably have more to do with measurement problems than, as the authors suggest "... relatively constant productivity and stagnant technology..." (Bates & Santerre [7], p. 386). Yet, in addition to the obvious microeconomic and econometric issues that are still to be resolved in respect of the drivers of health expenditure, there are also some important macroeconomic dimensions of health expenditure growth that are yet to be explored. The purpose of this paper is to use recent developments in the economic growth literature to address the question of whether or not health expenditure growth across nations tends to converge over time. This question is of interest because if the rate of health expenditure

---

*Correspondence: hongson.nghiem@gmail.com; son.nghiem@qut.edu.au
[1]The Australian Research Centre for Health Services Innovation, Institute of Health and Biomedical Innovation, School of Public Health and Social Work, Queensland University of Technology, Kelvin Grove, Brisbane QLD 4059, Australia
Full list of author information is available at the end of the article

growth for countries does converge over time, this effect may attenuate (or exacerbate) the rates of growth that might otherwise be estimated and predicted from microeconometric work on this topic. Clearly, if such a phenomenon were at work, it may have important implications for public policy and planning with respect to the health sector. Health expenditures account for a large proportion of the Gross Domestic Products (GDP) in each of the Organization for Economic Cooperation and Development (OECD) countries and have grown considerably over the past few decades. For instance, the median health expenditure in the OECD increased from 3.8% in 1960 to 7.9% in 1990 [2]. Our observations from OECD health data in the 1975–2004 period also reveal that the growth of health expenditure per capita consistently exceeds the growth of GDP per capita. In addition, health expenditure growth is faster in more affluent countries, and the health sector accounts for a greater proportion of GDP in those countries. For example, the proportion of health expenditures in GDP of the United States– the richest country in the OECD– in 1960 and 1998 was 5.2 and 14.0%, respectively. The level of total health expenditure per capita (measured in purchasing power parity) of the United States also consistently among the highest in the OECD for the period 1975–2004.

Common features of developed countries (e.g., aging population, technological advancement, high coverage of health insurance), all of which positively affect the cost of health care, lead us to form a hypothesis that health expenditure in countries of similar economic development level converge over time. To the best of our knowledge, only a limited number of previous studies, including Hitiris [36]; Barros [6]; Nixon [50]; Hitiris & Nixon [37]; Narayan [44]; Panopoulou & Pantelidis [53]; Lau et al. [41]; Pekkurnaz [55], have examined the convergence of health expenditure among OECD countries. However, the standard convergence tests in the economic growth literature (i.e., $\beta-$ and $\sigma-$convergences) applied in Barros [6] and Nixon [50] assume that all countries follow the same growth path. The unit root test procedure applied by Narayan [44] is more flexible but it was focused on structural breaks at the level (rather than on the growth) of health expenditure and accommodates no more than two breaks.

This study contributes to the literature by examining the convergence of the growth in health expenditure in OECD countries using the dynamic growth model by Phillips & Sul [58]. The advantage of this approach is that it allows individual countries to follow distinctive growth paths. In addition, we examine the determinants of health expenditure growth using panel data methods, which confer several further econometric advantages over some of the previous work on this topic.

A brief review of the literature

It is expected, based on the available literature, that technology will be the major determinant of health expenditure. Much of the existing literature on this topic, though, suffers from the use of econometric techniques—such as standard ordinary least-squares (OLS) regression—to analyse time-series data. This is now known to be problematic as, typically, health expenditure (HE) and GDP are cointegrated [27]. Modern time-series econometric techniques are able to overcome the possibly spurious results [76] that can be associated with regressing non-stationary cointegrated time-series. Given the statistical problems that beset the historical literature on this topic, it is interesting that research tends to confirm its long-standing and somewhat counter-intuitive result: technically (according to the standard economic definition), health care is a "luxury". Specifically, spending in the health sector tends to rise at a faster rate than national income. Indeed the "income elasticity of HE" (i.e., the percentage change in HE for a percentage change in GDP) usually well exceeds unity at the national level for the Organization for Economic Cooperation and Development (OECD) countries (see e.g., [17]). The most recent contribution to the applied literature [73] for example, estimates that the income elasticity of HE in the US over a 40-year period was approximately 1.388 to 1.445. The most recent results for Australia were based on OECD data from 1960 to 1997 and produced a similar point estimate of 1.47 (Clemente et al. [17], Table 2, p.598).

There are considerable differences in the size of the health sector among OECD countries: in 2010, HE comprised 6.9% of GDP in Mexico and 17.4% of GDP in the USA [39]. On a per capita basis too, the US is an outlier, with the US spending in more per capita than the mean of other high-income countries [19]. Given these differences and the remarkable heterogeneity of insurance arrangements, practitioner remuneration arrangements, regulatory controls and so forth, it is also astounding that the rate of growth of HE per capita has long been shown to be similar across the developing world (see, e.g. [17, 21, 48, 49]). This has led economists to question whether or not the rates of health expenditure growth across countries might tend to converge over time [6, 36, 51]. The most recent study in this genre [44] examined the health expenditure growth of six countries (not including Australia) for the period 1960–2000. It found that there was evidence of the convergence of per capita health expenditures of the UK, Canada, Japan, Switzerland and Spain to that of the USA.

The trends and determinants of health expenditure in developed countries have been widely examined and revealed that main determinants of health expenditure growth include: income growth [1, 6, 14, 30, 49], the ageing of the population [31, 43, 68], technological progress

[3, 15, 16, 52, 75], and the widespread availability of health insurance [13, 22, 24, 29, 57, 70]. Newhouse [48] is the most cited study examined the relationship between income and health expenditure. In particular, Newhouse [48] showed that GDP per capita explained more than 90 percent of the variations in health expenditure per capita in OECD countries, and hence health services belong to the group of "luxury" goods (i.e., income elasticity is greater than one). However, results of other studies were mixed: the income elasticity of health expenditure was found to be above one [63], around unity [67], or less than one [4]. Roberts [60] argued that possible reasons for different estimates of income elasticity of health expenditure include: model specifications (e.g., cross-sectional vs panel; and static vs dynamic); variable selections; and treatments for the unobserved heterogeneity across countries. Getzen [32] argued that the income elasticity of health care has the characteristics of a necessity goods at the individual and household levels and that of a luxury goods at national levels. The main reason for a lower income elasticity of health care at the individual level is due to the availability of health insurance. At the same time, insured consumption also then contributes to the rapid growth of health expenditure at the aggregate level [49]. Parkin et al. [54] suggested that purchasing power parity (PPP), instead of exchange rates, should be used to compare health spending and GDP per capita among nations. They also showed that the elasticity estimated varied considerably using different functional forms, some of which produced income elasticity estimates of less than one.

The convergence of health expenditure in developed countries have been examined in only a limited number of previous studies: Hitiris [36]; Barros [6]; Nixon [50]; Hitiris & Nixon [37]; Narayan [44]; Panopoulou & Pantelidis [53]; Lau et al. [41]; Pekkurnaz [55]. In the first study Hitiris [36] argued that convergence in economic development and standard of living among countries can lead to the convergence of health expenditure. However, the author found that health care spending and GDP per capita of European countries in the 1960–1990 period actually diverged (based on significant variations of these variables among countries).

Barros [6] found that cross-sectional dispersions in health spending decrease over time (i.e., evidence of σ−convergence) and negative correlation between the growth rate and the initial level of health spending (i.e., evidence of β− convergence). However, the characteristics of the health system (e.g., the availability of a gatekeeper, public reimbursement or public integrated system) were found to have no significant effects on either the growth or level of health expenditure. The share of public spending in total health expenditure (negative effects) and the proportion of the population over 65 years

of age (positive effects) significantly determined the *level* of health expenditure despite having no significant effect the *growth* of health spending.

Nixon [50] tested for the presence of σ−convergence (i.e., less variation in growth rates among countries over time) and β−convergence (i.e., countries with lower starting point grow at faster rates) in health expenditure among OECD countries in the 1960–1995 period. The author found that health expenditure of OECD countries indeed converged in the study period for both β− and σ− convergence measures. Similar findings were also obtained by Hitiris & Nixon [37] using data of EU member countries for the period of 1980–1995.

Narayan [44] applied the Lagrange multiplier unit root test procedure, which allows up to two structure breaks, to explore the stationarity of differences in health spending per capita of the United Kingdom, Canada, Japan, Switzerland, and Spain with the USA over the period 1960–2000. The author found significant evidence that health expenditures in the six countries converged. However, he did not find evidence of convergence when applying standard unit root tests with no structural breaks.

Panopoulou & Pantelidis [53] was the first study that applied the Phillips & Sul [58]'s approach to examine the convergence of health expenditure of 19 OECD countries in the period of 1972–2006. They found no evidence of overall convergence, which was mainly due to the faster growth of health expenditure in the USA. The authors also conducted a convergence test for five components of the health expenditure per capita: health expenditure per GDP, labour productivity, employment rate, activity rate, and the proportion of working age population. They found full convergence in employment rate, activity rate and the proportion of working age population but divergence in the proportion of health expenditure in GDP and labour productivity. The authors also applied the test on health outcomes, macroeconomic, demographic, and lifestyle indicators. Their results reveal that overall convergence only arose for selected factors, including the infant mortality rate (health outcomes), GDP per capita, inflation (macroeconomic indicators), the dependency ratio, the labour participation rate for females (demographic indicators), and alcohol consumption (lifestyle indicators). Although testing for the convergence of health expenditure determinants empirically has been useful investigations, we believe that theoretical foundations are required to link the convergence tests in these factors.

Lau et al. [41] applied a non-linear panel unit root test to examine the convergence of health expenditure among 14 EU countries during the 1970–2008 period. The authors did not find significant evidence that health expenditure in the selected EU countries converge, which is in contrast to the simpler β− and σ− convergence tests by Nixon [50] and Hitiris & Nixon [37]. Pekkurnaz [55] also applied a non-linear panel unit root test to investigate the convergence of health expenditure of 22 OECD countries in the 1980–2012 period. Similar to Lau et al. [41], the author could not reject the null hypothesis of a unit root in health expenditure, indicating no overall convergence. The findings from these studies highlight the importance of taking into account the non-linearity and dynamics in health expenditure.

In summary, there were only a limited number of previous studies that examined the convergence of health expenditures among developed countries. The test procedure in most previous studies included $\beta-$ and $\sigma-$ convergence which were based on restrictive assumptions that countries follow the same growth path due to, for example, having common technology, similar preference, policies and potential for growth. The unit root test approach applied by Narayan [44] was more flexible but it only allows up to two structural breaks in the form of dummy variables (i.e., level breaks). More recent studies include the dynamic convergence test by Panopoulou & Pantelidis [53] and non-linear panel unit root tests by Lau et al. [41] and Pekkurnaz [55] but they did not follow-up with analysis on determinants of health expenditure growth. This study contributes to the literature by applying a dynamic economic growth model proposed by Phillips & Sul [58] followed by panel analysis on factors determining the growth of health expenditure in OECD countries.

Methods
Economic growth and health care expenditure
Despite the extensive body of literature on health expenditure growth[1], very few studies have specified a specific theoretical model to test [60, 72]. This study discusses the inter-connectedness between health expenditure and economic development and applies a dynamic economic growth model to examine the sources of growth in health spending, and the (null) hypothesis of (no) growth convergence among developed countries.

Health care plays an important role in economic development because it may help to ensure a healthy and productive labor force for the economy [34]. It is obvious that when workers have good health, they are less likely to be absent from work due to sickness, and hence, become more productive at producing goods and services, *cereris paribus*.[2] Microeconomic theory (see, for example, Baumol & Blinder [8]) suggests that increased income raise the demand for health services (via income and substitution effects), especially in respect of elective services such as cosmetic surgery. This behavior can also be explained by the health capital concept proposed by Grossman [33], which suggests that individuals tend to invest for further health improvement when income increases such that their improved health stock would be

available to generate more wealth in the future. Ironically, income increases may also lead to further increases in health care consumption due to the emergence of "diseases of affluence" such as obesity, strokes and cancer (see, for example, Van de Poel et al. [69]). Economic development may lead to an aging population because life expectancy increases [42] and fertility declines due to, for example, increases in the direct and opportunity costs of having children [12, 25, 64]. Since people often incur high health expenditure at the end of their lifetimes, an aging population is one of the factors contributing to the rising health spending, especially in developed countries [40]. Health expenditure is also affected by lifestyle factors in affluent societies such as the over-consumption of high-energy food, and the lack of physical activity. However, the main factor that drives both economic development and health expenditure is technological progress because, for example, new technologies offer firms, including health services providers, an opportunity to earn monopoly profits [26, 52, 65].

Based on economic growth models (e.g., Solow [66]), the production of health services can be represented as a function of labor (e.g., doctors, nurses and allied health workers) and capital (e.g., buildings, beds and medical equipment). In the early stage of economic development, labor and capital are the main contributors to the amount of health care services provided. Based on this concept, indicators such as ratios of doctors and number of hospital beds per 1000 population are still used to measure the development of health services. Endogenous growth models (e.g., Nelson & Phelps [46]; Romer [61, 62]), however, suggested that technological progress is more important to economic growth, especially in the long-term. In the health sector, technological progress allows the treatment of new diseases or makes current treatments more effective, and hence more health care services are produced. However, the process of inventing new technologies often involves more time and resources than the process of learning from existing technologies, and hence health expenditure growth rates of countries can converge over time as developing countries adopt new technological advances in their production process. Other factors that drive the convergence of health expenditure growth are the diminishing returns to capital and labor: the amount of output produced increase at decreasing rates as labor and capital increases [5, 10, 11, 23].

The economic growth literature refers mainly to two types of convergence: $\beta-$ convergence and $\sigma-$ convergence which, together, explain how developing economies can "catch up" (e.g., by adopting existing technologies) with developed economies. The $\beta-$convergence refers to a negative correlation between the initial level of real income per capita (a proxy for economic development) and its growth over time, which occurs when economic growth rates of developed countries tend to be slower than that of developing countries. The σ−convergence refers to the reduced dispersion of growth across countries over time (as measured by the coefficient of variation). Another approach to examine the convergence of growth is testing for the stationarity of the differences in growth rates between countries. If the difference in the growth rate of two countries is stationary, the pair converges. In this study, we follow the economic growth model by Phillips & Sul [58] which allows heterogeneity with different transition paths among countries and also enables one to identify convergence among sub-groups of countries.

The *log t* convergence test

Based on the dynamic growth model developed by Phillips & Sul [58] we argued that the growth rates of health expenditure of a country are determined by accessibility to common technology (which is available to all countries) and the individualised factors of the country (e.g., the ability to conduct research and development to extend technological progress in the health care sector). This argument can be represented as:

$$y_{it} = \delta_{it}\mu_t + \varepsilon_{it} \qquad (1)$$

where y_{it} is a measure of growth in health expenditure for country i at time period t, μ_t is the growth contributed by the common technology, δ_{it} is the individual growth factor of country i, and ε_{it} represent random shocks. The health expenditure growth of countries converge when the individual growth factor (δ_{it}) converges. Assume that the cross-sectional average growth rate of all countries at any period represents the common growth factor (μ_t), we can isolate δ_{it} by taking the ratio of a growth rate of a country and the average rate:

$$h_{it} = \frac{y_{it}}{N^{-1}\sum_{i=1}^{N} y_{it}} = \frac{\delta_{it}}{N^{-1}\sum_{i=1}^{N} \delta_{it}} \qquad (2)$$

The coefficient h_{it}, which was referred to by Phillips and Sul as the 'relative transition path', measures the performance of country i relative to the growth rate achieved by using the common technology μ_t. In this formulation, the overall convergence of all countries is achieved when $h_{it} \to 1$ for all i as $t \to \infty$. In particular, this condition states that convergence is achieved at the long run ($t \to \infty$) when the difference between common growth factors and individualised growth factors is minimal. This convergence condition can also be expressed as the mean squared of relative transition differences:

$$H_t = N^{-1}\sum_{i=1}^{N}(h_{it} - 1)^2 \qquad (3)$$

In this representation, the growth rate of countries converges if $H_t \to 0$ as $t \to \infty$. When H_t remains positive as $t \to \infty$ it is possible for the growth rates of all countries diverge or some countries converge despite divergence occur among all countries. To formulate the test for the hypothesis of convergence, Phillips and Sul [58] employed a semiparametric model for the transition coefficients that allows for heterogeneity over time and across countries as:

$$\delta_{it} = \delta_i + \sigma_i\xi_{it}L(t)^{-1}t^{-\alpha} \qquad (4)$$

where δ_i is a time-invariant growth factor for country i, ξ_{it} is identically and independently distributed with mean of zero and variance of one across i, but weakly dependent over t, and $L(t)^{-1}$ is a slow decay function such as the logarithm of t for which $L(t)^{-1} \to 0$ as $t \to \infty$; σ_i is an idiosyncratic scale parameter; and $\alpha \geq 0$ is the decay rate. Equation (4) suggests that the condition for convergence is a slow decay component in the growth rate trajectories of individual countries. Under this specification, the null (convergence) and the alternative (non-convergence) hypotheses are expressed as:

$$\begin{cases} H_0 : \delta_{it} = \delta \text{ for all } i \\ H_A : \delta_{it} \neq \delta \text{ for some } i \end{cases} \qquad (5)$$

The alternative hypothesis can also be specified to test for the formation of sub-convergence groups. For example, the alternative hypothesis for the formation of two sub-convergence groups is specified as:

$$H_A : \delta_{it} \to \begin{cases} \delta_1 \text{ if } i \in G_1 \\ \delta_2 \text{ if } i \in G_2 \end{cases} \qquad (6)$$

where $\delta_1 = \lim_{N\to\infty} N_1^{-1}\sum_{i\in G_1}\delta_{it}$ and $\delta_2 = \lim_{N\to\infty} N_2^{-1}\sum_{i\in G_2}\delta_{it}$, N_1 and N_2 are the number of countries in Group 1 and Group 2 such that $N_1 + N_2 = N$, which is the total number of countries.

Using the limiting form for the quadratic difference $H_t \sim \frac{A}{L(t)^2 t^{2\alpha}}$ as $t \to \infty$ for a constant $A > 0$ and setting the decay function $L(t) = log(t)$, Phillips and Sul [58] proposed the test for convergence in the form of a regression of 'log t' as:

$$log\frac{H_1}{H_t} - 2log(log\, t) = \omega + \gamma\, log\, t + u_t \qquad (7)$$

where u_t is the random error. The null hypothesis of convergence is rejected (i.e., health expenditure growth rates of countries diverge or only converge among sub-groups) if γ is less than zero, while a non-negative γ suggests that convergence occurs among all countries. Thus, the test for convergence is now simply a heteroscedasticity and autocorrelation consistent (HAC) one-sided t-test for the null hypothesis that $\gamma \geq 0$ by estimating Eq. (7) with Newey & West [47] robust standard errors. In this study, we choose the five percent level of significance for the test, hence, the null hypothesis of convergence is rejected if t-value of parameter γ in Eq. (7) is less than or equal to -1.65. When the null hypothesis of overall convergence is rejected (i.e., γ is negative and significant), one can then test for the formation of sub-convergence groups using a four-step clustering algorithm by Phillips and Sul [58] as follows:

1. Order countries in the sample according to the health expenditure growth in the last period.
2. Form a core group of k^* countries by selecting the k countries with the highest health expenditure growth rate to form a sub-group G_k and run a convergence test. The optimal size of sub-groups is determined by maximizing the t-value of the γ coefficient using the k countries (t_k) such that $k^* = arg\,max_k\{t_k\}$ subject to $min\{t_k\} > -1.65$.
3. Add one country at a time to the core group and run the convergence test, the country is added if the t-value concludes that γ is non-negative.
4. Repeat the process in steps 1 to 3 for the remaining countries. If there is no k in step 2 that satisfies $t_k > -1.65$ then the remaining countries do not form any sub-convergence group.

Applying the above procedure we are able to test whether health expenditure of selected OECD countries in 1975–2004 converge, diverge totally or form convergence groups. To examine factors that may affect the trends and patterns of growth in health expenditures we apply panel data analysis.

Determinants of health expenditure

To examine the determinants of health expenditure, we propose a panel data specification as follows:

$$Hexp_{it} = \beta_0 + \beta_1 GDPcap_{it} + \gamma X_{it} + \delta\,trend + \alpha_i + \epsilon_{it} \quad (8)$$

where $Hexp_{it}$ is the logarithm of real health expenditure per capita of country i in period t; $GDPcap$ is the log of real GDP per capita (i.e., GDP per capita in 2000 prices); X_{it} is the set of other covariates (e.g., proportion of people over 65 years old, share of public expenditure in total health care spending) which are also expressed in natural logarithms; α_i are country-specific fixed-effects; $trend$ is the time trend representing technological progress in the study period; and ϵ_{it} are random errors. In order to obtain reliable estimates of Eq. 8, we apply panel data methods (e.g., random and fixed-effects estimators) to remove the effects of country unobserved characteristics (α_i). Because health expenditure and GDP per capita may be affected by the same source of external shocks, it is possible that cross-sectional correlations exist in the data set. We examine this issue by applying the cross-sectional dependence test by Pesaran [56]. It is also possible that the error term (ϵ_{it}) is serially correlated and has non-constant

variance, thus we apply the test for the serial autocorrelation by Wooldridge [74] and the likelihood ratio test for heteroscedasticity. Finally, we apply the Hausman specification test to select between the random effects and fixed effects estimators of Eq. 8.

Data and variable selections

Most variables for this study were selected from the OECD health data 2007 [18]. To form a balanced panel data for the analysis, we chose 21 countries and the period 1975–2004 based on the availability of data on health total expenditure per capita (a lot of missing data pre-1974 and in 2005, based on the 2007 version of OECD health data set) and lifestyle variables such as calories intake, fat intake and alcohol consumption (available only up to 2004). We also use data from the Penn World Table version 7.1 [35] to explore effects of macroeconomic indicators on the growth of health expenditure.

We selected health expenditure per capita measured as \$US in purchasing power parity (PPP) at 2000 prices to avoid the effect of exchange rates and inflation. Similarly, we selected the real GDP per capita (\$US PPP 2000 prices) to examine the relationship between health expenditure and income. It is expected that GDP per capita has a positive association with health expenditure per capita due to both the income and substitution effects discussed earlier. The proportion of people over 65 years of age is selected to represent the effects of population aging on health expenditure, which is also expected to be positive. The data set also contains information on life expectancy, but this variable is highly correlated with real GDP per capita, so we chose not to include it in our estimates. The unemployment rate is also included to capture the possible effects of economic activities on health. We expect higher rates of unemployment to be negatively associated with health due to, for example, stress and lower access to market inputs; and hence, the we expect the association between the unemployment rate and health expenditure to be positive. The consumption of food, as measured by calorie intake per capita, is another input at our disposal Since we believe that, in the OECD countries food shortage is by-and-large not a major problem, calories intake in this group of countries is expected to be positively associated with health expenditure, due to lifestyle-related health problems associated with obesity, for example. In this respect, the data set also contains information on the amount of sugar and fat consumption. We did not include these variables in the analyses because they are highly correlated with calorie intake. Finally, the dataset also indicates the public sector share of health expenditure. We include this variable as an indicator of the extent to which health sectors are "nationalised" or subsidised publicly. Such measures may be important for controlling health expenditure growth, as many countries that provide extensive public subvention of health care (e.g., Australia, New Zealand, Canada and the UK) also use centralised decision-making to determine which services and pharmaceuticals are eligible for subsidies. Furthermore, in some of these systems, the monopsony power of governments operating in the health sector may also serve as a brake on health expenditure growth.

The data show that health expenditure per capita experienced the highest growth in the study period, about double the growth of the consumer price index (CPI) and more than four times the growth of GDP per capita in the study period (see Fig. 1, right axis). For example, on average, health expenditure per capita in OECD countries in 2004 was 8 times larger than that in 1975. The relative figures for CPI and GDP per capita growth are five- and two- fold, respectively. The growth rate of other selected indicators are substantially lower: the proportion of people over 65 years old increased by 30% between 1975 and 2004, while the increase of life expectancy was 10 per cent (see Fig. 1, left axis). More importantly, the growth of health expenditure growth rate and CPI seems accelerate rapidly since 2000, while the growth of GDP per capita remained stable. In the analysis, we use CPI and exchange rate to adjust for monetary figure over time and across countries.

Results and discussion

Convergence

The "log t" test revealed that there is no significant evidence of overall convergence of real health expenditure per capita among OECD countries in the 1975–2004 period (i.e., γ is negative and significant) as the t-value of "log t" is –64.3 (see Table 1). One possible reason for no overall convergence is due to the substantial level of heterogeneity among OECD countries in both economic development and health expenditure. However, we found that there are three groups within which health spending of countries converge (i.e., $\gamma \geq 0$): the estimation of γ parameter is positive for Group 2 and not significantly different from zero for the remaining groups. The average annual growth rate of real health expenditure per capita is highest among countries in Group 1 (7.9%) and lowest in Group 3 (5.8%). With the exception of Luxembourg, Norway and the USA, countries in Group 1 are relatively poorer OECD countries. The presence of Norway and the USA in Group 1 is consistent with the finding by Panopoulou & Pantelidis [53] but we differ slightly in the ranking other countries, which could be due to the small differences in the number of countries and time period. Note that the convergence test conducted here is a univariate analysis. Thus, other factors such as ageing population, availability of new but expensive treatment options for complicated diseases such as viral hepatitis, HIV and tuberculosis are not taken into account.

For comparison with previous studies, we also conducted $\beta-$ and $\sigma-$ convergence tests. The results of all these tests show significant evidence of overall convergence. For example, cross-sectional dispersion in health expenditure of OECD countries reduce significantly over

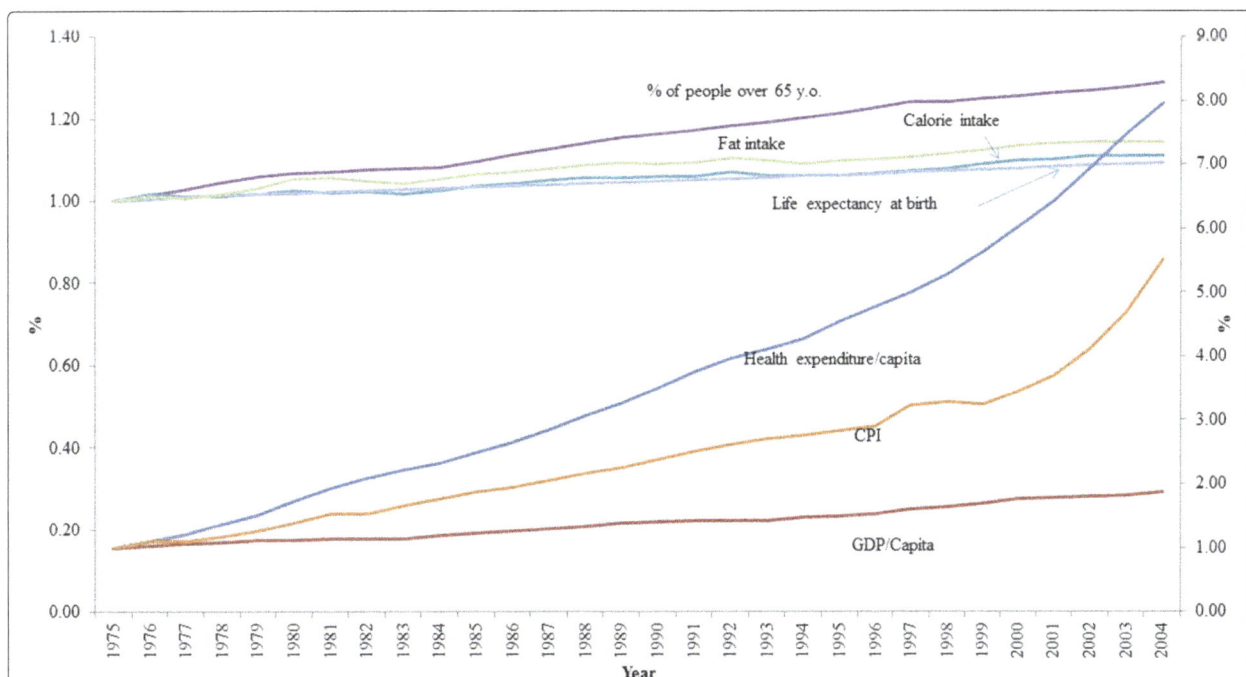

Fig. 1 Commutative growth rates of selected variables (secondary verticle axis is used for : health expenditure per capita, CPI and GDP per capita)

Table 1 The *log t* convergence test

Group	Countries	"log *t*" test		Average annual growth rate
		Coef. (γ)	t-stat	
1	Luxembourg, Norway, Portugal, Turkey, Iceland, Ireland, Spain, United States	-0.072	-1.010	***0.079
2	Austria, Belgium, Japan, United Kingdom	***1.969	8.477	***0.069
3	Australia, Canada, Finland, Netherlands, Switzerland, Denmark, Germany, New Zealand, Sweden	0.031	0.224	***0.058
	All countries	***-1.846	-64.332	***0.068

Note: ***, **, and * refers to 1%, 5% and 10% significant level, respectively

time, suggesting that σ−convergence is present (Fig. 2a). We also found a significant negative correlation between the average growth rate of health expenditure and the level of expenditure in the starting year of 1975, suggesting that β−convergence exists (Fig. 2b). A comparison of the results of the β−convergence test with that of the *log t* test in Fig. 2b confirms that countries in Group 1, with the exception of the USA, had the lowest health expenditure per capita in 1975, but the highest average growth rate. By contrast, the countries in Group 3 had highest

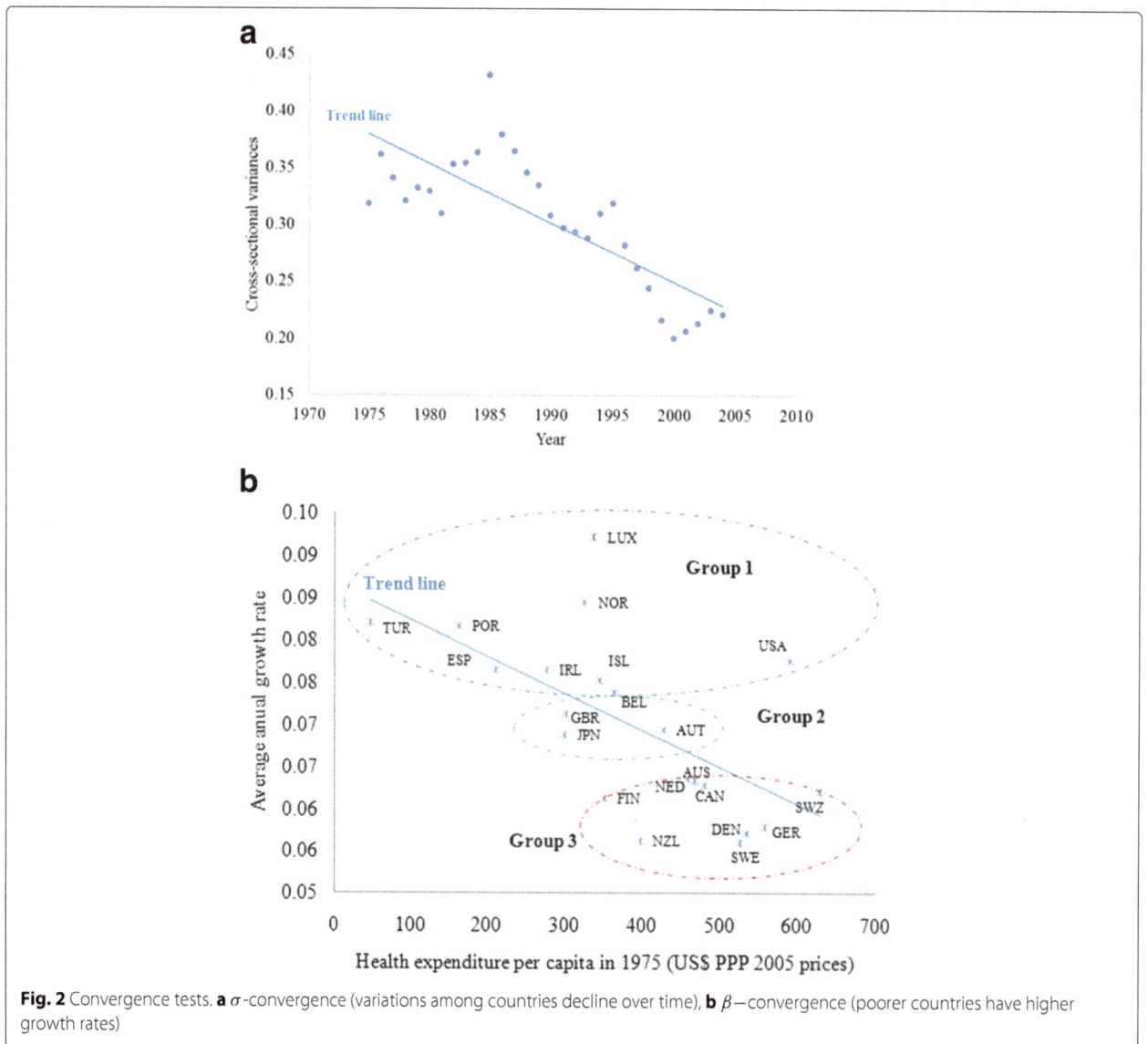

Fig. 2 Convergence tests. **a** σ-convergence (variations among countries decline over time), **b** β−convergence (poorer countries have higher growth rates)

starting health expenditure per capita in 1975, but the lowest average growth rate thereafter.

Determinants of health expenditure

We apply standard panel data econometric methods to examine the determinants of health expenditure. To explore the possible differences among convergence groups, we conducted the analysis separately for each group. An application of the Im et al. [38] test for unit roots rejected the null hypothesis that the panel contains a unit root (see Table 2). However, the test for serial correlation and cross-sectional dependent rejected the null hypothesis of no serial correlation and cross-sectional independent, respectively. Finally, the Hausman specification test rejected the null hypothesis that parameters of the random- and fixed-effects estimators are the same, suggesting that a fixed-effects estimator, which takes into account the effects of unobserved country characteristics, is preferred.

The regression results show that the income elasticity of health care expenditure is less than one. The random-effects estimator, however, produce an income elasticity of slightly greater than one. This result suggests that, ignoring unobserved country characteristics may over-estimate the income elasticity of health expenditure and conclude wrongly that health care is a luxury good. Thus, our results suggest that health care is a necessity, not a luxury, at the national level: a one percent increase in GDP per capita is associated with 0.9% increase in health expenditure per capita.

The results also show that the most significant parameter is the trend line, a proxy for technological progress over time. This result is consistent with the literature to date. In particular, parameters of the trend line show that the average growth rate of health expenditure per capita in the 1975–2004 period is four percent per year.

All remaining covariates are also significantly contribute to the increase of health expenditure. In particular, calorie intake is the most substantial determinant of health expenditure with the elasticity of 0.8. The most likely reason for this association may be due to the costs of obesity-related health problems. Public share of health expenditure also play an important role in the total health expenditure with the elasticity of 0.33, which is as expected for developed countries in the sample. Developed countries also face aging population, which may contribute to the rising costs of health care. In particular, an increase of the elderly ratio by one percent is associated with 0.17% increase in health expenditure. Unemployment is also significantly associated with health expenditure but the magnitude of elasticity is minimal, at 0.09.

Conclusions

This study has examined the trend of health care expenditure for OECD countries during the period 1975–2004. Adapting a dynamic economic growth model developed by Phillips and Sul [58], we tested the hypothesis that the growth of health spending per capita in these countries converge over time. We did not find significant evidence of overall convergence in the health spending growth among the countries for the study period, but identified three sub-groups of countries which tended to converge over this period. Using a fixed-effects estimator, we find that the rate of growth in health care expenditure per capita is less than that of GDP per capita (i.e., health care is a necessary goods). The main driver for increasing health expenditure is technological progress, which accounts for four percent per year and accelerated faster after each decade in the study period. This result is consistent with the existing literature on health expenditure growth. The results of our paper therefore suggest that the explanations and predictions of health expenditure growth based

Table 2 Factors determining health expenditures in OECD countries

Variables	Fixed-effects		Random-effects	
	Coef.	Std.err	Coef.	Std.err
Log of real GDP/capita	***0.900	0.067	***1.016	0.057
Log of elderly ratio	**0.167	0.068	***0.237	0.062
Log of calories consumption	***0.800	0.154	***0.820	0.151
Log of unemployment rate	***0.092	0.013	***0.100	0.012
Log of public share of total health expenditure	***0.339	0.049	***0.308	0.048
Trend line	***0.042	0.002	***0.039	0.002
Constant	***-11.215	1.520	***-12.549	1.433
	Unit root test	Auto- correlation test	Cross-sectional independent	Hausman test
Test statistics	254.6	65.5	23.2	151.1
p-value	0.00	0.00	0.00	0.00

Note: Significant levels are ***=1%, **=5% and *=10%

on existing models is unlikely to be affected by convergence. This result is important, because it suggests that policy-makers in lower health expenditure countries need not be concerned about convergence *per se* frustrating attempts to contain health expenditures. Yet it also means that policy-makers in high health-expenditure countries should not depend on convergence to help contain health expenditure growth at home. Rather, microeconomic initiatives that target the modifiable sources of health expenditure growth–particularly health technology diffusion and insurance–are likely the only solutions to containing the growth of health expenditure in high-income nations.

Endnotes

[1] See, for example, Gerdtham & Jonsson [28] for a comprehensive review of these studies.

[2] The *ceteris paribus* condition assumes that other factors (e.g., proportion of elderly people and their higher share of health expenditure) among OECD countries remain constant.

Acknowledgements
The authors acknowledge valuable comments received from participants of the 35th Australian Conference of Health Economics, Canberra, Australia.

Funding
None.

Authors' contributions
SN collected and analysed data, reviewed the literature and drafted the manuscript. LC designed the analysis, provided feedback on results and edited the manuscript. Both authors read and approved the final manuscript.

Competing interests
The authors declare that they have no competing interests.

Author details
[1] The Australian Research Centre for Health Services Innovation, Institute of Health and Biomedical Innovation, School of Public Health and Social Work, Queensland University of Technology, Kelvin Grove, Brisbane QLD 4059, Australia. [2] Centre for the Business and Economics of Health, Faculty of Health and Behavioural Sciences, The University of Queensland, Brisbane QLD 4072, Australia.

References

1. Alcalde-Unzu J, Ezcurra R, Pascual P. Cross-country disparities in health-care expenditure: a factor decomposition. Health Econ. 2009;18(4): 479–85.
2. Anderson GF, Hurst J, Hussey PS, Jee-Hughes M. Health spending and outcomes: trends in OECD countries, 1960-1998. Health Aff. 2000;19(3): 150–7.
3. Anderson GF, Frogner BK, Johns RA, Reinhardt UE. Health care spending and use of information technology in OECD countries. Health Aff. 2006;25(3):819–31.
4. Baltagi BH, Moscone F. Health care expenditure and income in the OECD reconsidered: Evidence from panel data. Econ Model. 2010;27(4):804–11.
5. Barro RJ, Sala-i Martin X. Economic growth and convergence across the United States. NBER Working Paper No. 3419. 1990. doi:10.3386/w3419, http://www.nber.org/papers/w3419. Accessed 5 May 2016.
6. Barros PP. The black box of health care expenditure growth determinants. Health Econ. 1998;7(6):533–44.
7. Bates LJ, Santerre RE. Does the US health care sector suffer from Baumol's cost disease? Evidence from the 50 states. J Health Econ. 2013;32(2): 386–91.
8. Baumol W, Blinder A. Microeconomics: Principles and policy. Boston: Cengage Learning; 2015.
9. Baumol WJ. Macroeconomics of unbalanced growth: the anatomy of urban crisis. Am Econ Rev. 1967;57(3):415–26.
10. Baumol WJ. Productivity growth, convergence, and welfare: what the long-run data show. Am Econ Rev. 1986;76(5):1072–85.
11. Bernard AB, Jones CI. Technology and Convergence. Econ J. 1996;106(437):1037–44.
12. Borg MO. The income-fertility relationship: Effect of the net price of a child. Demography. 1989;26(2):301–10.
13. Bustamante AV, Chen J. Health expenditure dynamics and years of U.S. residence: analyzing spending disparities among Latinos by citizenship/nativity status. Health Serv Res. 2012;47(2):794–818.
14. Carrion-i Silvestre JL. Health care expenditure and GDP: are they broken stationary? J Health Econ. 2005;24(5):839–54.
15. Chandra A, Skinner J. Technology growth and expenditure growth in health care. J Econ Lit. 2012;50(3):645–80.
16. Chernew ME, Hirth RA, Sonnad SS, Ermann R, Fendrick AM. Managed care, medical technology, and health care cost growth: a review of the evidence. Med Care Res Rev. 1998;55(3):259–88.
17. Clemente J, Marcuello C, Montañés A, Pueyo F. On the international stability of health care expenditure functions: are government and private functions similar? J Health Econ. 2004;23(3):589–613.
18. CREDES-OECD. OECD health data 2007. 2007. SUB-17293S1, http://www.fedpubs.com/subject/health/oecdhealth.htm. Accessed 10 Mar 2016.
19. Cutler DM, Ly DP. The (paper) work of medicine: understanding international medical costs. J Econ Perspect. 2011;25(2):3–25.
20. Cutler DM, McClellan M. Is technological change in medicine worth it? Health Aff. 2001;20(5):11–29.
21. Cutler DM, McClellan M, Newhouse JP. What has increased medical-care spending bought? Am Econ Rev. 1998;88(2):132–6.
22. Danzon PM, Pauly MV. Health Insurance and the Growth in Pharmaceutical Expenditures. J Law Econ. 2002;45(S2):587–613.
23. Dowrick S, Nguyen DT. OECD comparative economic growth 1950-85: catch-up and convergence. Am Econ Rev. 1989;79(5):1010–30.
24. Frank RG, Goldman HH, McGuire TG. Trends in mental health cost growth: an expanded role for management? Health Aff. 2009;28(3):649–59.
25. Freedman DS. The relation of economic status to fertility. Am Econ Rev. 1963;53(3):414–26.
26. Galor O, Tsiddon D. Technological progress, mobility, and economic growth. Am Econ Rev. 1997;87(3):363–82.
27. Gerdtham UG, Lothgren M. On stationarity and cointegration of international health expenditure and GDP. J Health Econ. 2000;19(4): 461–75.
28. Gerdtham U-G, Jonsson B. International comparisons of health expenditure: theory, data and econometric analysis. Handb Health Econ. 2000;1:11–53.
29. Gerdtham U-G, Ruhm CJ. Deaths rise in good economic times: evidence from the OECD. Econ Hum Biol. 2006;4(3):298–316.
30. Gerdtham U-G, Sogaardb J, Andersson F, Jonsson B. An econometric analysis of health care expenditure: a cross-section study of the OECD countries. J Health Econ. 1992;11(1):63–84.
31. Getzen TE. Population aging and the growth of health expenditures. J Gerontol. 1992;47(3):S98–104.
32. Getzen TE. Health care is an individual necessity and a national luxury: applying multilevel decision models to the analysis of health care expenditures. J Health Econ. 2000;19(2):259–70.
33. Grossman M. On the concept of health capital and the demand for health. J Polit Econ. 1972;80(2):223–55.
34. Gupta S, Verhoeven M, Tiongson ER. The effectiveness of government spending on education and health care in developing and transition economies. Eur J Polit Econ. 2002;18(4):717–37.

35. Heston A, Summers R, Aten B. Penn World Table Version 7.1. Center for International Comparisons of Production, Income and Prices at the University of Pennsylvania. 2012. https://fred.stlouisfed.org/categories/33100. Accessed 11 June 2016.

36. Hitiris T. Health care expenditure and integration in the countries of the European Union. Appl Econ. 1997;29(1):1–6.

37. Hitiris T, Nixon J. Convergence of health care expenditure in the EU countries. Appl Econ Lett. 2001;8(4):223–28.

38. Im KS, Pesaran MH, Shin Y. Testing for unit roots in heterogeneous panels. J Econ. 2003;115(1):53–74.

39. Jurd A. Expenditure on Healthcare in the UK, 1997-2010. 2012. http://webarchive.nationalarchives.gov.uk/20160109181813/http://www.ons.gov.uk/ons/dcp171766_264293.pdf. Accessed 15 Mar 2016.

40. Koizumi A. Longevity and health care: a cost-benefit type analysis of life expectancy and medical expenditure. Jinkogaku Kenkyu. 1984;7:9–14.

41. Lau CKM, Fung KWT, Pugalis L. Is health care expenditure across Europe converging? Findings from the application of a nonlinear panel unit root test. Eurasian Business Rev. 2014;4(2):137–56.

42. Lichtenberg FR. Sources of US longevity increase, 1960–2001. Q Rev Econ Financ. 2004;44(3):369–89.

43. Mendelson DN, Schwartz WB. The effects of aging and population growth on health care costs. Health Aff. 1993;12(1):119–25.

44. Narayan PK. Do health expenditures 'catch-up'? Evidence from OECD countries. Health Econ. 2007;16(10):993–1008.

45. Narayan S, Narayan PK, Mishra S. Investigating the relationship between health and economic growth: Empirical evidence from a panel of 5 Asian countries. J Asian Econ. 2010;21(4):404–11.

46. Nelson RR, Phelps ES. Investment in humans, technological diffusion, and economic growth. Am Econ Rev. 1966;56(1/2):69–75.

47. Newey WK, West KD. A Simple Positive Semi-Definite, Heteroskedasticity and Autocorrelation Consistent Covariance Matrix. Econometrica. 1987;55(3):703–8.

48. Newhouse JP. Medical expenditure: a cross-sectional survey. J Hum Resour. 1977;12(1):115–25.

49. Newhouse JP. Medical care costs: how much welfare loss? J Econ Perspect. 1992;6(3):3–21.

50. Nixon J. Convergence analysis of health care expenditure in the EU countries using two approaches. The University of York Discussion Papers in Economics No. 1999/03. 1999. https://www.york.ac.uk/media/economics/documents/discussionpapers/1999/9903.pdf. Accessed 31 Mar 2016.

51. Okunade AA, Karakus MC. Unit root and cointegration tests: timeseries versus panel estimates for international health expenditure models. Appl Econ. 2001;33(9):1131–7.

52. Okunade AA, Murthy VNR. Technology as a "major driver" of health care costs: a cointegration analysis of the Newhouse conjecture. J Health Econ. 2002;21(1):147–59.

53. Panopoulou E, Pantelidis T. Convergence in per capita health expenditures and health outcomes in the OECD countries. Appl Econ. 2012;44(30):3909–20.

54. Parkin D, McGuire A, Yule B. Aggregate health care expenditures and national income: is health care a luxury good? J Health Econ. 1987;6(2):109–27.

55. Pekkurnaz D. Convergence of Health Expenditure in OECD Countries: Evidence from a Nonlinear Asymmetric Heterogeneous Panel Unit Root Test. J Rev Glob Econ. 2015;4:76–86.

56. Pesaran MH. General diagnostic tests for cross section dependence in panels. CESifo Working Paper Series No. 1229; IZA Discussion Paper No. 1240. 2004. https://doi.org/10.17863/CAM.5113. Accessed 18 Mar 2016.

57. Pfaff M. Differences in health care spending across countries: statistical evidence. J Health Polit Policy Law. 1990;15(1):1–68.

58. Phillips PCB, Sul D. Transition modeling and econometric convergence tests. Econometrica. 2007;75(6):1771–855.

59. Pradhan RP. The long run relation between health spending and economic growth in 11 OECD countries: Evidence from panel cointegration. Int J Econ Perspect. 2010;4(2):427–38.

60. Roberts J. Sensitivity of elasticity estimates for OECD health care spending: analysis of a dynamic heterogeneous data field. Health Econ. 1999;8(5):459–72.

61. Romer PM. The origins of endogenous growth. J Econ Perspect. 1994;8(1):3–22.

62. Romer PM. Endogenous technological change. J Polit Econ. 1990;98:s71–102.

63. Schieber GJ, Puollier JP. International health care spending. Health Aff. 1986;5(3):111–22.

64. Simon JL. The effect of income on fertility. Popul Stud. 1969;23(3):327–41.

65. Smith S, Newhouse JP, Freeland MS. Income, insurance, and technology: why does health spending outpace economic growth? Health Aff. 2009;28(5):1276–84.

66. Solow RM. A contribution to the theory of economic growth. Q J Econ. 1956;70(1):65–94.

67. Suku SN, Caner A. Health care expenditures and gross domestic product: the Turkish case. Eur J Health Econ. 2011;12(1):29–38.

68. Tchoe B, Nam S-H. Aging risk and health care expenditure in Korea. Int J Environ Res Public Health. 2010;7(8):3235–54.

69. Van de Poel E, O'Donnell O, Van Doorslaer E. Urbanization and the spread of diseases of affluence in China. Econ Hum Biol. 2009;7(2):200–16.

70. Vander Stichele RH, Peys F, Van Tielen R, Van Eeckhout H, van Essche O, Seys B. A decade of growth in public and private pharmaceutical expenditures: the case of Belgium 1990-1999. Int J Clin Lab Med. 2003;58(5):279–89.

71. Willem P, Dumont M. Machines that go 'ping': medical technology and health expenditures in OECD countries. Health Econ. 2015;24(8):1027–41.

72. Wilson RM. Medical care expenditures and gdp growth in OECD nations. Am Assoc Biobehav Soc Sci J. 1999;2:159–171.

73. Woodward RS, Wang Le. The Oh-So Straight And Narrow Path: Can The Health Care Expenditure Curve Be Bent?. Health Econ. 2012;21(8):1023–9.

74. Wooldridge JM. Econometric analysis of cross section and panel data. Cambridge: The MIT Press; 2002.

75. Wu S, Chaudhry B, Wang J, Maglione M, Mojica W, Roth E, Morton SC, Shekelle PG. Systematic review: impact of health information technology on quality, efficiency, and costs of medical care. Ann Intern Med. 2006;144(10):742–52.

76. Yule GU. Why do we sometimes get nonsense-correlations between Time-Series?–a study in sampling and the nature of time-series. J R Stat Soc. 1926;89(1):1–63.

16

Costs of productivity loss due to occupational cancer in Canada: estimation using claims data from Workers' Compensation Boards

W. Dominika Wranik[1][*] [iD], Adam Muir[2] and Min Hu[3]

Abstract

Introduction: Cancer is a leading cause of illness globally, yet our understanding of the financial implications of cancer caused by working conditions and environments is limited. The goal of this study is to estimate the costs of productivity losses due to occupational cancer in Canada, and to evaluate the factors associated with these costs.

Methods: Two sources of data are used: (i) Individual level administrative claims data from the Workers Compensation Board of Nova Scotia; and (ii) provincial aggregated cancer claims statistics from the Association of Workers Compensation Boards of Canada. Benefits paid to claimants are based on actuarial estimates of wage-loss, but do not include medical costs that are covered by the Canadian publicly funded healthcare system. Regional claims level data are used to estimate the total and average (per claim) cost of occupational cancer to the insurance system, and to assess which characteristics of the claim/claimant influence costs. Cost estimates from one region are weighted using regional multipliers to adjust for system differences between regions, and extrapolated to estimate national costs of occupational cancer.

Results/Discussion: We estimate that the total cost of occupational cancer to the Workers' Compensation system in Canada between 1996 and 2013 was $1.2 billion. The average annual cost was $68 million. The cancer being identified as asbestos related were significantly positively associated with costs, whereas the age of the claimant was significantly negatively associated with costs. The industry type/region, injury type or part of body affected by cancer were not significant cost determinants.

Conclusion: Given the severity of the cancer burden, it is important to understand the financial implications of the disease on workers. Our study shows that productivity losses associated with cancer in the workplace are not negligible, particularly for workers exposed to asbestos.

Background

The incidence of cancer in Canada was higher than the global average in 2012; more than 290 individuals per 100,000 population were diagnosed with cancer, as compared to a global average of approximately 190 per 100,000 [1] This can create an emotional and financial burden on patients and their families, the latter in the form of health care costs, and also costs of missed employment.

Health care costs to individuals are defrayed in Canada by virtue of the health care system being predominantly publicly funded from general taxation revenues. While drugs are typically not included on the public reimbursement list, many cancer drugs are funded publically [2]. Costs of lost earnings can also be partially defrayed for workers whose cancer diagnosis can be attributed to their working conditions or environment. In those cases, workers can lay claims against their employer.

The Workers' Compensation system in Canada is an insurance system that protects employers against the risk of work-related injury claims. It was established in the early parts of the 20th century. The general premise behind the

---

* Correspondence: dwl@dal.ca
[1]School of Public Administration, Department of Community Health and Epidemiology, Dalhousie University, Halifax, NS, Canada
Full list of author information is available at the end of the article

program is that workers relinquish their right to sue employers in the event of workplace injury, but gain compensation benefits in exchange [3]. Each injury/fatality claim is carefully reviewed to establish attribution of the injury or illness to workplace conditions. The Workers' Compensation system in Canada has been characterized as parallel to the publicly funded provincial insurance [3].

When workers in Canada develop cancer that is attributable to the conditions or environments of their workplace, typically referred to as occupational cancer [4], they may file a claim with the Workers' Compensation Board (WCB). Even though several types of industry have been identified as posing a higher risk of cancer for their workers (construction, fire-fighting, mining, etc.) [5], the specific causes of any individual's cancer can be challenging to identify, however. Multiple factors can contribute to the illness, and there is often latency between cause and diagnosis [6, 7]. Claims may therefore be rejected.

Canada has 12 WCBs, individually representing each of the provinces and territories, with the exception of Northwest Territories and Nunavut, which share a program. Table 1 outlines the characteristics of these provincial boards. The Workers' Compensation system has been developing and evolving over the majority of the previous century. Not unlike other national systems in Canada, it has evolved at different speeds and in different directions in the various jurisdictions. The status quo is such that the features of the WCB vary across provinces in the amounts that a worker can expect to receive in compensation, the percentage of regular earnings recovered, and the requirements placed on employers in the case of a workplace injury.

The amounts of benefits paid to workers by a Workers' Compensation Board are based on an actuarial estimation of earnings losses that occur as a result of the injury or illness. As such, the amount of benefits can serve as a proxy to understanding the amount of wage loss, which in turn signals productivity loss resulting from a specific injury or illness.

Literature

Occupational cancer is the leading cause of work-related death in Canada and rates of accepted claims have generally increased since 1997 in Canada [8, 9] and the United Kingdom [10]. Moreover, asbestos-related cancer accounted for nearly 70% of all compensated deaths and most typically affect those with manual labour professions [8, 11]. While the incidence of these reports are clear, measuring the cost of occupational cancer remains difficult.

Little is known about the costs of occupational cancer to a health care system, or any of its components. Estimates in the literature rely on administrative records, national aggregate statistics, and/or questionnaires to estimate occupational cancer costs. All rely on assumptions made about the transferability of incomplete or imperfect data to estimate the incidence and/or prevalence of occupational cancer and/or its cost. For this reason, there is a limited number of published studies that estimate the burden and/or costs of occupational cancer (Additional file 1: Appendix A1).

The creativity of some approaches published in the literature signals the difficulty of finding reliable data regarding the costs of occupational cancer. For example, Fritschi and Driscoll [12] use Finnish estimates of the proportion of cancers caused by occupation to estimate occupational cancer rates in Australia. They use EU estimates of the proportion of workers exposed to carcinogens and apply to Australian industry profiles [12]. Other studies of occupational cancer do not contain cost estimates.

Table 1 Characteristics of Workers' Compensation Boards in Canada

Province	Name of board	Year	Max. compensated earnings	% of earnings (basis for benefits)
Alberta	Workers' Compensation Board of Alberta	1918	$95,300	90% net
British Columbia	WorkSafeBC	1917	$78,600	90% net
Manitoba	Workers' Compensation Board of Manitoba	1917	$121,000	90% net
New Brunswick	WorkSafeNB	1919	$60,900	85% loss of earnings
Newfoundland and Labrador	Workplace Health, Safety and Compensation Commission	1951	$61,615	90% net
Northwest Territories/Nunavut	Workers' Safety & Compensation Commission	1977	$86,000	90% net
Nova Scotia	Workers' Compensation Board of Nova Scotia	1915	$56,800	75% net (26 weeks) then 85% net
Ontario	Workplace Safety and Insurance Board	1915	$85,200	85% net
Prince Edward Island	Workers' Compensation Board of Prince Edward Island	1949	$52,100	80% net (38 weeks) then 85% net
Quebec	Commission de la santé et de la sécurité du travail	1931	$70,000	90% net
Saskatchewan	Workers Compensation Board of Saskatchewan	1929	$65,130	90% net
Yukon	Yukon Workers' Compensation Health & Safety Board	1973	$77,610	75% gross

Despite limited academic study, especially in Canada, some conclusions can be drawn regarding the nature of occupational cancer and its labour impact, and provide the basis for exploring new methods to estimate costs.

Internationally, the impact of occupational cancer is significant when measured in terms of mortality. Two studies use national mortality data to estimate the number of potential or expected years of life and/or working life lost due to occupational cancer. Binazzi et al. (2013) estimate that on aggregate 170,000 potential years of life and 16,000 potential years of working life were lost due to occupational cancer in Italy in 2006 [13]. Lee et al. (2012) estimate that in Taiwan, between 1997 and 2005, the expected years of life lost per individual were between 5 and 18 on average, depending on the type of cancer [14].

The financial cost of occupational cancer to health systems internationally is also extensive. Estimations of the monetized costs of cancer vary across regions, years, and the specific types of costs included in the calculation. For example, work attributable cancers are estimated to have cost the Spanish Basque health system close to €10 million in 2008 [15]. Costs for all of France in 2010 are estimated between €917 million and €2.18 billion, including direct and indirect social costs [16]. In contrast, O'Neill estimates the cost of work-related cancers in the UK to be in the order of £30 to £60 billion per year, which is a much higher estimate [17].

The cost of occupational cancer in Canada is comparable to international estimates, but the Canadian literature employs a multitude of measurement strategies, particularly at the provincial levels. For example, Hopkins et al. [18] use data from the Canadian Community Health Survey, as well as published numbers from the literature to estimate the national-level cost of occupational cancer in terms of wage loss in 2009. They estimate that workers (patients) and their families have lost $ 3.18 billion [18]. Orenstein et al. [19] estimate that the indirect costs (loss of economic resources and reduced productivity) in Alberta alone are approximately $64 million per year, and that the province incurs approximately $16 million per year in medical system costs. While Quebec estimates that occupational diseases account for approximately $834 million dollars annually in worker's compensation claims and occupational disease related deaths cost approximately $128 million, exact figures regarding the cost of occupational cancer were unclear [11]. Additionally, the number of compensated occupational cancer claims has also grown progressively in Ontario, however the true burden of occupational cancer is yet to be properly estimated [8]. Due to the lack of literature focusing on all Canadian provinces, particularly Nova Scotia, understanding the cost of occupational cancer is relatively unknown. Estimating and exploring the determinants of the cost of occupational cancer claims in Nova Scotia, as well as nationally by province must be attempted.

Methods

The goal of this study is twofold: (i) to understand the structure of occupational cancer costs borne by the WCB in Nova Scotia, and (ii) to estimate the national burden of occupational cancer using the NS data.

Two models are developed, a regional model and a national model. The regional model estimates the total costs and average costs per cancer related claim, and the determinants of costs at the level of the province (Nova Scotia). The national model extrapolates national level costs from the regional level using NS average cost per claim, the number of claims per province/territory per year, and a weighing technique to account for differences in the provincial/territorial WCB systems.

Data

We use two sources of data: (i) the Nova Scotia Workers' Compensation Board (WCB) administrative claims records, and (ii) the Association of Workers' Compensation Boards of Canada (AWCBC) aggregated statistics available online or through customized order.

The Nova Scotia WCB records were made available at the individual claims level from 1957 to 2015 and includes all claims with and without time-loss. The records include the short and long term earnings loss benefits paid to individuals up until September 22nd, 2015. Other variables available were age in years at the time of the biopsy (<50, 51–64, 65+), industry that the incident occurred (government, construction, manufacturing, and other), type of cancer (occupational, asbestos, fire fighter, and missing), type of injury (Asbestosis, Leukemias, Lymphosarcoma and Reticulosarcoma, neoplasms and tumors, Mesothelioma, other, and unknown), region injury occurred (Halifax-East Shore-West Hants, Annapolis Valley-South Shore-South West, Colchester-East Hants-Cumberland-Pictou, Cape Breton-Guysborough-Antigonish, other, and missing), and type of body part affected (abdomen/digestive, urinary systems, body systems, respiratory system, circulatory system, head and neck, pelvic region, other, and missing). The categorization within variables was exploratory and largely dictated by the nature of the WCB records. Where appropriate categories within variables were collapsed. There were 385 occupational related cancer claims accepted by the Nova Scotia WCB. Claims were dropped from analysis if there was no cost accrued or reported by the WCB (21.0%). Overall, 304 claims with 298 men and six women were included in this study.

For the national model, we used two data-sets from the AWCBC:

1. The total annual costs of all claims and the number of time-loss claims per province/territory for the years 1996 to 2013 was obtained through the online request (http://awcbc.org/?page_id=14). Cost per

claim per province per year was calculated (not cancer specific).

2. The number of time-loss claims per province/territory per year for the years 1996 to 2013 for each injury/fatality type, including cancer was obtained through customized order. The full list of cancer types included is in Additional file 1: Appendix A2.

Disaggregated claims-level data are not available through the AWCBC.

Analysis
Regional model
Total cancer cost in Nova Scotia (TC_{NS}) included individual short term disability benefits, long term disability benefits, and medical costs. The total cost per claim was calculated as the summation of annual costs per claim discounted by inflation.

$$TC_{NS} = \sum TC_{NS,t}^{pc} * \pi_t \qquad (1)$$

Where TC_{NS} is the total cost in Nova Scotia, $TC_{NS,t}^{pc}$ is the total cost per claim in Nova Scotia in year t, and π_t is inflation in year t.

To account for inflation, we used the Consumer Price Index (CPI) base year 2014 data from Statistics Canada [20]. Assumptions about the region and composition of the CPI were required. Furthermore, assumptions about the year(s) of payout for each claimant were required, as this was missing from the data. As a result, we provide eight estimates of TC_{NS} (Table 2) for comparison of the implications of assumptions.

First, the CPI is available at the national level, and since 1979 it is also at the provincial/territorial levels. Cost calculations using provincial CPI values are therefore challenging for years prior to 1979, and the national CPI is used in those years. This is compared to cost calculations using the national CPI for all years 1957 to 2015. Second, the CPI is available for all goods and services, and it is also available specifically for goods and services related specifically to health and personal care. Estimates using both are compared. Third, for purposes of inflation adjustment, assumptions had to be made about the year in which benefits were paid to claimants. Dates of payments were not available from WCB, and dates when claims were closed were deemed unreliable,

because claims were often re-opened. We assumed that short term disability benefits were paid in full in the year the claim was filed and inflation adjustment was done in that year. Long term disability benefits are paid out over a number of years after the claim is filed, however. Two different years of payout were assumed for purposes of inflation adjustment: the first year the claim was filed, and the median year between the first and last years that the claim was open.

Regional model – determinants of total costs per cancer-related claim
The determinants of total costs per claim were assessed by estimating the associations between total costs and claim characteristics. Total cost $\left(TC_{NS}^{pc}\right)$ did not have a normal distribution and required a natural log transformation to satisfy assumptions necessary to perform linear regression. Univariate analyses, full-model multiple linear regression, and a parsimonious- multiple regression model on natural log transformed total cost were conducted. Equation [2] shows the approach used to estimate the drivers of inflation adjusted total cost per cancer claim.

$$Ln\left(TC_{NS}^{pc}\right) = \alpha + X'\beta + \varepsilon \qquad (2)$$

Where α is the intercept, X' are the claims characteristics (injury type, cancer type, body part affected, age of claimant at biopsy, industry type, region), β is a vector of estimated coefficients, and ε is the error term.

National model
The WCB benefits costs related to occupational cancer in Canada were estimated in a series of three steps: (1) regional model estimation of average cost per claim (NS WCB data); (2) estimation of provincial multipliers to capture the relative differences between Provinces (AWCBC data); and (3) estimation of annual and total costs of occupational cancer in Canada by province/territory (NS WCB and AWCBC data).

The average cost per claim in Nova Scotia was calculated using the estimates from the regional model. Equation [1] shows the approach used to estimate the average cost (AC) per claim in Nova Scotia.

Table 2 Combinations of assumptions used for inflation adjustment of costs

	CPI – national level		CPI – national level	
	CPI – all items	CPI – health and personal care	CPI – all items	CPI – Health and personal care
Year (First Year of Claim)	Cost Estimate 1	Cost Estimate 2	Cost Estimate 5	Cost Estimate 6
Year (Median Year of Claim)	Cost Estimate 3	Cost Estimate 4	Cost Estimate 7	Cost Estimate 8

$$AC_{NS}^{pc} = \frac{TC_{NS}}{n_{NS}} \tag{3}$$

Where AC_{NS}^{pc} is the average cost per claim, TC_{NS} is the total cost per claim, and n_{NS} is the number of claims in Nova Scotia. The confidence interval for the AC_{NS}^{pc} is found as follows:

$$95\% \ CI_{NS} = AC_{NS}^{pc} \pm 1.96 * \frac{\sigma_{NS}}{\sqrt{n_{NS}}}$$

Provincial multipliers introduced here are weighted indices developed to account for general differences in the WSB systems across provinces, specifically for the systemic relative differences in the costs of claims. Systemic relative differences refer to those outlined in Table 1, namely differences in the maximum compensated earnings, and the percentages of earnings considered as a basis for benefits. The multipliers are calculated using the average cost per claim in each province for all types of claims, not restricted to cancer, including short term and long term benefit costs, but not administrative costs (using AWCBC data).[1] For each province, we calculate an annual average cost per claim $AAC_{it^{pc}}$, where i is the province and t is the year. The multiplier reflects the relative size of the average cost per claim in province i in relation to Nova Scotia in each year (Eq. 4).

$$AAC_{it}^{pc} = \frac{TC_{it}}{n_{it}} \tag{4}$$

The multiplier is calculated as per equation [5], where we have designated Nova Scotia as the numeraire province:

$$M_{it} = \frac{AAC_{it}^{pc}}{AAC_{NS,t}^{pc}} \tag{5}$$

The approach that was used to estimate the average cost of time-loss claims related to occupational cancer from the perspective of the WCB per claim per province is shown in equations [6] and [7]. We assume that all claims in Canada are independent and identically distributed, and follow the same distribution as claims in Nova Scotia, with the same mean and standard deviation. To derive mean and standard deviation for province i, we adjust for the mean provincial multiplier.

$$AC_i = \overline{M_{it}} * AC_{NS} \tag{6}$$

$$\sigma_i = \overline{M_{it}} * \sigma_{NS} \tag{7}$$

This is the average cost per claim in Nova Scotia discounted by the provincial multiplier. The average cost per claim, standard deviation, and 95% confidence intervals for Canada as a whole are found as per equations [8], [9] and [10].

Table 3 Characteristics of Nova Scotia Workers' Compensation Board administrative cancer claims records from 1957–2015 ($N = 304$)

	Proportion (%)
Age at biopsy	
<=50	11.84
51–64	44.41
65+	43.75
Industry	
Government	32.24
Construction	6.25
Manufacturing	50.99
Other	10.53
Cancer type	
Occupational	49.01
Asbestos	26.97
Fire Fighter	22.70
Missing	1.32
Injury type	
Asbestosis	8.55
Leukemias	2.63
Lymphosarcoma and Reticulosarcoma	2.30
Neoplasms and Tumors	50.66
Mesothelioma	11.84
Other	14.47
Unknown	9.54
Region	
Halifax, East shore, West Hants	17.43
Annapolis Valley, South Shore, South West	1.97
Colchester-East Hants, Cumberland, Pictou	3.62
Cape Breton, Guysborough, Antigonish	35.86
Other	0.66
Missing	40.46
Body part affected	
Abdomen/Digestive	10.86
Urinary System	3.62
Body Systems	3.29
Respiratory System	55.92
Circulatory System	5.26
Circulatory SystemHead and Neck	4.93
Pelvic Region	2.96
Other	3.95
Missing	9.21

$n = 304$

$$AC_{canada} = \frac{\sum_i (AC_i * n_i)}{\sum_i n_i} \qquad (8)$$

$$\sigma_{canada} = \sqrt{\sum_i \left(\frac{n_i}{\sum_i n_i} * \sigma_i \right)^2} \qquad (9)$$

$$95\% \ CI_i = AC_i \pm t_{0.95,n_i} * \frac{\sigma_i}{\sqrt{n_i}} \qquad (10)$$

This approach to the calculation of national level costs is unique and to the best of our knowledge, has not been used in the literature.

Results

Regional model

Descriptive statistics are reported for the full set of Nova Scotia WCB administrative claims related to occupational cancer. Table 3 shows the characteristics of the 304 records from 1957 to 2015. The majority of claims (88.16%) were made at a biopsy age of over 50 years, approximately half (50.99%) were from the manufacturing sector, and claims typically came from the Nova Scotia regions of Cape Breton, Guysborough, and Antigonish. Government workers (32.24%) made a higher percentage of claims than workers in construction (6.25%) and other industries (10.53%). The public sector in Nova Scotia employs many occupations, including construction, therefore the distinction may be blurred. The most common type of occupational cancer is unspecified (49.01%), most often affects the respiratory system (55.92%) and the cancer usually manifests as neoplasms and tumours (50.66%). Asbestos exposure was the most common (26.97%) form of unspecified cancer claim.

Estimates of the total costs (TC_{NS}) and average cost per claim (AC_{NS}^{pc}) of occupational cancer in Nova Scotia are presented in Table 4. Eight estimates are presented according to the assumptions made about inflation, as discussed above (figure 1). The range of total cost

estimates was between \$36.5 million (CPI regional, health and personal care, last year) and \$44.0 million (CPI regional, all items, median year). The range of average cost per claim was between \$120,182 and \$145,807. Assumptions about the CPI influenced the estimates, but differences in estimates were not statistically significant. It is important to note that the cost estimates may change over time, because several claims are still open and continue to accrue costs.

The analysis of the determinants of the cost per claim in Nova Scotia presented here focuses on cost estimate 8, based on the regional health related CPI and using the midpoint year. Results do not appear to be sensitive to the choice of cost estimate (Additional file 1: Appendix A3). Results of unadjusted (univariate) and adjusted (multivariate) linear regression models of natural log transformed cost estimates are provided in Table 5 for both a full and a parsimonious model. The full-model included, age in years at the time of the biopsy, industry that the incident occurred, type of cancer, type of injury, region, and type of body part affected. The parsimonious model includes age at the time of the biopsy, industry that the incident occurred, and cancer type. All models indicate p-values including, $p < 0.01$, $p < 0.05$, and $p < 0.1$. All beta-coefficients are exponentiated and expressed as a percentage of the effect on total cost compared to the referent.

Overall, our results suggest that the average costs per WCB cancer claim are influenced by the age of the claimant and the cancer type being related to asbestos.

Specifically, results show that the costs of claims of individuals who were 65 years and older at time of biopsy were significantly lower compared to individuals 50 years or younger. Cost were lower by approximately 67% in the unadjusted model ($p < 0.1$), and 82% in the adjusted full model ($p < 0.01$) and 80% in the parsimonious model ($p < 0.01$). Furthermore, claims for asbestos related cancer were substantively more costly than the general unspecified occupational cancer type. Costs were higher by 363% in the unadjusted model ($p < 0.01$), 1309% higher

Table 4 Nova Scotia - total cost of all cancer claims and the average cost of cancer claims (95% confidence intervals, adjusted for inflation using combinations of three assumptions: CPI region; CPI composition; year of claim)

Cost estimate	CPI assumptions (2014 base year)			Total cost ($ '000)	Average cost ($ '000)	95% CI ($ '000)
1	National	Last Year	All Items	37 500	123	107 – 140
2			Health[b]	36 800	121	105 – 137
3		Median Year	All Items	43 100	142	122 – 162
4			Health[b]	41 400	136	117 - 155
5	Regional[a]	Last Year	All Items	37 900	125	108 – 141
6			Health[b]	36 500	120	104 – 136
7		Median Year	All Items	44 000	145	124 – 165
8			Health[b]	40 500	133	115 – 152

[a]Combination of the National CPI until 1979 and the Nova Scotia CPI in 1979 and thereafter
[b]Health and Personal Care Items

Table 5 Determinants of occupational cancer costs in Nova Scotia – cost estimate 8

	Unadjusted	Adjusted full model	Adjusted parsimonious model
Age at biopsy			
<=50	1	1	1
51–64	4.13%	−21.69%	−21.11%
65+	**−67.08%***	**−81.83%***	**−79.81%***
Industry			
Government	1	1	1
Construction	173.74%	173.22%	163.21%
Manufacturing	−0.32%	6.30%	55.19%
Other	**−71.96%***	−61.38%	−64.75%
Cancer type			
Occupational	1	1	1
Asbestos	**362.61%***	**1308.63%***	**555.68%***
Fire Fighter	94.57%	165.25%	140.73%
Missing	513.98%	619.51%	759.43%
Injury type			
Asbestosis	1	1	
Leukemias	158.78%	377.98%	
Lymphosarcoma and Reticulosarcoma	−30.25%	96.03%	
Neoplasms and Tumors	5.13%	84.67%	
Mesothelioma	82.63%	13.10%	
Other	201.89%	**620.30%**	
Unknown	−46.15%	72.77%	
Region			
Halifax, East shore, West Hants	1	1	
Annapolis Valley, South Shore, South West	114.26%	26.59%	
Colchester-East Hants, Cumberland, Pictou	−59.90%	−2.97%	
Cape Breton, Guysborough, Antigonish	−36.17%	16.88%	
Other	**−98.58%***	**−98.92%***	
Missing	**−73.96%***	−50.63%	
Body part affected			
Abdomen/Digestive	1	1	
Urinary System	126.23%	126.42%	
Body Systems	185.17%	26.36%	
Respiratory System	8.94%	2.99%	
Circulatory System	−31.00%	−52.84%	
Head and Neck	−73.36%	−74.76%	
Pelvic Region	−37.69%	−3.41%	
Other	−38.65%	−69.28%	
Missing	−63.66%	−81.03%	

Unadjusted and adjusted linear regression models were log transformed. Values shown are exponentiated to estimate the geometric mean, expressed as a percentage of change in total cost compared to the referent

Estimates are adjusted for the national (1957–1978) and Nova Scotia (1979–2015) Consumer Price Index for Health and Personal Care

Inflation was determined using year of biopsy

***$p < 0.01$, **$p < 0.05$, *$P < 0.1$

$N = 304$

Total cost: $40 500 000

The bold-face entries are highlighting those results that are statistically significant in the full adjusted model ($p < 0.01$), and 556% higher in the adjusted parsimonious model ($p < 0.01$) relative to unspecified occupational cancer claims. Costs were also influenced by injury type and region within Nova Scotia being reported as 'other'. The effects of industry type were statistically significant only in the unadjusted model, but became insignificant after adjustment for covariates. Cost did not depend on the body part affected. Cost per claim by gender was not examined because there were too few women in the sample (fewer than 10).

National model

Results of the estimation of Provincial multipliers are reported in Table 6. Multipliers show the interprovincial variation in the costs of benefits paid by Provincial WCBs across all claims, including but not limited to cancer. A multiplier lower than one indicates that the Province's WCB typically has lower benefits when compared to Nova Scotia, for example Alberta, British Columbia, Quebec, and Manitoba. A multiplier higher than one indicates that the Province's WCB typically has higher benefits when compared to Nova Scotia, for example Ontario and New Brunswick.

The burden of occupational cancer is captured in Table 7 showing the number of claims made in each Province between 1996 and 2013, as well as Canada wide. Nunavut/NWT, New Brunswick and Prince Edward Island had the lowest number of claims, and Ontario, Quebec and British Columbia had the highest number of claims.

The estimated costs of work-related cancer to the WCB system in Canada and by province are shown in Table 8. The average cost of per claim in Nova Scotia is estimated on the basis of the claims-level Nova Scotia data. The average costs per claim for other provinces are estimated using the multiplier approach (based on

Table 6 Provincial WCB multipliers

Province	Multiplier in 2013	Average multiplier (1996–2013)
Alberta	0.69	0.87
British Columbia	0.78	0.78
Manitoba	0.41	0.39
New Brunswick	0.99	1.22
Newfoundland	0.90	1.09
Nova Scotia	1.00	1.00
Nunavut/NWT	0.87	1.24
Ontario	1.03	1.50
Prince Edward Island	0.85	0.69
Quebec	0.83	0.73
Saskatchewan	0.61	0.54
Yukon	1.24	1.45

Table 7 Time-loss claims by province

Province	Number of new claims	Claims in 2013[a]
Alberta	758	83
British Columbia	1242	92
Manitoba	127	12
New Brunswick	17	5
Newfoundland	115	18
Nova Scotia	57	6
Nunavut/NWT	4	-
Ontario	3540	150
Prince Edward Island	10	-
Quebec	2314	175
Saskatchewan	28	-
Yukon	49	-
Total for Canada	8261	541

[a]Provincial reporting is not complete for 2013, some values are missing

AWCBC data). Table 8 also reports on the total cost of occupational cancer between 1996 and 2003 for each province, as well as for Canada as a whole. The total cost in Canada between 1996 and 2003 was approximately $1.2 billion, and the average cost per year was approximately $68 million.

Discussion

Our study explores the determinant of cost of cancer claims in Nova Scotia and provides insight into an area little investigated. Our estimates from the parsimonious model suggest that claims with asbestos related cancer have a fivefold increase in cost compared to unspecified occupational cancer claims. Del Bainco and Demers [8] observed that in Ontario, the number of accepted claims for occupational cancer-related deaths have increased between 1997 and 2010, and that it was most often as a result of exposure to asbestos, commonly experienced in high risk industries. Our results complement their findings, suggesting that while asbestos related cancers are becoming more commonly reported, they are also significantly more costly than other occupational cancer claims. This association is independent of the type of industry in which the claimant acquired the illness. Further investigations into the mechanisms by which asbestos exposure claim increase costs are needed.

We also find that older claimants accrue significantly (80%) lower costs than younger claimants. We have not found comparable findings in the literature. Given that long term benefits primarily reflect lost wages, the likely explanation is that many claimants over the age of 65 do not qualify for wage replacement benefits due to retirement.

Our estimates are conservative estimates of the costs of occupational cancer in Canada as faced by the WCB

Table 8 Cost of work-related cancer by province (1996 to 2013)[a]

Province	Total cost ($ '000)	95% CI of total cost ($ '000)	Average cost per year ($ '000)	95% CI of average cost per year ($ '000)	Average cost per case ($ '000)	95% CI of cost per case ($ '000)
Alberta	87,839	(80,138 – 95,539)	4,879	(3,065 – 6,695)	116	(106 – 126)
British Columbia	129,037	(120,199 – 137,874)	7,169	(5,086 – 9,252)	104	(97 – 111)
Manitoba	6,597	(5,184 – 8,010)	439	(75 – 805)	52	(41 – 63)
New Brunswick	2,763	(1,022 – 4,503)	691	(−179 – 1,561)	163	(60 – 265)
Newfoundland	16,696	(12,939 – 20,454)	1,518	(385 – 2,651)	145	(113 – 178)
Nova Scotia	40,492	(38,065 – 42,929)	4,049	(3,282 – 4,817)	133	(91 – 176)
Nunavut/NWT	660	(−469 – 1,789)	661	(−469 – 1,789)	165	(−117 – 447)
Ontario	707,281	(678,589 – 735,973)	39,293	(32,531 – 46,056)	199	(192 – 208)
Prince Edward Island	919	(122 – 1,716)	919	(122 – 1,716)	92	(12 – 172)
Quebec	225,001	(213,711 – 236,289)	12,500	(9,839 – 15,161)	97	(92 – 102)
Saskatchewan	2,014	(1,054 – 2,974)	403	(−26 – 832)	72	(38 – 106)
Yukon	9,464	(6,134 – 12,793)	3,155	(1,232 – 5,077)	193	(125 – 261)
Total for Canada	1,228,763	(1,208,669 – 1,248,856)	68,265	(63,529 – 73,001)	149	(146 – 151)

[a]Rounded to nearest 1000 Canadian dollars, including only years for which data were available. Negative confidence interval caused by small number of observations, and high variance of specific provinces, e.g. NU. There are only 1 year data for both NU and PEI, so their total cost equal average cost per year

system. Our results likely underestimate the true costs, because the data available through the AWCBC is not complete, given that it relies on provincial reporting. It is also a conservative estimate, since all claims approved by WCB have been reviewed and determined to be cancers attributed to work conditions. More cases of occupational cancer may exist, but remain unclaimed, or claims are rejected due to insufficient evidence. Discrepancies between the average 1996–2013 costs and the total costs are present, because data are not reported for all years for all provinces. Estimations are based only on reported data. For example, the average cost per year in Manitoba is based on 15 years of data, not 18.

Our estimates of the cancer burden, in terms of number of claims accepted, are relatively lower than those reported in the literature. There are three reasons. First, the AWCBC reports only time-loss claims, and does not include claims of individuals who continue to work while ill. This difference could be substantial. For example, the Nova Scotia dataset records 248 new claims between 1996 and 2013, whereas the AWCBC database records 57 time-loss claims in that same time period, i.e. only 23% of all claims were time-loss claims. Second, the number of claims filed and claims approved by the insurance is naturally lower than the number of cases of occupational cancer, since some patients do not file a claim, and some claims are not approved.

Since 1996, the Canadian WCB system has paid approximately $ 1.2 billion for work related cancer claims, at an average annual cost of approximately $66 million. Ontario faced the highest cost in total and on average, followed by Quebec, British Columbia and Alberta. This is not surprising, given that Ontario has the highest

number of approved claims, and pays the highest benefits relative to other provinces. Quebec pays relatively lower benefits, but faces a higher number of approved claims compared to Ontario.

The cost to the WCB insurer does not account for the costs to the health care system that were incurred outside of the WCB claim. Many claimants living with cancer bring their claim to the WCB after the illness has progressed and treatment has begun or has been completed. The WCB does not reimburse the public health system for the costs of care retroactively.

The cost to the WCB insurer serves as a meaningful proxy to the estimation of wage loss due to occupational cancer for workers. It does not account for wage loss due to cancer that is not work-related, nor does it account for the wage loss of family members affected. Furthermore, the payments made by the WCB have upper limits based on the maximum insurable earnings threshold and insure less than 100% of earnings (Table 1). Therefore, our national level estimate of $1.2 billion is lower than the $3 billion estimated by Hopkins et al. [18]. Similarly, our estimate for Alberta is $4.9 million, which is lower than the $64 million estimated by Orenstein et al. [19]. This is consistent with our discussion, since the other studies define productivity and wage loss to include the loss experienced by workers afflicted with cancer directly, and also indirectly through the loss experienced by others in the system, e.g. caregivers. Furthermore, Orenstein et al. rely on an attributable risk approach to estimate the proportion of cancer cases in the province that are liked to working conditions, whereas our study focuses on the number of claims made by workers and accepted by the insurer.

The limitations of our study are twofold. First, we have a relatively small number of the WCB individual claims data from Nova Scotia. Claims due to occupational cancer as a proportion of total WCB claims are less than 1% in most years. Second, the aggregate records available through the AWCBC appear to be incomplete, in particular for the Territories, Saskatchewan and Prince Edward Island, where data is not available for most of the years between 1996 and 2013.

Conclusion

We find that the Canadian WCB insurance system spends approximately $68 million on occupational cancer claims annually, and has spent approximately $1.2 billion between 1996 and 2013. The study contributes to a very limited body of literature and expands our understanding of the size and determinants of the costs of occupational cancer. The study is based on claims of lost wages laid against employers through the Canadian worker's compensation insurance system, which serve as an approximation of productivity losses with high face validity.

The need for programs to prevent occupational cancer has long been recognized in Canada [21, 22] and internationally [23]. Yet our data suggest that the number of occupational cancer claims has not been declining over the years, and neither have the costs of claims. Increased funding of for programs to prevent occupational cancer may be a best strategy to cost-savings, not to mention a reduction in the incidence of cancer.

Endnote

[1]The average cost per claim for all claims is likely to be lower than the average cost per claim for cancer claims only. Reliance on all claims in this calculation is likely to introduce bias. Our approach overestimates the costs of cancer for regions with a proportion of cancer cases higher than in Nova Scotia, and vice versa.

Acknowledgement
The authors wish to acknowledge the contribution of the Workers Compensation Board of Nova Scotia. Specifically, we would like to express our gratitude to Daniel Makhan, Kimberly Eldridge, and Michael White, who have spent many hours preparing the data, fielding data related concerns, and reviewing for accuracy. The authors take full responsibility for any and all remaining errors and omissions.

Funding
The study was funded by the Canadian Institutes for Health Research Grant number PHE 129912. The granting agency was not involved in the design of the study, data collection, analysis nor interpretation.

Authors' contributions
DW holds a PhD in Health Economist and is a health policy researcher. AM holds a Masters degree in Epidemiology and Community Health. MH is a PhD candidate in Economics. DW is the lead author responsible for the conceptualization of the study, the development of estimation methods, interpretation of results and discussion. Methods and interpretation of results were discussed face-to-face by all three authors extensively. AM and MH were responsible for the manipulation of data, estimation of results, and preparation of parts of the manuscript. DW and AM were responsible for the literature review. All authors read and approved the final manuscript.

Competing interest
The authors declare that they have no competing interests.

Author details
[1]School of Public Administration, Department of Community Health and Epidemiology, Dalhousie University, Halifax, NS, Canada. [2]Department of Community Health and Epidemiology, Dalhousie University, Halifax, NS, Canada. [3]Department of Economics, Dalhousie University, Halifax, NS, Canada.

References
1. Cancer Research UK. Worldwide cancer incidence statistics. London: Cancer Research UK; 2014. Available at: http://www.cancerresearchuk.org/cancer-info/cancerstats/world/incidence/#By. [Accessed 10 Apr 14].
2. Wranik D. Gambold L. Hanson N. Levy A. The evolution of the cancer formulary review in Canada: Can centralization improve the use of economic evaluation? Int J Health Plann Manage. 2016. doi:10.1002/hpm.2372.
3. Hurley J, Pasic D, Lavis JN. Parallel lines do intersect: Interactions between the Workers' Compensation and provincial publicly financed healthcare systems in Canada. Healthc Policy. 2008;3(4):100–12.
4. Canadian Centre for Occupational Health and Safety. http://www.ccohs.ca/oshanswers/diseases/occupational_cancer.html. Accessed 1 Nov 2016.
5. LeMasters GK, Geniady AM, Succop P, Deddens J, Sobeih T, Barriera-Viruet H, Dunning K, Lockey J. Cancer risk among firefighters: A review and meta-analysis of 32 studies. J Occup Environ Med. 2006;48(11):1189–202.
6. Clapp RW, Jacobs MM, Loechler EL. Environmental and occupational causes of cancer new evidence, 2005–2007. Res Environ Health. 2008;23(1):1–37.
7. Bofetta P. Epidemiology of environmental and occupational cancer. Oncogene. 2004;23:6392–403.
8. Del Bianco A, Demers P. Trends in compensation for deaths from occupational cancer in Canada: A descriptive study. Can Med Assoc J. 2013;1(3):91–6.
9. Labreche F, Duguay P, Boucher A, Arcand R. But other than mesothelioma? An estimate of the proportion of work-related cancers in Quebec. Curr Oncol. 2016;23(2):144–9.
10. Rushton L, Bagga S, Brown T, Cherrie J, Holmes P, Fortunato L, Slack R, Van Tongeren M, Young C, Hutchings S. Occupation and cancer in Britain. Br J Cancer. 2010;102(9):1428–37.
11. Lebeau M, Duguay P, Boucher A. Costs of occupational injuries and diseases in Quebec. J Saf Res. 2014;50:89–98.
12. Fritschi L, Driscoll T. Cancer due to occupation in Australia. Aust N Z J Public Health. 2006;30(3):213–9. doi:10.1111/j.1467-842X.2006.tb00860.x.
13. Binazzi A, Scarselli A, Marinaccio A. The burden of mortality with costs in productivity loss from occupational cancer in italy. Am J Ind Med. 2013;56(11):1272–9.
14. Lee LJ, Chang Y, Liou S, Wang J. Estimation of benefit of prevention of occupational cancer for comparative risk assessment: Methods and examples. Occup Environ Med. 2012;69(8):582–6.
15. García Gómez M, Castañeda López R, Urbanos Garrido R, López Menduiña P, Markowitz S. Medical costs of cancer attributable to work in the basque country (spain) in 2008. Gac Sanit. 2013;27(4):310–7.
16. Serrier H, Sultan-Taieb H, Luce D, Bejean S. Estimating the social cost of respiratory cancer cases attributable to occupational exposures in france. Eur J Health Econ. 2014;15(6):661–73.

17. O'Neill R, Pickvance S, Watterson A. Burying the evidence: How Great Britain is prolonging the occupational cancer epidemic. Int J Occup Environ Health. 2007;13(4):428–36.

18. Hopkins RB, Goeree R, Longo CJ. Estimating the national wage loss from cancer in Canada. Curr Oncol. 2010;17(2):40–9.

19. Orenstein MR, Dall T, Curley P, Chen J, Tamburrini AL, Petersen J. The economic burden of occupational cancers in Alberta. Calgary: Alberta Health Services; 2010.

20. Statistics Canada Tables. http://www.statcan.gc.ca/tables-tableaux/sum-som/l01/cst01/econ46a-eng.htm. Accessed 14 Oct 2015.

21. King A, Whate R. Occupational Health Clinics for Ontario Workers Inc. Preventing Occupational and Environmental Cancer. 2001. http://www1.toronto.ca/city_of_toronto/toronto_public_health/healthy_public_policy/tcpc/files/pdf/tcpc_occupational_enviro_carcinogens.pdf. Accessed 10 Oct 2015.

22. Occupational Cancer Research Centre (current website) Interventions. http://www.occupationalcancer.ca/topics/research/interventions/. Accessed 10 Oct 2015.

23. International Labour Office. Occupational Cancer Prevention and Control. 1977. http://www.ilo.org/wcmsp5/groups/public/—ed_protect/—protrav/—safework/documents/publication/wcms_236179.pdf. Accessed 10 Oct 2015.

17

Hepatocellular carcinoma after prior sorafenib treatment: incidence, healthcare utilisation and costs from German statutory health insurance claims data

Johannes Clouth[1][*] (iD), Astra M. Liepa[2], Guido Moeser[3], Heiko Friedel[4], Magdalena Bernzen[4], Jörg Trojan[5] and Elena Garal-Pantaler[4]

Abstract

Objective: To estimate both the number of patients with hepatocellular carcinoma (HCC) eligible annually for second-line therapy following sorafenib in Germany and the healthcare costs accrued by patients meeting eligibility criteria.

Methods: Patients with an HCC diagnosis and one or more sorafenib prescription were identified from samples of > 3 million insured persons in each of 2012, 2013 and 2014 using the anonymised Betriebskrankenkasse health insurance scheme database. Incidence rates from 2013 were extrapolated to the German population using data from the statutory health insurance system database and Robert Koch Institute. Resource use and cost data were collected for a subset of patients with follow-up data post-sorafenib.

Results: Between 1032 and 1484 patients with HCC in Germany (893–1390 publicly insured patients) were estimated as likely to be eligible for second-line therapy after sorafenib annually. For post-sorafenib analyses, 117 patients were identified with HCC, one or more sorafenib prescription and considered potentially eligible for second-line treatment, 15 of whom were alive after 12 months' follow-up. Total mean costs per patient accrued in the 12 months after sorafenib treatment ended were €11,152 (hospital care, €6483 [58.1%]; outpatient prescriptions, €3137 [28.1%]).

Conclusion: The estimated number of publicly insured HCC patients annually eligible for second-line therapy in Germany was < 1400 and mean total costs accrued in the year after completion of sorafenib therapy were approximately €11,000 per patient for the German statutory healthcare system. These estimates can be used when evaluating the budgetary impact of new second-line therapies for advanced HCC in Germany.

Keywords: Hepatocellular carcinoma, Germany, Second line, Sorafenib, Health economics, German statutory health insurance claims data

Background

Liver cancer is one of the most common cancers worldwide (annual incidence: 10.1 cases per 100,000), with 70.8% of cases occurring in men [1]. The prognosis of liver cancer is poor, and it is the second most common cause of cancer-related deaths worldwide [1]. Hepatocellular carcinoma (HCC) accounts for approximately 70–85% of the total liver cancer burden worldwide [2]. Around

80% of HCC cases are associated with chronic hepatitis B or C viral infections [3, 4]. However, the risk of HCC is increased in diabetic populations, particularly those with type 2 diabetes mellitus [5], as well as in patients with the metabolic syndrome who can present with non-alcoholic steatohepatitis and no cirrhosis [6, 7]. Since the metabolic syndrome is highly prevalent, even small increases in obesity- or diabetes-related risk could result in a large number of HCC cases [8]. In Germany, the age-adjusted incidence rates of liver cancer in 2012 [1] and 2013 [9], respectively, were 2.3 and 3.5 per 100,000 population in females and 7.2 and 10.3 per 100,000 population in males;

* Correspondence: johannes.clouth@gmx.de
[1]Medical Affairs, Lilly Deutschland GmbH, Werner-Reimers-Str. 2-4, 61352 Bad Homburg, Germany
Full list of author information is available at the end of the article

crude rates were 6.4 per 100,000 population in females and 15.6 per 100,000 population in males in 2013 [9]. Recent estimates of HCC incidence in Germany were not identified in the literature.

Staging of HCC is important for determining prognosis and planning therapy and includes an assessment of tumour stage, underlying liver function and clinical performance status. A number of different staging systems are used in HCC, although the Barcelona Clinic Liver Cancer (BCLC) classification is the only system that takes into account all of these factors and is endorsed for prognostic prediction and treatment allocation [10, 11]. Treatment options for HCC include surgical resection, liver transplantation and local ablation for early-stage disease, locoregional treatments (e.g. transarterial chemoembolisation and radioembolisation) for intermediate-stage disease, and systemic therapies for advanced-stage disease. Current treatment guidelines recommend that patients with advanced HCC (BCLC stage C; defined as disease with vascular invasion or metastases) should receive sorafenib [10, 12]. Best supportive care or the inclusion of patients in clinical trials after disease progression or intolerance to sorafenib is recommended [10, 12], as there are no approved second-line treatments for HCC at the time of these analyses.

In Germany, incidence and prevalence data are required to assess the potential benefits and financial impact of any new treatment according to the Act on the Reform of the Market for Medicinal Products [13]. Currently, the size of the potential population of patients with advanced HCC eligible for second-line therapy is unknown as relevant epidemiologic data are not available. Thus, the present study was performed to estimate the number of patients with advanced HCC eligible for second-line therapy annually in Germany and the healthcare costs accrued by patients with HCC eligible for second-line therapy based on data from the German statutory health system.

Methods
Study design and data source
This was a retrospective, observational study of data from the Betriebskrankenkasse (BKK) health insurance scheme in Germany over a 7-year period (2008 to 2014). The BKK includes data from insured persons registered at company health insurance funds. Although initially for employees of companies or enterprises, these funds have been open to all German citizens since 1996 and have become more representative of the entire statutory health insurance scheme. We requested and obtained access to these strictly regulated data from the BKK who had no other involvement in these analyses. After BKK approval, data from the electronic databases of six different anonymised statutory health insurance funds were

made available from central data service providers (Bitmarck Service for BitInfonet, and Bitmarck-Beratung for ISKV 21c) and participating company health insurance funds directly. These data were gathered under naturalistic conditions and anonymised by the providers in accordance with an approved data privacy concept. The raw data were then imported, prepared and checked by the authors using previously established processes.

The target patient population, i.e. patients with advanced HCC who had received sorafenib and were potentially eligible for second-line therapy, was identified. The data extracted for the present study were demographic information, utilisation of health services (e.g. hospitalisation, inpatient and outpatient care, prescriptions, sickness and other benefits) and associated costs. No ethics approval or consent to use the included information was required because of the anonymised nature of all data.

Identification of the target populations
The source sample population consisted of > 3 million insured persons in each of the study index years (2012 to 2014) and was representative of the German statutory health insurance population in terms of gender and age group distributions (Additional file 1: Table S1).

Two different approaches were used to identify target populations so that the two study objectives could be met. The first approach identified all patients with advanced HCC potentially eligible for second-line therapy during the analysis period. The second approach identified patients with the required follow-up data to allow estimation of healthcare costs accrued by patients with HCC eligible for second-line therapy. The details are shown in the study flowchart (Fig. 1), with the two methodological approaches indicated with orange and blue arrows.

First, to estimate the number of patients with advanced HCC eligible for second-line therapy after sorafenib (Fig. 1, orange arrows), patients with a diagnosis of liver cancer, and HCC in particular, were identified using the *International Classification of Diseases and Related Health Problems, tenth revision* (ICD-10) codes C22 and C22.0, respectively, every year from 2012 to 2014 (each was considered an index year). Diagnoses made in the inpatient and/or ambulatory care setting were permitted. Inpatients with HCC were identified using primary or secondary inpatient C22.0 diagnoses, whereas outpatients with HCC were identified using the 'assured' (gesichert) and 'status after' ("Zustand nach") C22.0 diagnosis. Patients who had no relevant ICD-10 diagnosis during 1 year preceding the index year were considered incident in the corresponding index year. Patients younger than 18 years (in the corresponding index year) and those who had undergone liver transplantation at any time over the study period were excluded. Patients with a diagnosis of HCC together with at least one prescription for sorafenib in

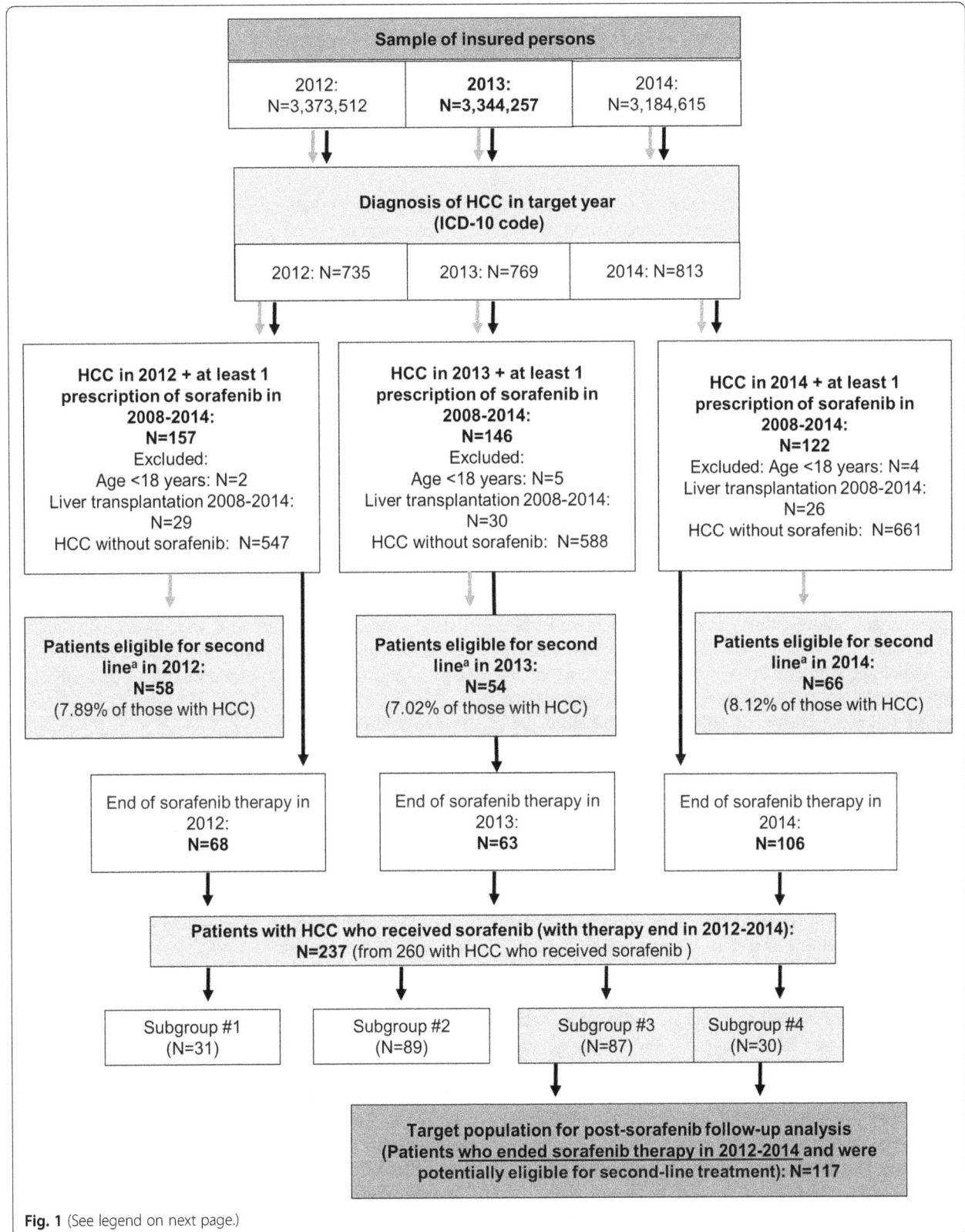

Fig. 1 (See legend on next page.)

(See figure on previous page.)
Fig. 1 Flowchart of HCC patient selection for epidemiological analysis and post-sorafenib follow-up analysis. Subgroup #1: patients still alive at the end of the observation period but with fewer than 70 observation days from the last sorafenib prescription; Subgroup #2: patients who died while on sorafenib therapy; Subgroup #3: patients who died within the observation period but not under sorafenib therapy (i.e. more than 70 days between the last sorafenib prescription and death); Subgroup #4: patients who were still alive at the end of the observation period and for whom at least 70 days had passed between the last prescription of sorafenib and the end of the observation period. [a]Patients alive after sorafenib therapy end/failure. *HCC* hepatocellular carcinoma, *ICD-10* International Classification of Diseases and Related Health Problems, tenth revision

each index year were then identified. Sorafenib prescriptions were identified using ATC code L01XE05 for outpatient prescriptions and OPS codes 6–003.b* for inpatient treatment. Patients who were alive after the end of sorafenib therapy for each index year were considered to be the target population, i.e. patients with advanced HCC previously treated with sorafenib who were eligible for second-line therapy.

To obtain a population with sufficient follow-up data post-sorafenib therapy for determination of healthcare costs (Fig. 1, blue arrows), we identified patients with a diagnosis of HCC who had received at least one prescription for sorafenib and who had ended sorafenib therapy in the timeframe 2012 to 2014. No maximum end date for sorafenib therapy in 2014 was designated, acknowledging that some patients may have less follow-up data. Clinically accepted markers for identifying treatment failure either could not be identified from the database because of missing or unspecific coding (i.e. radiologic findings or symptomatic progression) or were thought to be unreliable (i.e. discontinuation of therapy following treatment failure). We therefore performed a series of exploratory analyses to identify the target group of patients who had failed sorafenib therapy and who were possible candidates for second-line therapy (Additional file 2). An explorative approach was used that combined potentially distinguishing markers to detect failure of first-line therapy. Markers considered were the frequency and duration of sorafenib prescriptions, the pattern of sorafenib prescriptions (i.e. full dose, dose reductions and dose interruptions), observation time and adverse events. The data were stratified to examine potential influences of, and differences between, these markers and to find an adequate definition of treatment failure. From these analyses, the following four subgroups were identified:

- Subgroup #1: Patients still alive at the end of the observation period (31 December 2014) and with fewer than 70 observation days (allowing for a 56-day intake of a reduced dosage [two tablets daily instead of four tablets daily as is recommended [14]] plus 14 days of follow-up) from the last sorafenib prescription.
- Subgroup #2: Patients who died while on sorafenib therapy.

- Subgroup #3: Patients who died within the observation period (i.e. before 31 December 2014) and no longer received sorafenib therapy (i.e. more than 70 days of follow-up between the last sorafenib prescription and death).
- Subgroup #4: Patients who were still alive at the end of the observation period (31 December 2014) and for whom at least 70 days of follow-up had passed between the last prescription of sorafenib and the end of the observation period.

Patients in subgroup #1 had insufficient follow-up to allow meaningful analysis. Patients in subgroup #2 died while on sorafenib treatment and could not have received a second-line agent. Therefore, subgroups #1 and #2 were not considered for further analysis. Patients in subgroups #3 and #4 were considered to have failed first-line sorafenib therapy and were potentially eligible for second-line treatment and therefore constituted the target population for post-sorafenib follow-up analysis.

Data collection
Data from the target population for post-sorafenib follow-up analysis were examined retrospectively for up to 4 years from the first prescription of sorafenib to identify pre-existing and concomitant conditions diagnosed in the inpatient and/or outpatient settings, and especially risk factors for HCC (e.g. cirrhosis of the liver, hepatitis B and C). Treatments received prior to initiation of sorafenib therapy in inpatient and/or outpatient care were also captured.

Starting from the end of sorafenib therapy (defined as last prescription + 56 days) and until 31 December 2014 or death, resource use (i.e. hospital stays and care, including ambulatory treatments; outpatient visits; outpatient prescriptions; work disability; remedies; and other benefits) and associated cost data were gathered for the target population. Cost data were for all healthcare utilisations classified into the listed resource use categories that had been refunded or paid by the sickness funds. A so called "Orientierungspunktwert" (reference point value) according to the Uniform Evaluation Scale catalogue, also known as EBM (Einheitlicher Bewertungsmaßstab), was used for monetarisation of patient-physician contacts in outpatient care. Survival data from the last sorafenib prescription were also collected.

Data analysis

Crude incidence and prevalence rates of HCC for 2013 in Germany were estimated using data from two different sources:

(i) German statutory health insurance system database (Gesetzliche Krankenversicherung [GKV]) (2013) and
(ii) Robert Koch Institute (2013) [9, 15].

Calculations were based on the annual number of HCC diagnoses reported for the stated year. The crude incidence rate of HCC was calculated as the number of new disease diagnoses/sample population × 100,000 [16].

To calculate the crude incidence rate for the GKV, the study sample population (BKK) estimates underwent age- and gender-adjusted extrapolation to the total GKV population using published methods [17].

The Robert Koch Institute reported only diagnoses of liver cancer (C22). Therefore, the number of HCC cases reported by the Robert Koch Institute was estimated using two sources: the first based on the Robert Koch Institute report that 66% of liver cancers in Germany are HCC [15] and the second based on a published paper that reported a value of 80% [18]. Numbers for the total population in Germany, used for estimating crude incidence rates, were as stated by the German Federal Statistical Office/eurostat [19, 20].

The mean (standard deviation; 95% confidence interval [CI]) proportion of patients in the BKK with HCC eligible for second-line treatment from each of the index years (2012 to 2014) was calculated and then applied to the estimated populations of patients with HCC in Germany as identified from the two sources mentioned above.

Resources and costs were analysed from the perspective of the German statutory healthcare system (i.e. public healthcare provider). Mean real (unweighted) estimates of resource use and costs were calculated for the target population for each type of resource for the first year after the end of sorafenib therapy. Data from all eligible insured patients were included, independent of individual length of follow-up i.e., the yearly costs of the target population were evaluated from the payer perspective. Utilisation of inpatient care was measured from the documented admission date and included ambulatory and hospital treatments. All costs were expressed in euros, using the values recorded without correction.

Results

Incidence and prevalence

The numbers of patients with diagnoses of HCC in our study population in 2012 to 2014 are shown in Fig. 1 (orange arrows); 769 such diagnoses were recorded in 2013. The estimated crude incidence and prevalence rates of HCC for the present sample population in 2013

and the total GVK in 2013, as well as crude estimates for the German population based on data from the Robert Koch Institute, are shown in Table 1 [9].

The mean (standard deviation; 95% CI) proportion of the study population with HCC that was eligible for second-line therapy, based on findings from 2012 to 2014, was 7.68% (0.58; 7.02–8.33). Extrapolating this to the total German population, we estimated that, annually, between 1171 and 1390 patients with HCC were potentially eligible for second-line therapy based on the statutory health system (GKV) data, and between 1032 and 1484 patients were eligible based on Robert Koch Institute data (Table 1). As 86.5% of the population in Germany is covered by public health insurance [19–21], the Robert Koch Institute value would decrease to between 893 and 1284 for publicly insured patients.

Post-sorafenib follow-up analysis
Target population

For the post-sorafenib follow-up analysis, we identified 237 patients with a diagnosis of HCC who had received at least one prescription for sorafenib and who had ended sorafenib therapy in the timeframe 2012 to 2014 (Fig. 1; blue arrows). Of these 237 patients, 31 were in Subgroup #1 and 89 were in Subgroup #2; these patients were not considered further. The target population for post-sorafenib follow-up analysis was the remaining 117 patients in subgroups #3 ($n = 87$) and #4 ($n = 30$) who were considered to have failed first-line sorafenib therapy and were potentially eligible for second-line treatment. The baseline characteristics, comorbidities (including diagnoses of conditions considered to be risk factors) and pre-existing medications of these 117 patients are shown in Table 2.

The mean (standard deviation) duration of follow-up of the target population was 170.4 (202.8) days (median 90 days, range 15–1043); 15 patients were still alive after 12 months of follow-up.

Resource utilisation and costs

A summary of mean resource use and costs for the 12 months after the end of sorafenib treatment for the target population is presented in Table 3. Mean costs accrued by month in the target population are shown in Fig. 2.

In the target population, mean total costs in the 12 months after the end of sorafenib therapy were €11,152 per patient. Hospital care and outpatient prescriptions were the two highest contributing cost groups to the total, accounting for 58.1% (€6483) and 28.1% (€3137) of the total mean costs per patient over the 12-month period, respectively. Mean hospital care costs were also among the highest contributing cost groups for subgroups #3 and #4 when analysed separately, accounting for 68.7% of total mean costs per patient

Table 1 Estimated incidence and prevalence data for HCC in Germany in 2013

Population/parameter	Total
Study sample population (insured for ≥1 day in 2013)	3,344,257
New HCC diagnoses	407
Crude HCC incidence (per 100,000)	12.17
HCC diagnoses (throughout 2013)	769
Crude HCC prevalence (per 100,000)	22.99
Proportion of population with HCC eligible for second-line therapy, mean % (95% CI)[a]	7.68% (7.02–8.33)
German statutory health system population (at 1 July 2013)	69,854,922
New HCC diagnoses (extrapolated incidence)[b]	8841
Crude HCC incidence (extrapolated) (per 100,000)[b]	12.66
HCC diagnoses (extrapolated throughout 2013)	16,685
Crude HCC prevalence (extrapolated) (per 100,000)[b]	23.89
Number eligible for second-line therapy, low–high limit[c]	1171–1390
Germany – RKI (2013)	
New HCC diagnoses[d]	5801–7032
Crude HCC incidence (per 100,000)[e]	7.18–8.71
HCC diagnoses (estimated throughout 2013)[f]	14,697–17,814
Crude HCC prevalence (estimated throughout 2013) (per 100,000)[f]	18.20–22.06
Number eligible for second-line therapy, low–high limit[g]	1032–1484

C22 International Classification of Diseases, tenth revision code for liver cancer, *CI* confidence interval, *HCC* hepatocellular carcinoma, *RKI* Robert Koch Institute
[a]Mean of estimates for 2012 (7.89% [58/735]), 2013 (7.02% [54/769]) and 2014 (8.12% [66/813])
[b]Patients with a diagnosis of HCC in 2013, extrapolated from the German Betriebskrankenkasse (BKK) health insurance scheme data (present study sample), age- and gender-adjusted to the entire German statutory health insurance system
[c]Based on 95% CI for study sample estimate (i.e. 7.02–8.33)
[d]Assumes that HCC accounts for 66–80% of total liver cancer burden (RKI estimate [15] – reported value in literature [18]) and based on total number of new liver cancer cases reported in 2013 by the RKI (male: 6160; female: 2630)
[e]Calculated using number of new HCC cases estimated to be reported in 2013 by the RKI [9] as a proportion of the German population reported by the German Federal statistical office/eurostat [19, 20] in 2013 (N = 80,767,463)
[f]Prevalence of insured patients with C22 diagnosis was the sum of 5-year prevalence in 2012 (n = 10,800) and incidence in 2013 (n = 8790) = 19,590. Since the 10-year prevalence of C22 reported in 2013 (n = 14,990) exceeded the 5-year prevalence for the same year (n = 12,010) by 1.248 times, this factor (1.248) was used to estimate 10-year prevalence in 2012 and correct calculations as follows: NC22 in Germany = (10,800 × 1.248 = 13,478) + 8790 = 22,268 individuals with C22 diagnosis in the course of 2013. Corrections to estimate HCC prevalence were based on the assumption that HCC accounts for 66–80% of total liver cancer burden (RKI estimate – reported value in literature [18])
[g]Assumes that HCC accounts for 66–80% of the total liver cancer burden (RKI estimate – reported value in literature [18]) and 95% CI for study sample estimates (i.e., 7.02–8.33)

(€6556; $n = 87$) in subgroup #3 and 39.6% of the total mean costs per patient (total costs €6272; $n = 30$) in subgroup #4 over the 12-month period. Mean costs of prescriptions accounted for 50.7% (€8026) of the total costs per patient in subgroup #4 but only for 15.2% (€1452) in subgroup #3 over the 12-month period.

Monthly mean total costs for both subgroups generally declined over time during the first 12 months after the end of sorafenib treatment, with some spikes in cost observed at arbitrary months (Fig. 2). When examining subgroup #4 in more detail ($n = 30$), as this subgroup had longer follow-up data available, there was a general downward trend over time following sorafenib treatment that was reflected in all areas of the statutory health system. Mean monthly costs of hospital care per patient were €2044.89 in the first month and fluctuated between €8 and €3051 in the first 12 months; the costs for appointments with physicians in the outpatient setting were €121 in the first month and declined to €66 in month 12. Similarly, the mean number of monthly prescriptions per patient was 4.20, costing €1412 in the first month, and 4.50 prescriptions, costing €226, at month 12. No costs relating to sick pay and inability to work were reported.

Discussion

In the present study, we used data from two different sources to estimate the incidence and prevalence of HCC in Germany. Using the statutory health system database, which includes a sample of publically insured persons in Germany, the estimated annual crude incidence rate of HCC for 2013 was 12.17 per 100,000, whereas the annual crude incidence using relevant data from the Robert Koch Institute ranged from 7.18 to 8.71 per 100,000. The higher incidence rate in the statutory health system population as compared with the Robert Koch Institute estimates may be due in part to the predominantly urban population in the former sample, a trend noted in other reports of liver cancer incidence rates in rural and urban populations from Germany [22, 23]. In addition, we cannot be certain that we identified only incident cases of HCC in our analysis; however, we believe that a one-year period is sufficient to exclude patients with ongoing disease given the high mortality of this cancer. Differences in prevalence rates (23.89 per 100,000 in the GKV vs 12.25–14.85 per 100,000 in the Robert Koch Institute data [value directly calculated based on the Robert Koch Institute 10-year prevalence of liver cancer for 2013]) could have been because the statutory health system data are based on claims data and do not consider mortality, whereas the prevalence data from the Robert Koch Institute considered the patients who survived until 31 December 2013. Recalculating the Robert Koch Institute prevalence estimate considering all HCC cases over the course of 2013 resulted in a prevalence rate of

Table 2 Available patient and disease characteristics for patients with HCC potentially eligible for second-line therapy

	Subgroups #3 and #4	Subgroup #3[a]	Subgroup #4[b]
N	117	87	30
Sex, n (%)			
Men	100 (85)	75 (86)	25 (83)
Women	17 (15)	12 (14)	5 (17)
Age, years			
Mean	71.87	71.52	72.90
Pre-existing confirmed diagnoses (ICD code)[c], n (%)			
Hypertension (I10.x)	96 (83)	70 (81)	26 (53)
Diabetes mellitus (E11, E14)	66 (56)	50 (58)	16 (53)
Liver cirrhosis (K74.3, K74.4, K74.5, K74.6, K70.3, K71.7, P78.8)	62 (53)	45 (52)	17 (57)
Liver cirrhosis and fibrosis (K74.x)	57 (49)	41 (47)	16 (53)
Other liver diseases (K76.x)	46 (39)	30 (26)	16 (53)
Disorders of lipoprotein metabolism and other lipidaemias (E78.x)	51 (44)	35 (40)	16 (53)
Disorders of refraction and accommodation (H52.x)	46 (39)	31 (36)	15 (50)
Obesity (E66.x)	39 (33)	26 (30)	13 (43)
Dorsalgia (M54.x)	37 (32)	28 (32)	9 (23)
Gastritis and duodenitis (K29.x)	35 (30)	28 (32)	7 (23)
Chronic ischemic heart disease (I25.x)	36 (31)	26 (30)	10 (33)
Disorders of purine and pyrimidine metabolism (E79.x)	32 (27)	24 (28)	8 (27)
Cataract (H25.x)	26 (22)	19 (22)	7 (23)
Pre-existing medications (ATC code)[c], n (%)			
β-blocking agents (C07A)	69 (59)	54 (62)	15 (50)
Loop diuretics (C03C)	45 (38)	36 (41)	9 (30)
ACE inhibitors, plain (not in combination) (C09A)	45 (38)	31 (36)	14 (47)
Lipid-modifying agents, plain (C10A)	33 (28)	21 (24)	12 (40)
Antithrombotic agents (B01A)	33 (28)	24 (28)	9 (30)
Agents for peptic ulcer and gastro-oesophageal reflux disease (A02B)	64 (55)	46 (53)	18 (60)
Anti-inflammatory and antirheumatic products, non-steroids (M01A)[d]	42 (36)	31 (36)	11 (37)
Other analgesics and antipyretics (N02B)	35 (30)	26 (30)	9 (30)
Opioids (N02A)	17 (15)	15 (17)	2 (7)
Antibacterials for systemic use (J01)[e]	41 (35)	30 (34)	11 (37)
Diagnostic agents (V04B, V04C)	33 (28)	25 (29)	8 (27)
Anti-gout preparations (M04A)	31 (26)	23 (26)	8 (27)
Antidiabetes medications, excl. insulins (A10B)	29 (25)	22 (25)	7 (23)
Patients who received chemotherapy prescriptions[f] (L01)	2 (2)	1 (1)	1 (3)
Mean duration of sorafenib therapy, days		223.6	230.0
Standard deviation		307.3	376.0
Range		28–1630	28–1972

ACE angiotensin-converting enzyme, *ATC* anatomical therapeutic chemical, *ICD* International Classification of Diseases

[a]Patients who died during the observation period but not on sorafenib therapy (i.e. more than 70 days between the last sorafenib prescription and death)

[b]Patients who were still alive at the end of the observation period and at least 70 days had passed between the last prescription of sorafenib and the end of the observation period

[c]During the year prior to sorafenib therapy (diagnoses during the quarter in which patients were identified were not included but those of prior quarters were); reported by at least 20% of patients in at least two of the three groups (study population, subgroup #3, subgroup #4), with the exception of opioids, which were an important contributor to the analgesic category

[d]Value may be underestimated because many of these medications are available without prescription (i.e. over the counter)

[e]Patients may have received more than one cycle of treatment with antibiotics

[f]During the year prior to sorafenib therapy

Table 3 Resource use and costs for patients with HCC potentially eligible for second-line therapy[a]

Variable	Subgroup #3[b] [n = 87]		Subgroup #4[c] [n = 30]		Subgroup #3 and #4 [n = 117]	
	Utilisation, n (SD)	Cost per patient (€)	Utilisation, n (SD)	Cost per patient (€)	Utilisation, n (SD)	Cost per patient (€)
Hospital care[d]	1.86 (2.37)	6556.25	1.30 (1.58)	6271.95	1.72 (2.20)	6483.36
Outpatient visits	19.05 (19.43)	862.54	26.77 (23.11)	789.69	21.03 (20.61)	843.86
Outpatient prescriptions	24.94 (24.41)	1451.77	27.90 (27.56)	8025.81	25.70 (25.17)	3137.42
Other benefits[e]	5.60 (6.75)	671.12	5.37 (11.12)	730.96	5.54 (8.04)	686.46
Remedies	0.03 (0.18)	0.64	0.00 (0.00)	0.00	0.03 (0.16)	0.48
Total	–	9542.32	–	15,818.41	–	11,151.58

Data are presented as mean (standard deviation, SD) values

HCC hepatocellular carcinoma

[a]Resource utilisation and costs in the 12 months after the end of sorafenib treatment

[b]Patients who died within the observation period but not under sorafenib therapy (i.e. more than 70 days between the last sorafenib prescription and death)

[c]Patients who were still alive at the end of the observation period and at least 70 days passed between the last prescription of sorafenib and the end of the observation period

[d]Costs include all hospital-related costs – admissions and ambulatory treatments in hospital

[e]Additional benefits paid by the German statutory health insurance (e.g. statutory pension fund benefits, therapeutic appliances, travelling costs, nursing care benefits, home healthcare)

18.20–22.06 per 100,000 (Table 1), which is much closer to the GKV estimation. We further applied these data to estimate the number of patients in Germany with advanced HCC likely to be candidates for second-line therapy after prior sorafenib treatment. From a payer's perspective in Germany, we estimated this number to range between 893 and 1390 patients per year based on the GKV and Robert Koch Institute data.

Epidemiological data from the present study also allowed us to characterise patients with advanced HCC likely to be candidates for second-line therapy after prior sorafenib. Of the 117 patients identified in our study with sufficient data for the follow-up analysis, most were

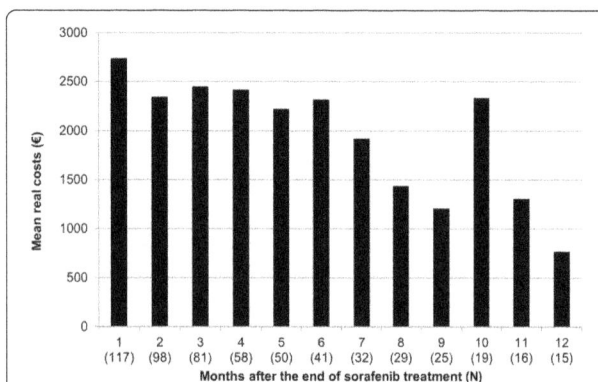

Fig. 2 Monthly costs[a] for patients with HCC previously treated with sorafenib (subgroups #3[b] and #4[c]). [a]At values reported for each index year 2012 to 2014; all patients who were insured for at least one day in the corresponding month contributed to costs. [b]Patients who died within the observation period but not under sorafenib therapy (i.e. more than 70 days between the last sorafenib prescription and death). [c]Patients who were still alive at the end of the observation period and for whom at least 70 days had passed between the last prescription of sorafenib and the end of the observation period. HCC hepatocellular carcinoma

men (85%), with a mean age of 72 years. Of the potential risk factors for HCC, liver cirrhosis (53.0%), often with accompanying fibrosis, and diabetes mellitus (56.4%) were observed most commonly; obesity and other metabolic disorders were also documented. The high prevalence of non-insulin-dependent diabetes in our population is consistent with systematic reviews and meta-analyses, which have reported that diabetes is associated with an increased risk of HCC [5, 24].

The German statutory health system included detailed real-life cost data, which allowed us to estimate costs for the target population from the perspective of the public healthcare provider. The mean total estimated healthcare costs accrued by the target population in the first year after sorafenib were €11,152 per patient. Mean monthly costs generally decreased over this time, which suggests that patients received more treatments and healthcare in the first few months following sorafenib therapy. For patients who were still alive at the end of the observation period (subgroup #4), mean total costs per patient for the first year after sorafenib discontinuation were €15,818, which were accounted for mainly by inpatient care (hospital stays) (€6272) and prescriptions (€8026). In patients who died during the observation period (subgroup #3) and likely were alive for a shorter period than patients in subgroup #4, total costs over the same timeframe were predictably lower (€9542), with inpatient care (€6556) accounting for most of the total. No costs relating to sick pay or inability to work were reported, possibly because most patients were retired and would have been receiving pension funds.

At the time of these analyses, no second-line therapies were approved for patients with HCC, representing an unmet need for patients who progress on sorafenib treatment. However, based on positive trial results, regorafenib (RESORCE trial [25]) was approved in both Europe and the USA in 2017, and nivolumab (Check-Mate-040 trial [26]) was approved in the USA in 2017, for the second-line treatment of patients with HCC who had previously received sorafenib. In addition, a survival benefit versus placebo has been reported for ramucirumab following first-line treatment with sorafenib in patients with advanced HCC and elevated baseline alpha-fetoprotein levels (REACH-2 [27]) and for cabozantinib in patients with advanced HCC previously treated with sorafenib (CELESTIAL [28]). All studies evaluating potential second-line therapies had stringent inclusion criteria regarding adequate organ function, including liver function, and performance status. In the RESORCE trial, patients were also required to have documented radiographic progression and to have tolerated sorafenib [25]. These criteria, if applied in clinical practice, would likely limit the target population for second-line treatment.

Limitations

The present study had several limitations, including the retrospective nature of the study design, the relatively small study sample and the limited medical information available from the database (e.g. information was not available on disease staging or treatment failure). For this reason, we needed to use an explorative approach to identify potential candidates for second-line therapy from the overall study population. In addition, data were not available concerning the status of patients with respect to their performance status and organ functioning. Because potential second-line therapies have only been evaluated in patients for whom these clinical factors were adequate, the numbers of patients eligible for post-sorafenib therapy may be lower than estimated. Our study sample was derived from the BKK health insurance scheme and included > 3 million persons insured with company health insurance in each index year. Although our source sample (the BKK database) was only ~ 5% of the total statutory healthcare population in Germany in 2013, basic demographic data suggested it was representative of the total insured population. Cost estimates may have had a slight downward bias because of incomplete coverage of services and incomplete cost data for ambulatory care. However, only about 5% of treatments charged in ambulatory care could not be linked with costs. A lack of more specific data meant we assumed sorafenib was used as first-line treatment, even though it appears cytotoxic chemotherapy was given instead in a few cases (2%).

Conclusion

From a payer's perspective in Germany, we estimate that approximately 893–1390 publicly insured patients with advanced HCC are potential candidates for second-line

post-sorafenib therapy annually. The estimated total healthcare costs for this patient group are approximately €9500–16,000 per patient in the first year after completing sorafenib treatment. Hospital stays are the main contributing factor to these costs. These estimated costs will help decision makers determine the potential budgetary impact of new second-line therapies for advanced HCC.

Abbreviations
ACE: Angiotensin-converting enzyme; ATC: Anatomical therapeutic chemical; BCLC: Barcelona Clinic Liver Cancer; BKK: Betriebskrankenkasse; CI: Confidence interval; GKV: Gesetzliche Krankenversicherung; HCC: Hepatocellular carcinoma; ICD-10: *International Classification of Diseases and Related Health Problems, tenth revision*; SD: Standard deviation

Acknowledgements
Raw anonymised data for these analyses were obtained from the German Betriebskrankenkasse (BKK) health insurance scheme.
The authors would like to acknowledge Rx Communications (Mold, UK) for medical writing assistance with the preparation of this article, funded by Eli Lilly and Company.

Funding
This work was supported by Eli Lilly and Company, who played a role in the design of the study; collection, analysis and interpretation of the data; and preparation, review, and approval of the manuscript.

Authors' contributions
JC, AML, GM and HF were involved in the conception and design of the work. JC, HF, MB and EG-P were involved in the acquisition of data for the work, and MB and EG-P analysed the data. JC, AML and JT interpreted the data for the work. All authors critically revised the manuscript for important intellectual content. All authors read and approved the final manuscript.

Competing interests
Johannes Clouth and Astra M Liepa are employees and stockholders of Eli Lilly and Company. Jörg Trojan has received consulting fees from Eli Lilly and Company, Bayer HealthCare and Bristol-Myers Squibb. Guido Moeser works for masem research institute GmbH, which received consulting fees from Eli Lilly and Company as well as from other healthcare companies. Heiko Friedel was responsible for the analysis and was paid by Eli Lilly and Company. Elena Garal-Pantaler and Magdalena Bernzen performed the analyses and were paid by Eli Lilly and Company.

Author details
[1]Medical Affairs, Lilly Deutschland GmbH, Werner-Reimers-Str. 2-4, 61352 Bad Homburg, Germany. [2]Eli Lilly and Company, Lilly Corporate Center, Indianapolis, IN 46285, USA. [3]masem Research Institute GmbH, Unter den Eichen 5/G, D-65195 Wiesbaden, Germany. [4]Team Gesundheit GmbH, Rellinghauser Straße 93, 45128 Essen, Germany. [5]Universitätsklinikum Frankfurt, Medizinische Klinik 1, Theodor-Stern-Kai 7, 60590 Frankfurt, Germany.

References

1. GLOBOCAN fact sheets. International Agency for Research on Cancer. 2012. http://globocan.iarc.fr/Pages/fact_sheets_cancer.aspx. Accessed June 2014.

2. International Agency for Research on Cancer (IARC). Pathology and genetics of tumours of the digestive system. In: Hamilton SR, Aaltonen LA, editors. World Health Organisation Classification of Tumours. Lyon: IARC Press; 2000. http://publications.iarc.fr/_publications/media/download/1434/ba29d0c2989141bdd262de18f557c0a402a965df.pdf.

3. Perz JF, Armstrong GL, Farrington LA, et al. The contributions of hepatitis B virus and hepatitis C virus infections to cirrhosis and primary liver cancer worldwide. J Hepatol. 2006;45:529–38.

4. El-Serag HB. Epidemiology of viral hepatitis and hepatocellular carcinoma. Gastroenterology. 2012;42:1264–73. e1

5. El-Serag HB, Hampel H, Javadi F. The association between diabetes and hepatocellular carcinoma: a systematic review of epidemiologic evidence. Clin Gastroenterol Hepatol. 2006;4:369–80.

6. Ertle J, Dechêne A, Sowa J-P, et al. Non-alcoholic fatty liver disease progresses to hepatocellular carcinoma in the absence of apparent cirrhosis. Int J Cancer. 2011;128:2436–43.

7. Paradis V, Zalinski S, Chelbi E, et al. Hepatocellular carcinomas in patients with metabolic syndrome often develop without significant liver fibrosis: a pathological analysis. Hepatology. 2009;49:851–9.

8. El-Serag HB. Hepatocellular carcinoma. N Engl J Med. 2011;365:1118–27.

9. Bericht zum Krebsgeschehen in Deutschland 2016. Berlin: Robert Koch Institut; 2016. http://www.krebsdaten.de/Krebs/DE/Content/Publikationen/Krebsgeschehen/Krebsgeschehen_download.pdf?__blob=publicationFile. Accessed May 2017.

10. European Association for the Study of the Liver, European Organisation for Research and Treatment of Cancer. EASL–EORTC clinical practice guidelines: management of hepatocellular carcinoma. J Hepatol. 2012;56:908–43.

11. Bruix J, Sherman M, American Association for the Study of Liver Diseases. Management of hepatocellular carcinoma: an update. Hepatology. 2011;53:1020–2.

12. Verslype C, Rosmorduc O, Rougier P, ESMO Guidelines Working Group. Hepatocellular carcinoma: ESMO-ESDO clinical practice guidelines for diagnosis, treatment and follow-up. Ann Oncol. 2012;23(Suppl 7):vii41–8.

13. Federal Ministry of Health. The act on the reform of the market for medicinal products (Gesetz zur Neuordnung des Arzneimittelmarktes). 2011. https://www.bundesgesundheitsministerium.de/?id=1017. Accessed June 2014.

14. Bayer Pharma AG. Nexavar. Summary of product characteristics. http://www.ema.europa.eu/docs/en_GB/document_library/EPAR_-_Product_Information/human/000690/WC500027704.pdf. Accessed Jul 2017.

15. Robert Koch Institut und der Gesellschaft der epidemiologischen Krebsregister in Deutschland e. V. Krebs in Deutschland 2011/2012. Berlin: Robert Koch-Institut; 10 Ausgabe, 2015.http://www.gekid.de/Doc/krebs_in_deutschland_2015.pdf. Accessed Mar 2017.

16. Bonita R, Beaglehole R, Kjellström T. Basic epidemiology. 2nd ed. Geneva: World Health Organisation; 2006.

17. Friedel H, Clouth J, Brück P, Nicolay C, Garal-Pantaler E, Moeser G, Liepa AM, Taipale KL, Kiiskinen U. A retrospective observational study of the epidemiology of advanced gastric cancer in Germany. An analysis of health insurance data from a central database. Gesundh Ökon Qual Manag. 2015; 20:108–13.

18. Marquardt JU, Andersen JB, Thorgeirsson SS. Functional and genetic deconstruction of the cellular origin in liver cancer. Nat Rev Cancer. 2015;15: 653–67. https://doi.org/10.1038/nrc4017.

19. Destatis Statistisches Bundesamt. Population based on the 2011 census https://www.destatis.de/EN/FactsFigures/SocietyState/Population/CurrentPopulation/Tables/Census_SexAndCitizenship.html. Accessed Jul 2017.

20. eurostat. Bevolkerung am 1. Januar http://ec.europa.eu/eurostat/tgm/table.do?tab=table&init=1&language=de&pcode=tps00001&plugin=1. Accessed Jul 2017.

21. Federal Health Reporting – joint service by RKI and destatis. Number of members and jointly insured family members of the statutory health insurance on July 1st of the respective year. http://www.gbe-bund.de/oowa921-install/servlet/oowa/aw92/dboowasys921.xwdevkit/xwd_init?gbe.isgbetol/xs_start_neu/&p_aid=3&p_aid=30570531&nummer=249&p_sprache=D&p_indsp=-&p_aid=31712643. Accessed Aug 2017.

22. Muir CS, Waterhouse J, Mack T, Powell J, Whelan SL. Cancer incidence in five continents volume V. IARC scientific publication no. 88. Lyon: IARC; 1987.

23. Parkin DM, Muir CS, Whelan SL, Gao YT, Ferlay J, Powell J. Cancer incidence in five continents volume VI. IARC scientific publication no. 120. Lyon: IARC; 1992.

24. Wang P, Kang D, Cao W, et al. Diabetes mellitus and risk of hepatocellular carcinoma: a systematic review and meta-analysis. Diabetes Metab Res Rev. 2012;28:109–22.

25. Bruix J, Qin S, Merle P, et al. RESORCE investigators. Regorafenib for patients with hepatocellular carcinoma who progressed on sorafenib treatment (RESORCE): a randomised, double-blind, placebo-controlled, phase 3 trial. Lancet. 2017;389:56–66.

26. El-Khoueiry AB, Sangro B, Yau T, et al. Nivolumab in patients with advanced hepatocellular carcinoma (CheckMate 040): an open-label, non-comparative, phase 1/2 dose escalation and expansion trial. Lancet. 2017;389:2492–502.

27. Zhu AX, Kang Y-K, Yen C-J, et al. REACH-2: A randomized, double-blind, placebo-controlled phase 3 study of ramucirumab versus placebo as second-line treatment in patients with advanced hepatocellular carcinoma (HCC) and elevated baseline alpha-fetoprotein (AFP) following first-line sorafenib. J Clin Oncol. 2018;36(suppl 15):4003.

28. Abou-Alfa GK, Meyer T, Cheng A-L, et al. Cabozantinib versus placebo in patients with advanced hepatocellular carcinoma who have received prior sorafenib: Results from the randomized phase III CELESTIAL trial. 2018 Gastrointestinal Cancers Symposium. Abstract 207. Presented January 2018.

18

"Market withdrawals" of medicines in Germany after AMNOG: a comparison of HTA ratings and clinical guideline recommendations

Thomas R. Staab[1,5], Miriam Walter[2], Sonja Mariotti Nesurini[2], Charalabos-Markos Dintsios[3], J.-Matthias Graf von der Schulenburg[4], Volker E. Amelung[5] and Jörg Ruof[5,6*] (iD)

Abstract

Background: According to the AMNOG act, the German Federal Joint Committee (G-BA) determines the additional benefit of new medicines as a basis for subsequent price negotiations. Pharmaceutical companies may withdraw their medications from the market at any time during the process. This analysis aims to compare recommendations in clinical guidelines and HTA appraisals of medicines that were withdrawn from the German market since the introduction of AMNOG in 2011.

Methods: Medications withdrawn from the German market between January 2011 and June 2016 following benefit assessment were categorized as opt-outs (max. 2 weeks after start of price negotiations) or supply terminations (during or after further price negotiations). Related guidelines were systematically analyzed. For all withdrawals, therapeutic area, additional benefit rating and recommendation status in relevant clinical guidelines were assessed.

Results: Among 139 medications, 10 opt-outs and 12 supply terminations were identified. Twenty-one out of 22 withdrawn medicines (95%) received 'no additional benefit' appraisal by the G-BA (average 'no additional benefit' rating for all AMNOG products: 47%). Of the 22 medicines, 15 (68%) were recommended by at least one guideline at the time of benefit assessment and 18 (82%) on 1 June 2016. Heterogeneity among guidelines was high. Acceptance of clinical trial endpoints was different between G-BA appraisals and clinical guidelines.

Conclusion: Our analysis revealed considerable differences across clinical guidelines as well as between clinical guidelines and HTA appraisals of the medicines that were withdrawn from the German market. Better alignment of the clinical perspective and close collaboration between all involved parties is required to achieve and maintain optimization of patient care.

Keywords: AMNOG, Early benefit assessment, Product recalls and withdrawals, Opt-out

Background

Health technology assessments (HTA) of innovative medicines are a common feature all across Europe. A key challenge for all healthcare systems is how to decide which medicines should be covered under the national reimbursement scheme. In the United Kingdom, a predefined cost-effectiveness ratio determines a threshold for reimbursement [1]. In France, the SMR ('service médical rendu', actual clinical benefit) and ASMR ('amélioration du service médical rendu', improvement in actual clinical benefit) determine the price level and the rate of reimbursement by the national health insurance [2].

In Germany, the manufacturer has to submit a benefit dossier at the time of market entry. Thereafter, the IQWIG ('Institut für Qualität und Wirschaftlichkeit im Gesundheitswesen') reviews the dossier before the Federal Joint Committee ('Gemeinsamer Bundesausschuss', G-BA) conducts the appraisal of the additional benefit of the

* Correspondence: joerg.ruof@r-connect.org
[5]Medical School of Hanover, Hanover, Germany
[6]r-connect ltd, Hauensteinstr. 132, 4059 Basel, Switzerland
Full list of author information is available at the end of the article

innovative medicine versus the current standard of care. Based on the outcome of the benefit appraisal, the National Association of the Statutory Health Insurance Funds ('GKV Spitzenverband', GKV-SV) and the manufacturer enter into price negotiations. A mutually agreed price is in place 1 year after market entry. During the initial 12 months after market entry, the medication is sold at a price set by the manufacturer, i.e. newly licensed drugs are available without restriction in the German health care system as soon as they enter the German market. Should the parties not come to an agreement on the sales discount, an arbitration board is called in. The legal basis for this procedure is anchored in the Act on the Reform of the Market for Medical Products ('Arzneimittelmarktneuordnungsgesetz', AMNOG), introduced in 2011 [3–5].

The manufacturer has the legal right to resign from price negotiations at the latest 2 weeks after the first negotiation meeting; this is referred to as opt-out. Termination of supplies can be chosen as a second option either before, during or after price negotiations. In both cases, the medicine is then withdrawn from the German market [6]. Although after official withdrawal of a specific medicine from the German market, patients may be able to continue receiving it via individual imports, this is usually associated with high administrative effort [7].

A particular challenge to any HTA body are accelerated approval procedures for innovative medicines that are applied both in the US and in Europe [8]. Available data at the time of market entry are often immature, making the assessment of the additional benefit difficult.

It has been shown that in clinical practice, the possibility of a medicine being withdrawn has a major impact on individual decision making. This is particularly relevant in the context of AMNOG: a German federal state association of panel doctors urged their members to account for the possibility of market withdrawals when prescribing newly approved medicines for which no reimbursed price had been agreed on yet [9]. In line with this, in a survey of 150 German physicians, 67% reported considering the possibility of market withdrawal when making therapeutic decisions. This indicates that physicians may be hesitant to initiate therapies with novel medicines because these might be withdrawn from the market and a therapy change would be required in all patients receiving them [10].

While HTA procedures are mandatory and fully justified in an environment of steadily increasing health care costs, the respective appraisals, subsequent price negotiations, and optional withdrawal decisions by the pharmaceutical manufacturers should not lead to a deterioration of treatment options for patients. It is the authors' position that medicines that are recommended in clinical guidelines should be available as an option for treating patients.

Our analysis therefore aims to compare clinical guideline recommendations and HTA appraisals of medicines that were withdrawn from the German market.

Methods
Analysis set
Opt-outs and supply terminations since introduction of the benefit assessment in 1 January 2011 up until 1 June 2016 were identified in the AMNOG Report, the GKV-SV database, the German medicine atlas, the German prescription report and by manual search [10–13].

Up until January 2014, when changes in policy were put in place, the G-BA also assessed the benefit of medications which had already been on the German market. This assessment of the existing market covered therapeutic areas of chronic pain, osteoporosis, cardiovascular diseases, and diabetes mellitus [14]. Market withdrawals from both early benefit assessments and assessments of the existing markets were taken into account. Medicines that were temporarily withdrawn from the market but reintroduced before June 1st 2016 were reviewed but excluded from the systematic analysis. Products that changed their brand name, were excluded from the analysis if supply of the molecule was continuously guaranteed throughout the observation time. Moreover, orphan medicines were reviewed but not included in the systematic analysis as the G-BA does not determine an appropriate comparative therapy for orphan medicines and therefore no systematic analysis of guidelines is performed.

Therapeutic areas
All therapeutic areas were included. Medication assignment to therapeutic areas was done in line with the G-BA [15].

Benefit assessments
Details on the benefit assessments including date of decision, extent of granted additional benefit, and reason for no additional benefit, if applicable, were obtained from the G-BA database [15]. In cases where the G-BA re-assessed certain medications in the same indication, only the latest benefit assessment was evaluated. As a conservative approach, if a drug was assessed in several patient groups, the best rating was used for the analysis. The reasons for not granting an additional benefit were considered in the following order (corresponding to decreasing levels of demonstrated clinical advantage): medicine judged as showing insufficient clinical superiority according to the G-BA appraisal, no appropriate data according to the G-BA appraisal (e.g. because an inappropriate comparator was used), or no dossier submitted. If several reasons were provided for a given drug due to several indications and/or subgroups, the first

applicable reason (corresponding to the highest level of demonstrated clinical advantage) was considered.

Arbitration procedures

Medications that underwent the arbitration procedure were extracted from a recent publication [5]. As this publication only included documents up to January 2016, a manual search for further procedures was conducted.

Approval and withdrawal dates

The date of approval by the European Medicines Agency (EMA) was extracted from the database of European public assessment reports [16]. To assess the date of withdrawal, the latest entry in the German pharmaceutical catalogue, the *Lauer-Taxe*, was consulted [17].

Guideline recommendations

The G-BA chooses the appropriate comparative therapy for the benefit assessment based on, among other factors, relevant literature and guidelines identified in a systematic literature search prior to the assessment (according to the G-BA Rules of Procedure, par. 7.2) [4].

Recommendation status at the time of benefit assessment was analyzed using the guidelines identified by the G-BA's systematic literature search. Guidelines may recommend either 'specific medicines' or a 'class' of medicines only. Within our analysis we discriminated between those two levels of recommendations with the latter being considered the weaker level of recommendation. In cases where the G-BA re-assessed certain medications in the same indication, the earliest benefit assessment was evaluated. To assess recommendation status at the time of analysis (1 June 2016), guidelines were identified by a) a search for the version that was current on 1 June 2016 for all guidelines used by the G-BA, and b) a manual search, using the G-BA algorithm, for evidence-based guidelines newly published until 1 June 2016 (Additional file 1: Figure S1). If a guideline used by the G-BA was not available anymore, the information provided in the G-BA documentation was analyzed. Guidelines were analyzed in terms of the methodology applied, i.e. whether they included i) a systematic rating of evidence, which allowed for a ranking of recommendations, and ii) a graphical display of a suggested treatment algorithm. Country of origin was determined for each guideline, and for German guidelines, we also evaluated whether guidelines adhered to the S3 category, reflecting the highest methodological standard, according to the classification of the Association of the Scientific Medical Societies in Germany [18].

Recommendation status was assessed as follows:

- Medications, or their class, were defined as *recommended* if at least one of the identified guidelines issued a positive recommendation, i.e. if a medicine or class was either included in a recommendation or specifically mentioned as a valid treatment option in the text.
- If a guideline recommended the specific medicine as well as the class, this was counted as a *recommendation for the specific medicine* only.

Results

Analysis set

In total, 139 products were evaluated by the G-BA in 14 different therapeutic areas in the period between January 2011 and June 2016. Of these, 22 products (16%) were withdrawn from the market. Three additional products (bosutinib, dapagliflozin and pitavastatin) were only temporarily withdrawn from the market and were therefore not included in the full analysis:

- For pitavastatin, a medicine for the treatment of hypercholesterolemia, no dossier was submitted to the G-BA. The medicine was temporarily withdrawn from the market but reintroduced after a fixed reference price had been determined.
- Bosutinib, an orphan medicine for the treatment of chronic myelogenous leukemia, received a non-quantifiable benefit rating from the G-BA. During price negotiation, it was temporarily withdrawn from the market but reintroduced before finalization of the final rounds of price negotiation.
- Dapagliflozin, indicated for the treatment of diabetes, was not granted an additional benefit by the G-BA. It was temporarily withdrawn from the market but reintroduced after price agreement has been reached.

Figure 1 provides an overview of the complete analysis set.

Detailed information on the 22 withdrawn products is summarized in Table 1. Only 2 of the 22 medications, vildagliptin and vildagliptin/metformin, underwent an assessment of the existing market by the G-BA; all other 20 products passed through the early benefit assessment.

Ataluren was the only orphan medicine within our sample. It is indicated for Duchenne muscle dystrophy, a rare disease with < 100 patients in Germany. A guideline review was not part of the G-BA assessment and ataluren was therefore not included in the analysis. Nivolumab in the indication 'non-small cell lung cancer' was initially introduced leveraging the brand name 'Nivolumab BMS'. This brand was withdrawn from the market and marketing authorization shifted to 'Opdivo'. As the molecule was continuously available for patients it was not included in our analysis.

For 10 medications (45%), the manufacturers opted out from entering price negotiations, and for 12 products

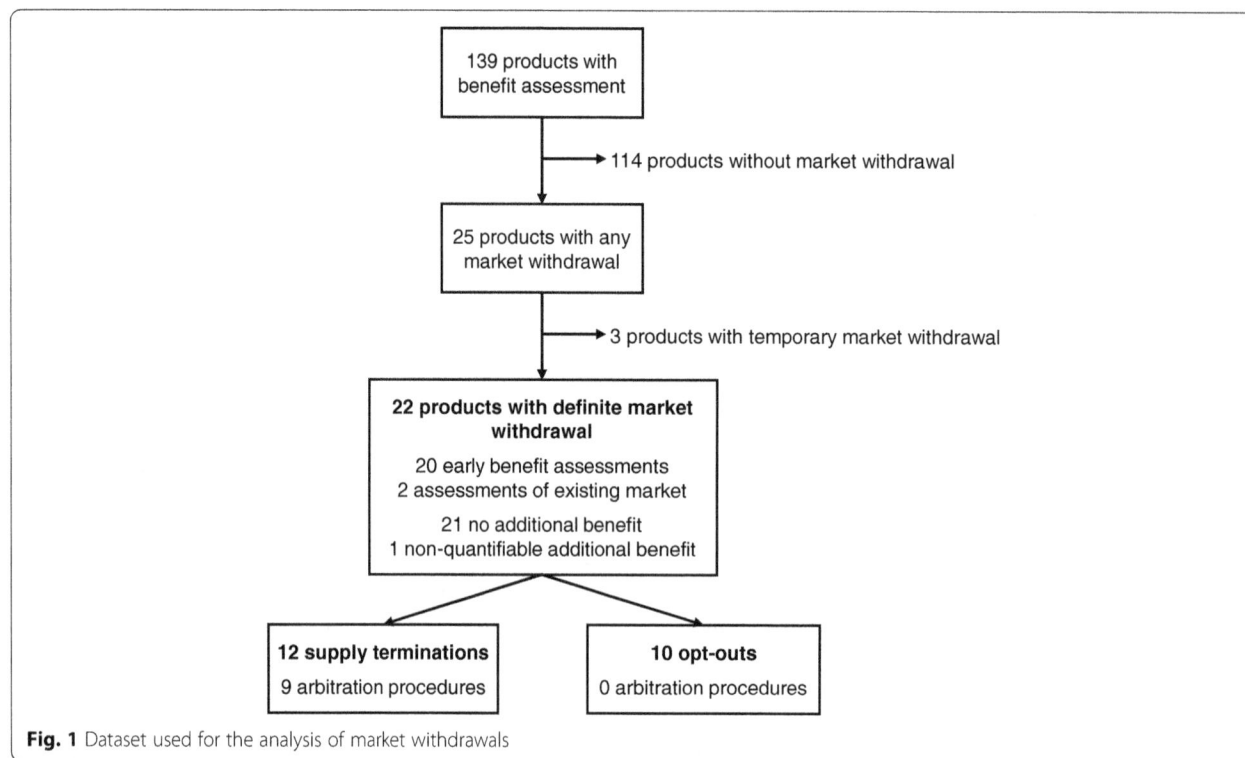

Fig. 1 Dataset used for the analysis of market withdrawals

(55%), the supply was terminated. For two medications (9%), supply was terminated not only in Germany, but across Europe: for both sipuleucel-T (Provenge), authorized for the treatment of prostate cancer, and colestilan (BindRen), authorized for the treatment of hyperphosphatemia in chronic kidney disease, the EMA (European Medicines Agency) withdrew marketing authorization at the request of the manufacturer for commercial reasons [19, 20]. Living larvae of *Lucilia sericata* were withdrawn from the outpatient market only and are still available in the hospital setting. Another product, retigabine, authorized for the treatment of drug-resistant partial onset epileptic seizures, has been discontinued worldwide by June 2017 due to limited usage [21]. Of the 12 medications that underwent supply terminations, 9 (75%) entered the arbitration procedure. For 9 of the 10 products with opt-out, there were no arbitration procedures as no price negotiations took place. For retigabine, price negotiations and an arbitration procedure were initiated by a parallel importer following the manufacturer's opt-out [5]; however, the parallel importer never marketed the product either.

On average (± standard deviation) and excluding assessments of the existing market, opt-outs occurred 401 ± 271 days after marketing authorization (range: 130–993), whereas medications with supply termination had been available on the market for 747 ± 218 days (range: 489–1089).

Therapeutic areas

Among the 139 medicines evaluated by the G-BA, the highest numbers of appraisals occurred in oncology (38 medicines) and metabolic disorders (30 medicines). In metabolic disorders, 9 out of 30 products (30%) were withdrawn from the market; in ophthalmic disorders, withdrawal rate was 33% (2 out of 6 medicines); in central nervous system disorders, it was 25% (2 out of 8 medicines); in cardiovascular diseases, 14% (1 out of 7 medicines); and in oncology, 5% (2 out of 38 medicines). No withdrawals occurred in the areas of infectious diseases ($N = 16$), respiratory diseases ($N = 9$), dermatology ($N = 3$), and hematology ($N = 2$), with N depicting the total number of assessed medications in these therapeutic areas.

Benefit assessment

Additional benefit ratings for all withdrawn products are shown in Table 2. Although only the highest benefit rating was considered in the analysis if the G-BA assessed more than one subgroup and/or indication, 95% (21 out of 22) of the withdrawn medications received a 'no additional benefit' rating. The only remaining medication, sipuleucel-T, received an additional benefit rating of 'not quantifiable'. The manufacturer had submitted data from three studies, which the G-BA determined as biased due to differences in post-progression therapies and the option of rescue therapy with a sipuleucel-T analogue specified in the protocol. The appraisal for sipuleucel-T was

Table 1 Medications withdrawn from the German market since the introduction of AMNOG benefit assessments

Active ingredient (brand name)	Manufacturer	Therapeutic area	EMA approval	Unlisted[a]	Type of withdrawal	Arbitration procedure
Aliskiren/amlodipine (Rasilamlo)	Novartis Pharma	Cardiovascular	14 Apr 2011	1 Sep 2011	Opt-out	NA[b]
Bromfenac (Yellox)	Bausch & Lomb/Dr. Mann Pharma	Ophthalmic	18 May 2011	1 May 2014	Supply termination	Yes
Canagliflozin (Invokana)	Janssen-Cilag	Metabolic	15 Nov 2013	15 Oct 2014	Opt-out	NA[b]
Canagliflozin/metformin (Vokanamet)	Janssen-Cilag	Metabolic	23 Apr 2014	1 Mar 2015	Opt-out	NA[b]
Colestilan (BindRen)	Mitsubishi Pharma	Other	21 Jan 2013	1 Apr 2015	Supply termination	No[c]
Gaxilose (LacTest)	Venter Pharma S.L.	Metabolic	NA[d]	1 Mar 2016	Opt-out	NA[b]
Insulin degludec (Tresiba)	Novo Nordisk Pharma	Metabolic	21 Jan 2013	15 Jan 2016	Supply termination	Yes
Living larvae from *Lucilia sericata* (BioBag)	BioMonde GmbH	Other	NA[d]	15 Jun 2015	Supply termination[i]	Yes
Linaclotide (Constella)	Almirall Hermal	Digestive	26 Nov 2012	15 Jul 2014	Supply termination	Yes
Linagliptin (Trajenta)	Boehringer Ingelheim Pharma	Metabolic	24 Aug 2011	1 Jan 2012	Opt-out	NA[b]
Lixisenatide (Lyxumia)	Sanofi-Aventis Deutschland	Metabolic	1 Feb 2013	15 Jun 2014	Supply termination	Yes
Lomitapide (Lojuxta)	Aegerion Pharmaceuticals	Metabolic	31 Jul 2013	1 Aug 2014	Opt-out	NA[b]
Lurasidone (Latuda)	Takeda GmbH	Psychiatric	21 Mar 2014	15 Nov 2015	Supply termination	No
Microbial collagenase (Xiapex)	Pfizer Pharma	Musculoskeletal	28 Feb 2011	15 Jun 2012	Opt-out	NA[b]
Mirabegron (Betmiga)	Astellas Pharma GmbH	Genitourinary	20 Dec 2012	1 Jun 2015	Supply termination	Yes
Perampanel (Fycompa)	Eisai	CNS	23 Jul 2012	1 Aug 2014	Supply termination	Yes
Regorafenib (Stivarga)	Bayer Vital	Oncology	26 Aug 2013	15 May 2016	Opt-out	NA[b]
Retigabine (Trobalt)	GlaxoSmithKline	CNS	28 Mar 2011	1 Jul 2012	Opt-out	NA[e]
Sipuleucel-T (Provenge)	Dendreon UK Limited	Oncology	6 Sep 2013	15 Jul 2015	Supply termination	No
Tafluprost/timolol (Taptiqom)	Santen	Ophthalmic	NA[d]	1 Aug 2015	Opt-out	NA[b]
Vildagliptin[f] (Galvus, Jalra, Xiliarx)	Novartis Pharma	Metabolic	26 Sep 2007	15 Sep 2014 1 Jul 2014[g]	Supply termination	Yes
Vildagliptin/metformin[f] (Eucreas, Icandra, Zomarist)	Novartis Pharma	Metabolic	14 Nov 2007	15 Sep 2014 1 Jul 2014[h]	Supply termination	Yes

[a]Date the medication was removed from the German pharmaceutical catalogue (Lauer-Taxe), which is updated bi-monthly
[b]Not applicable as opt-out medications do not enter price negotiations
[c]An arbitration procedure was initiated [42] but not completed [5]
[d]Not applicable as decentralized approval
[e]The manufacturer opted out before the price negotiations; however, price negotiations and eventually an arbitration procedure were subsequently initiated by a parallel importer [5]
[f]Assessment of the existing market
[g]For Galvus and Jalra, respectively (Xiliarx is marketed by foreign third parties)
[h]For Eucreas and Icandra, respectively (Zomarist is marketed by foreign third parties)
[i]Supply termination only for outpatient services, medicine still available in hospital settings
AMNOG: Act on the Reform of the Market for Medical Products; CNS: central nervous system; EMA: European Medicines Agency

conditional and benefit assessment was scheduled to be repeated in April 2018 [22]. However, with the Europe-wide market withdrawal of sipuleucel-T, a reassessment of its benefit seems unlikely.

Table 2 also displays the reasons why no additional benefit was granted (where applicable). For 15 of the 21 medications which were deemed without additional benefit, the G-BA determined that they demonstrated insufficient clinical superiority to the appropriate comparative therapy. Three dossiers did not report any appropriate data (aliskiren/amlodipine, retigabine, perampanel) and for three products, no dossier was submitted (bromfenac, gaxilose, living larvae of *Lucilia sericata*). Moreover, no appropriate data were reported for regorafenib in the second indication of gastrointestinal stromal tumor.

Guideline recommendations

For all products, the guidelines taken into account by the G-BA upon initiation of the respective benefit assessment were evaluated to assess whether or not they recommended the withdrawn medication and/or its class at the time. To additionally determine the perception of the clinical value of the medication on 1 June 2016, the versions of the guidelines selected by the G-BA that were current on 1 June 2016, as well as newly published guidelines before this date, were also analyzed.

Table 2 Extent of additional benefit and recommendation status for all withdrawn medicines

Medicine	Reason for 'no additional benefit' rating[a]	Number of guidelines with positive recommendation (total number of guidelines reviewed)			
		At time of benefit assessment		Additional guidelines June 2016	
		Guidelines	Recommendation[b]	Guidelines	Recommendation[b]
Aliskiren/ amlodipine	No appropriate data	1 (4)	Medicine (aliskiren)	1 (2)	Medicine (aliskiren)
Bromfenac	No dossier submitted	4 (7)	Class (NSAID)	1 (2)	Class (NSAID)
Canagliflozin	Insufficient clinical superiority	1 (4)	Class (SGLT-2 inhibitors)	3 (3)	Medicine (canagliflozin)
Canagliflozin/ metformin	Insufficient clinical superiority	1 (5)	Class (SGLT-2 inhibitors/ metformin)	3 (3)	Class (SGLT-2 inhibitors/metformin)
Colestilan	Insufficient clinical superiority	1 (1)	Class (phosphate binding agents)	1 (1)	Class (phosphate binding agents)
Gaxilose	No dossier submitted	n.a.	n.a.	n.a.	n.a.
Insulin degludec	Insufficient clinical superiority	7 (7)	Class (basal insulin analogues)	3 (3)	Medicine (insulin degludec)
Living larvae from *Lucilia sericata*	No dossier submitted	1 (1)	Medicine (living larvae)	n.a.	n.a.
Linaclotide	Insufficient clinical superiority	0 (4)	n.a.	1 (1)	Medicine (linaclotide)
Linagliptin	Insufficient clinical superiority	2 (3)	Class (DPP-4 inhibitors)	3 (3)	Medicine (linagliptin) and class (DPP-4 inhibitors)
Lixisenatide	Insufficient clinical superiority	5 (5)	Class (GLP-1 agonists)	3 (4)	Medicine (lixisenatide) and class (GLP-1 agonists)
Lomitapide	Insufficient clinical superiority	0 (2)	n.a.	1 (1)	Medicine (lomitapide)
Lurasidone	Insufficient clinical superiority	4 (4)	Medicine (lurasidone)	2 (2)	Class (second generation antipsychotic drugs)
Microbial collagenase	Insufficient clinical superiority	n.a.	n.a.	n.a.	n.a.
Mirabegron	Insufficient clinical superiority	0 (6)	n.a.	1 (1)	Medicine (mirabegron)
Perampanel	No appropriate data	0 (1)	n.a.	0 (1)	n.a.
Regorafenib	Insufficient clinical superiority	0 (7)	n.a.	3 (6)	Medicine (regorafenib)
Retigabine	No appropriate data	1 (1)	Medicine (retigabine)	1 (1)	Medicine (retigabine)
Sipuleucel-T	n.a.	4 (11)	Medicine (sipuleucel-T)	5 (9)	Medicine (sipuleucel-T)
Tafluprost/timolol	Insufficient clinical superiority	2 (2)	Class (preservative- free medicines)	n.a.	n.a.
Vildagliptin	Insufficient clinical superiority	5 (5)	Medicine (vildagliptin)	4 (4)	Medicine (vildagliptin) and class (DPP-4 inhibitor)
Vildagliptin/ metformin	Insufficient clinical superiority	5 (5)	Medicine (vildagliptin/metformin)	4 (4)	Class (DPP-4 inhibitors/metformin)

[a]All medicines had a 'no additional benefit' rating except Sipuleucel-T ('non quantifiable benefit')
[b]Recommendation of medicine or therapeutic class
DPP-4: dipeptidyl peptidase 4; GLP-1: glucagon-like peptide-1 receptor; n.a.: not applicable; NSAID: nonsteroidal anti-inflammatory drugs; SGLT-2: sodium-glucose co-transporter 2

An overview of guidelines, their country of origin, the inclusion of an evidence rating scheme, the display of a graphical treatment algorithm, and their recommendations at the time of benefit assessment and on 1 June 2016 is provided in Additional file 2: Table S1. A total of 94 guidelines were reviewed. Thirty four guidelines covered oncological conditions (i.e. colorectal carcinoma, gastrointestinal stromal tumor, prostate cancer), 19 covered metabolic conditions (i.e. diabetes, hypercholesterolemia), 11 covered ophthalmic conditions (i.e. postoperative management of cataract surgery and glaucoma), 7 covered overactive bladder, 6 guidelines

each covered hypertension and schizophrenia, 5 covered irritable bowel syndrome, 3 covered epilepsy, 2 covered hyperphosphatemia, and 1 covered wound healing.

Of those 94 guidelines, 82 (87%) were available as full publications. For the remaining guidelines, the G-BA documentation was analyzed as the documents were no longer available. Evidence ratings were applied by 72 (88%) of the 82 fully available guidelines. However, ratings were not consistent across guidelines. Graphically displayed treatment algorithms were available in 43 (52%) out of the 82 guidelines.

For gaxilose (metabolic diseases) and microbial collagenase (musculoskeletal disorders) no guidelines could be identified both by the G-BA and at the time of this analysis. For the benefit assessment of bromfenac (ophthalmic diseases), no systematic literature search was conducted by the G-BA. Instead, guidelines used for a German HTA rapid report in the relevant indication were used for this analysis [23].

Overall, 15 (68%) of the withdrawn medications had been recommended in at least one of the reviewed guidelines by name (*n* = 7; 32%) or class (*n* = 8; 36%) at the time of benefit assessment. Evaluation of the guidelines current as of 1 June 2016 showed an increase of overall recommended products to 18 (82%), of which 14 (64%) were recommended specifically and 4 (18%) by class. However, recommendation status of individual medicines remained inconsistent across guidelines and therapeutic classes (Table 3).

Discussion

The AMNOG act was not introduced to control and manage the supply/use of medicines. Its aim was to manage prices and total public expenditure of pharmaceutical products [24]. In order to achieve this, a link between the reimbursed price of newly approved drugs and the additional benefit that they offer is stipulated. Clinical guidelines, on the other hand, are focused on treatment options for patients. Considering the different goals of G-BA appraisals and clinical guidelines, it is not necessarily contradictory that a medicine is recommended within a guideline while being assessed as having no additional benefit by the G-BA. However, several years after its coming into effect, it is becoming increasingly clear that the new legislation impacts the traditionally high availability of newly approved drugs on the German market due to opt-outs following benefit assessments [25], and the recent discussion about including G-BA appraisals into the physicians' desk reference systems ('Arztinformationssystem') raises the question whether this may be to the disadvantage of patients and caregivers.

Our analysis showed that out of a total of 139 products evaluated by the G-BA between January 2011 and June 2016, 22 medicines (16%) were withdrawn from the German market. Twenty-one (95%) of those medicines received a 'no additional benefit' rating by the G-BA, a sharp contrast to the average of 43% of 'no additional benefit ratings' in all G-BA appraisals [10]. As both benefit appraisals and clinical guidelines rely on the principles of evidence-based medicine [26], those discrepancies are striking, raising the question of how these diverging evaluations of the same medicine fit together. The respective analysis reveals a couple of key features:

- An obvious heterogeneity between guideline recommendations and G-BA appraisals occurred in diabetes. The validity of HbA1C, a widely accepted primary endpoint in diabetes trials, is challenged by the G-BA [27], supporting the 'no additional benefit' decision by the G-BA for the majority of recently introduced diabetes drugs. The critical approach to widely accepted primary clinical trial outcomes by the G-BA is an example of a fundamental difference of German HTA appraisals and more clinically centered guidelines.

- Several of the 22 medicines such as linaclotide [28], lomitapide [29], lurasidone [30], mirabegron [31], retigabine [32], and regorafenib [33, 34] are recommended as later-line treatments in their respective disease area. While each of these medicines has to be considered individually, the unavailability of later-line treatment options generally carries a risk of suboptimal care, particularly in patients with advanced conditions.

- In some therapeutic areas, guidelines primarily support a class of products rather than specific medicines: nonsteroidal anti-inflammatory drugs are recommended for the postoperative management in cataract surgery, preservative-free medicines are supported for the subset of glaucoma patients allergic to preservatives, and phosphate binding medicines are recommended for the treatment of hyperphosphatemia. However, none of the respective products (bromfenac, colestilan, and tafluprost/timolol) are specifically recommended by guidelines, raising the question whether their unavailability really results in a major risk for public health, as long as appropriate alternatives from the same class with similar product characteristics are available. Furthermore, unavailable medicines that are specifically recommended in clinical guidelines might potentially be substituted by other medicines as long as comparators from the same class with similar product characteristics are available.

In addition to the inconsistencies between G-BA appraisals and guideline recommendations, our review also revealed major heterogeneities across guidelines. In two therapeutic areas (Dupuytren's contracture and hypolactasia), no guidelines were available at all and the only available guideline covering wound healing and the effect of living larvae of *Lucilia sericata* was developed in 2012 [35]. In contrast, 20 guidelines covered prostate cancer, 9 of which had included specific recommendations for sipuleucel-T in patients with asymptomatic metastatic prostate cancer prior to the withdrawal of the medicine due to bankruptcy of the manufacturer [36]. Heterogeneity between guidelines can partially been

Table 3 Summary table of key issues by therapeutic area

Therapeutic area indication	Medicines	Key issues within therapeutic class
Cardiovascular		
Hypertension	Aliskiren/amlodipine	Aliskiren is recommended within clinical guidelines both as monotherapy and in combination with other antihypertensives. However, the fixed combination of aliskiren and amlodipine that was appraised by the G-BA is not covered within the guidelines
Ophthalmic		
Postoperative management of cataract surgery	Bromfenac	Guidelines suggest the therapeutic class (NSAID) in the perioperative period in cataract surgery, but do not specify any medicine
Glaucoma	Tafluprost/timolol	Guidelines strongly support the use of preservative-free medicines if there is evidence that patients are allergic to the preservative, but do not specify any medicine
Metabolic		
Diabetes	Canagliflozin Canagliflozin/metformin Linagliptine Lixisenatide Vildagliptine Vildagliptine/metformin	Guidelines evolved over time. While metformin remains the gold standard for initial drug therapy, guidelines support other classes and products such as canagliflozin and its class (SGLT-2 inhibitors), linagliptin and vildagliptin (DPP-4 inhibitors), and lixisenatide and its class (GLP-1 agonists) i) as monotherapy (SGLT-2 and DPP-4 inhibitors) in patients who are not eligible for initial metformin treatment and ii) as combination therapy (SGLT-2 and DPP-4 inhibitors and GLP-1 agonists)
	Insulin degludec	Basal insulin analogues are recommended within guidelines. Within that class, insulin degludec is one option
Hypercholesterolemia	Lomitapide	Lomitapide and other new therapeutic options are part of the suggested treatment algorithm in patients with homozygous familiar hypercholesterolemia
Digestive		
Irritable bowel syndrome	Linaclotide	Only one updated guideline is available [28]. This guideline recommends linaclotide as second-line treatment if previous laxatives did not help and patients had constipations for at least 12 months
Psychiatric		
Schizophrenia	Lurasidone	Guidelines generally recommend second generation antipsychotic drugs, but the evidence base for appropriate comparisons is considered limited
Musculoskeletal		
Dupuytren's contracture	Microbial collagenase	Lack of relevant guidelines for the treatment of Dupuytren's contracture
Genitourinary		
Overactive bladder	Mirabegron	Guidelines evolved over time and included mirabegron as second-line treatment [31]
CNS		
Epilepsy	Perampanel	Guidelines are heterogeneous [44] and partially not updated, e.g. the American Epilepsy Society is still presenting a 2004 publication on their homepage as guidance for refractory epilepsy.
	Retigabine	Retigabine is recommended as adjunctive second line treatment [32]
Oncology		
Colorectal carcinoma	Regorafenib	Regorafenib is recommended both in US and EU clinical guidelines [33] as second/third line of therapy.
Gastrointestinal stromal tumor	Regorafenib	Regorafenib is recommended as second/third line of therapy [34]
Prostate cancer	Sipuleucel-T	Sipuleucel-T is recommended by various guidelines in patients with metastatic prostate cancer and asymptomatic or minimally symptomatic disease

Table 3 Summary table of key issues by therapeutic area *(Continued)*

Therapeutic area indication	Medicines	Key issues within therapeutic class
Other		
Hyperphosphatemia	Colestilan	Guidelines generally recommend phosphate binding agents but do not specify any medicine
Hypolactasia[a]	Gaxilose	No relevant guidelines were identified for hypolactasia.
Wound healing	Living larvae from *Lucilia sericata*	Only one guideline from 2012 is available [35]. Living larvae considered superior versus hydrogel therapy in terms of wound cleansing

[a]Hypolactasia was classified as a metabolic disorder by the G-BA

DPP-4 dipeptidyl peptidase 4, *G-BA* Federal Joint Committee, *GLP-1* glucagon-like peptide-1 receptor, *NSAID* nonsteroidal anti-inflammatory drugs, *SGLT-2* sodium-glucose co-transporter 2

explained by different standards of care across various countries. However, in contrast to HTA appraisals that are automatically initiated upon availability of an innovative medicine, clinical guidelines are often characterized by a lack of timely renewal and therefore may not always be up to date with the most recent developments.

A key discussion point in the current German HTA environment is the value of G-BA assessments in shaping treatment algorithms. In contrast to e.g. the UK, where most treatment guidelines are issued by NICE, the German Society of Hematology and Oncology makes an enormous effort to keep clinical guidelines i) under their influence and ii) always up to date. Clinical positioning statements are issued for each of the G-BA appraisals in oncology, and, despite criticism regarding insufficient methodological rigor, the 'Onkopedia' guidelines [37] aim towards clinically shaped treatment algorithms, thereby ensuring best clinical practice. A recently conducted comparative review of Onkopedia guidelines and G-BA appraisals revealed that 38% of patient groups established by the G-BA in the appraisal of oncological medicines partially or fully deviated from those mentioned in the Onkopedia guidelines, and 60% of additional benefit decisions by the G-BA showed a partial or complete discordance with the guidelines [38]. This indicates that many medicines might play an important role in a clinically optimized treatment algorithm despite a 'no additional benefit' appraisal by the G-BA.

Withdrawal from the market is particularly painful if a high utilization of the medicine had already occurred. The epilepsy treatment perampanel is considered a useful treatment option for patients with drug-resistant disease due to its unique mechanism of action [39]; moreover, the product is one of the few anticonvulsants with an explicit approval for use in adolescents above the age of 12 [15]. At the time of market withdrawal, more than 5.000 patients were receiving the medicine [7]. Also, when Novo Nordisk withdrew its basal insulin analogue insulin degludec from the German market in January 2016, health care professionals were asked to switch the approximately 40.000 patients receiving the product at that time to an alternative insulin [40]. Diabetes experts considered this mandated therapy change

to the disadvantage of patients, as insulin degludec offers a unique safety profile and a longer half-life [41]. Commenting on the recent withdrawal of osimertinib, a tyrosine kinase inhibitor for the treatment of non-small lung cancer carrying the T790 M mutation of the epidermal growth factor receptor (EGFR), the German Society for Hematology and Medical Oncology stated that "all parties involved are right but the damage is on the patients" [42, 43].

Interestingly, it has to be noted that there are several medicines that were re-introduced into the market after the initial withdrawal decision by the pharmaceutical manufacturer. For three medicines (bosuitinib, pitavastin, and dapagliflozin) the re-entry occurred within the time frame of our analysis (cut-off June 1st 2016). Also, ataluren, the only orphan medicine to be withdrawn from the market, as well as mirabegron, linaclotide, and perampanel, were reintroduced later on.

Within the German AMNOG environment the decision to withdraw a medicine from the market is taken by the manufacturer. An analysis of the reasons why the involved companies decided to withdraw the medicines (e.g. outcomes of the benefit assessment and/or the subsequent price negotiation), or why some of the medicines were reintroduced at a later time point, was beyond the scope of this analysis.

Our analysis compares HTA appraisals and clinical guidelines only. The determination of the appropriate comparative therapy within the G-BA procedures also includes systematic reviews and Cochrane reviews. Including those additional sources of evidence in this comparative analysis is therefore part of the future research agenda. An in-depth comparison of clinical guidelines, the recommendations for the various treatment lines and the rating systems of the guidelines is part of the upcoming research agenda.

Conclusions

Our analysis revealed considerable differences across clinical guidelines, as well as between clinical guidelines and HTA appraisals, for the medicines that were withdrawn from the German market. Better alignment of the clinical perspective in the determination of future treatment algorithms and close collaboration between all involved parties (G-BA, IQWiG, physician associations, and patient representatives) is required to achieve and maintain optimization of patient care in an increasingly HTA-shaped clinical environment.

Abbreviations
AMNOG: Act on the Reform of the Market for Medical Products ('Arzneimittelmarktneuordnungsgesetz'); EGFR: Epidermal growth factor receptor; EMA: European Medicines Agency; G-BA: Federal Joint Committee ('Gemeinsamer Bundesausschuss'); GKV-SV: National Association of the Statutory Health Insurance Funds ('GKV Spitzenverband'); HTA: Health Technology assessment; IQWIG: 'Institut für Qualität und Wirschaftlichkeit im Gesundheitswesen'; NICE: National Institute for Health and Care Excellence

Funding
Medical writing services were provided by nspm ltd, Meggen, Switzerland, with financial support from Roche Pharma AG.

Authors' contributions
TS and JR designed the research and MW and SMN performed the research and analyzed the data. All authors participated in the writing of the manuscript. All authors read and approved the final manuscript.

Competing interests
TS has been an employee of Roche Pharma AG, Grenzach-Wyhlen, Germany at the time of the preparation of this manuscript. MW and SMN received financial compensation from Roche Pharma AG for medical writing services provided for this manuscript. CMD is, in addition to his academic affiliation, employed by Bayer Vital GmbH, Leverkusen, Germany. VEA and JMS have no conflicts of interest to declare. JR has been an employee of Roche Pharma AG, Grenzach-Wyhlen, Germany at the time of manuscript preparation.

Author details
[1]Roche Pharma AG, Grenzach-Wyhlen, Germany. [2]nspm ltd, Meggen, Switzerland. [3]Health Services Research and Health Economics, Heinrich Heine University, Düsseldorf, Germany. [4]Leibniz University Hanover, Hanover, Germany. [5]Medical School of Hanover, Hanover, Germany. [6]r-connect ltd, Hauensteinstr. 132, 4059 Basel, Switzerland.

References
1. Cerri KH, Knapp M, Fernandez JL. Decision making by NICE: examining the influences of evidence, process and context. Health Econ Policy Law. 2014;9:119–41.
2. Maison P, Zanetti L, Solesse A, Bouvenot G, Massol J, ISPEP group of the French National Authority for Health. The public health benefit of medicines: how it has been assessed in France? The principles and results of five years'experience. Health Policy. 2013;112:273–84.
3. Deutscher Bundestag. [Sozialgesetzbuch (SGB) Fünftes Buch (V) - Gesetzliche Krankenversicherung - (Artikel 1 des Gesetzes v. 20. Dezember 1988, BGBl. I S. 2477, letzte Änderung durch Artikel 3 des Gesetzes vom 20. Dezember 2012 (BGBl. I S. 2781))]. 1988. https://www.gesetze-im-internet.de/bundesrecht/sgb_5/gesamt.pdf. Accessed 15 Sept 2016.
4. Ruof J, Schwartz FW, Schulenburg JM, Dintsios CM. Early benefit assessment (EBA) in Germany: analysing decisions 18 months after introductin the new AMNOG legislation. Eur J Health Econ. 2014;15:577–89.
5. Ludwig S, Dintsios CM. Arbitration board setting reimbursement amounts for pharmaceutical innovations in Germany when Price negations between payers and manufacturers fail: an empirical analysis of 5 Years' experience. Value Health. 2016;19:1016–25.
6. Verband Forschender Arzneimittelhersteller (vfa). [Das AMNOG im vierten Jahr]. 2014. https://www.vfa.de/download/amnog-4tes-jahr-lang.pdf. Accessed 13 Sept 2016.
7. Deutsche Apotheker Zeitung. [DAV beschwert sich über Fycompa]. 2016. https://www.deutsche-apotheker-zeitung.de/news/artikel/2016/04/28/dav-beschwert-sich-uber-fycompa. Accessed 13 Sept 2016.
8. Leyens L, Brand A. Early patient access to medicines: health technology assessment bodies need to catch up with new marketing authorization methods. Public Health Genomics. 2016;19:187–91.
9. Kassenärztliche Vereinigung Westfalen-Lippe. [Frühe Nutzenbewertung: Erfahrungen nach vier Jahren]. 2015. https://www.kvwl.de/arzt/verordnung/arzneimittel/info/invo/fruehe_nutzenbewertung_rueckblick_invo.pdf. Accessed 13 Sept 2016.
10. Greiner W, Witte J. In: Rebscher H, editor. AMNOG-Report 2016 - Nutzenbewertung von Arzneimitteln in Deutschland. Heidelberg: medhochzwei Verlag GmbH; 2016.
11. GKV-Spitzenverband. [Übersicht zu den Erstattungsbetragsverhandlungen nach § 130b SGB V]. 2016. https://www.gkv-spitzenverband.de/krankenversicherung/arzneimittel/verhandlungen_nach_amnog/ebv_130b/ebv_nach_130b.jsp?pageNo=3&submitted=true&sort=&descending=&searchterm=Suchbegriff+eingeben&status=Alle&specialFeature=#arzneimittelliste. Accessed 13 Sept 2016.
12. IGES Institut GmbH. [Arzneimittel-Atlas]. 2015. http://www.arzneimittel-atlas.de/im-fokus/amnog/versorgung/index_ger.html. Accessed 13 Sept 2016.
13. Schwabe U, Paffrath D. Arzneiverordnungs-Report. Berlin: Springer; 2015.
14. G-BA. [G-BA legt Kriterien für Bestandsmarktaufruf fest und bestimmt erste Wirkstoffgruppen für die Nutzenbewertung]. 2013. https://www.g-ba.de/institution/presse/pressemitteilungen/485/. Accessed 13 Sept 2016.
15. G-BA. Overview of products [Übersicht der Wirkstoffe]. 2016. http://www.g-ba.de/informationen/nutzenbewertung/. Accessed 16 Mar 2017.
16. European Medicines Agency. European public assessment reports. 2016. http://www.ema.europa.eu/ema/index.jsp?curl=pages/medicines/landing/epar_search.jsp&mid=WC0b01ac058001d124. Accessed 13 Sept 2016.
17. Lauer Fischer GmbH. Lauer-Taxe. 2016. https://www.cgm.com/lauer-fischer/loesungen_lf/lauer_taxe_lf/lauer_taxe.de.jsp. Accessed 13 Sept 2016.
18. Arbeitsgemeinschaft der Wissenschaftlichen Medizinischen Fachgesellschaften. [Aktuelle Leitlinien]. 2016. https://www.awmf.org/awmf-online-das-portal-der-wissenschaftlichen-medizin/awmf-aktuell.html. Accessed 27 Jan 2017.
19. European Medicines Agency. Provenge - Withdrawal of the marketing authorisation in the European Union (public statement). 2015. http://www.ema.europa.eu/docs/en_GB/document_library/Public_statement/2015/05/WC500186950.pdf. Accessed 13 Sept 2016.
20. European Medicines Agency. BindRen - Withdrawal of the marketing authorisation in the European Union (public statement). 2015. http://www.ema.europa.eu/docs/en_GB/document_library/Public_statement/2015/03/WC500184373.pdf. Accessed 13 Sept 2016.
21. GlaxoSmithKline. GlaxoSmithKline: Advance notification of Trobalt® discontinuation. 2016. https://assets.publishing.service.gov.uk/media/57fe4b6640f0b6713800000c/Trobalt_letter.pdf. Accessed 27 Jan 2017.
22. G-BA. [Sipuleucel-T - Nutzenbewertung gemäß §35a SGB V - Beschluss]. 2015. https://www.g-ba.de/downloads/40-268-3155/2015-03-19_AM-RL-XII_Sipuleucel-T_2014-10-01-D-139_TrG.pdf. Accessed 15 Sept 2016.
23. IQWiG. [Orientierende Aufbereitung für das Thema "Kataraktoperation"]. 2009. https://www.iqwig.de/download/V09-01C_Rapid-Report_Orientierende_Aufbereitung_Kataraktoperation.pdf. Accessed 19 Sept 2016.
24. Deutscher Bundestag. [Entwurf eines Gesetzes zur Neuordnung des Arzneimittelmarktes in der gesetzlichen Krankenversicherung (Arzneimittelmarktneuordnungsgesetz – AMNOG)]. 2010. http://dipbt.bundestag.de/dip21/btd/17/031/1703116.pdf. Accessed 3 Feb 2017.
25. Cassel D, Ulrich V. AMNOG auf dem ökonomischen Prüfstand - Funktionsweise, Ergebnisse und Reformbedarf der Preisregulierung für neue Arzneimittel in Deutschland. 1st ed. Baden-Baden: Nomos Verlagsgesellschaft; 2015.
26. Schlegl E, Durournau P, Ruof J. Different weights of evidence-based

medicine triad in regulatory, health technology assessment, and clinical decision making. Pharm Med. 2017;31:213–6.

27. Staab T, Isbary G, Amelung VE, Ruof J. Inconsistent approaches of the G-BA regarding acceptance of primary study endpoints as being relevant to patients - an analysis of three disease areas: oncological, metabolic, and infectious diseases. BMC Health Serv Res. 2016;16:651.

28. National Institute for Health and Care Excellence. Irritable bowel syndrome in adults: diagnosis and management. 2015. https://www.nice.org.uk/guidance/cg61/resources/irritable-bowel-syndrome-in-adults-diagnosis-and-management-975562917829. Accessed 20 Jan 2017.

29. Cuchel M, Bruckert E, Ginsberg HN, Raal FJ, Santos RD, Hegele RA, et al. Homozygous familial hypercholesterolaemia: new insights and guidance for clinicians to improved detection and clinical managment. A position paper from the consensus panel on familial Hypercholesterolaemia of the European atherosclerosis society. Eur Heart J. 2014;35:2146–57.

30. Hasan A, Falkai P, Wobrock T, Lieberman J, Glenthoj B, Gattaz WF, et al. World Federation of Societies of biological psychiatry (WFSBP) guidelines for biological treatment of schizophrenia, part 1: update 2012 on the acute treatment of schizophrenia and the management of treatment resistance. World J Biol Psychiatry. 2012;13:318–78.

31. Gormley EA, Lightner DJ, Burgio KL, Chai TC, Clemens JQ, Culkin DJ, et al. Diagnosis and Treatment of Overactive Bladder (Non-Neurogenic) in Adults: AUA/SUFU Guideline. 2014. http://www.auanet.org/guidelines/overactive-bladder-(oab)-(aua/sufu-guideline-2012-amended-2014). Accessed 18 Dec 2017.

32. National Institute for Health and Care Excellence. Epilepsies: diagnosis and management. 2016. https://www.nice.org.uk/guidance/cg137/resources/epilepsies-diagnosis-and-management-35109515407813. Accessed 20 Jan 2017.

33. Van Cutsem E, Cervantes A, Adam R, Sobrero A, Van Krieken JH, Aderka D, et al. ESMO consensus guidelines for the management of patients with metastatic colorectal cancer. Ann Oncol. 2016;27:1386–422.

34. ESMO/European Sarcoma Network Working Group. Gastrointestinal stromal tumours: ESMO clinical practice guidelines for diagnosis, treatment and follow-up. Ann Oncol. 2014;25(Suppl 3):iii21–6.

35. Deutsche Gesellschaft für Wundheilung und Wundbehandlung. [Lokaltherapie chronischer Wunden bei Patienten mit den Risiken periphere arterielle Verschlusskrankheit, Diabetes mellitus, chronische venöse Insuffizienz]. 2012. https://www.awmf.org/leitlinien/detail/ll/091-001.html. Accessed 20 Jan 2017.

36. Jaroslawski S, Caban A, Toumi M. Sipuleucel - T (Provenge®): autopsy of an innovative change in paradigm in Cancer treatment. Value Health. 2015;18:A479.

37. Deutsche Gesellschaft für Hämatologie und medizinische Onkologie (DGHO). Onkopedia guidelines. 2017. https://www.onkopedia-guidelines.info/en/onkopedia/guidelines. Accessed 25 Oct 2017.

38. Holzerny P, Werner S, Ruof J. Are FJC appraisals suitable to guide therapeutic decisions. Analysis of consistency between clinical guidelines and FJC appraisals in Oncology. Gesundh ökon Qual manag. 2018. https://doi.org/10.1055/s-0043-121590.

39. Frampton JE. Perampanel: a review in drug-resistant epilepsy. Drugs. 2015; 75:1657–68.

40. Deutsche Gesellschaft für Endokrinologie. [Insulin Degludec (Tresiba®) gestern von der Amerikanischen Arzneibehörde (FDA) zugelassen – und in Deutschland Ende dieses Monats trotz Zulassung von der Firma wieder vom Markt genommen]. 2015. http://blog.endokrinologie.net/insulin-degludec-trotz-zulassung-vom-markt-genommen-2278/. Accessed 13 Sept 2016.

41. Gallwitz B. [Für Patienten folgenreich]. 2015. https://www.aerzteblatt.de/pdf/112/43/p17.pdf?ts=20.10.2015+09%3A01%3A51. http://www.diabetologie-online.de/a/1753487. Accessed 13 Sept 2016.

42. AstraZeneca. TAGRISSO™ (osimertinib) approved in EU as first-in-class treatment for patients with EGFR T790M mutation-positive metastatic non-small cell lung cancer. 2016. https://www.astrazeneca.com/media-centre/press-releases/2016/tagrisso-osimertinib-approved-in-eu-as-first-in-class-treatment-for-lung-cancer-03022016.html. Accessed 16 Mar 2017.

43. Deutsche Gesellschaft für Hämatologie und medizinische Onkologie (DGHO). [Weiteres neues Krebsmedikament vom Markt genommen: Alle beteiligten Institutionen haben Recht, aber den Schaden haben die Patienten]. 2016. https://www.dgho.de/aktuelles/presse/pressearchiv/2016/weiteres-neues-krebsmedikament-vom-markt-genommen-alle-beteiligten-institutionen-haben-recht-aber-den-schaden-haben-die-patienten. Accessed 14 Nov 2016.

44. Sauro KM, Wiebe S, Dunkley C, Janszky J, Kumlien E, Moshe S, et al. The current state of epilepsy guidelines: a systematic review. Epilepsia. 2016;57:13–23.

Permissions

All chapters in this book were first published in HER, by BioMed Central; hereby published with permission under the Creative Commons Attribution License or equivalent. Every chapter published in this book has been scrutinized by our experts. Their significance has been extensively debated. The topics covered herein carry significant findings which will fuel the growth of the discipline. They may even be implemented as practical applications or may be referred to as a beginning point for another development.

The contributors of this book come from diverse backgrounds, making this book a truly international effort. This book will bring forth new frontiers with its revolutionizing research information and detailed analysis of the nascent developments around the world.

We would like to thank all the contributing authors for lending their expertise to make the book truly unique. They have played a crucial role in the development of this book. Without their invaluable contributions this book wouldn't have been possible. They have made vital efforts to compile up to date information on the varied aspects of this subject to make this book a valuable addition to the collection of many professionals and students.

This book was conceptualized with the vision of imparting up-to-date information and advanced data in this field. To ensure the same, a matchless editorial board was set up. Every individual on the board went through rigorous rounds of assessment to prove their worth. After which they invested a large part of their time researching and compiling the most relevant data for our readers.

The editorial board has been involved in producing this book since its inception. They have spent rigorous hours researching and exploring the diverse topics which have resulted in the successful publishing of this book. They have passed on their knowledge of decades through this book. To expedite this challenging task, the publisher supported the team at every step. A small team of assistant editors was also appointed to further simplify the editing procedure and attain best results for the readers.

Apart from the editorial board, the designing team has also invested a significant amount of their time in understanding the subject and creating the most relevant covers. They scrutinized every image to scout for the most suitable representation of the subject and create an appropriate cover for the book.

The publishing team has been an ardent support to the editorial, designing and production team. Their endless efforts to recruit the best for this project, has resulted in the accomplishment of this book. They are a veteran in the field of academics and their pool of knowledge is as vast as their experience in printing. Their expertise and guidance has proved useful at every step. Their uncompromising quality standards have made this book an exceptional effort. Their encouragement from time to time has been an inspiration for everyone.

The publisher and the editorial board hope that this book will prove to be a valuable piece of knowledge for researchers, students, practitioners and scholars across the globe.

List of Contributors

Tugba Büyükdurmus
Universität Duisburg-Essen, Essen, Germany

Hendrik Schmitz and Harald Tauchmann
CINCH - National Research Center for Health Economics, Essen, Germany

Harald Tauchmann
RWI - Leibniz-Institut für Wirtschaftsforschung, Essen, Germany

Tugba Büyükdurmus
Ruhr-Universität Bochum, Bochum, Germany

Thomas Kopetsch
Kassenärztliche Bundesvereinigung, Berlin, Germany

Hendrik Schmitz
Universität Paderborn, Paderborn, Germany

Harald Tauchmann
Friedrich-Alexander-Universität Erlangen-Nürnberg, Findelgasse 7/9, 90402 Nürnberg, Germany

Hirotaka Kato
Graduate School of Economics, Kyoto University, Yoshida-honmachi, Sakyo, Kyoto 6068501, Japan

Rei Goto
Graduate School of Business Administration, Keio University, Yokohama, Japan

Lee R. Mobley, Mei Zhou and Srimoyee Bose
Georgia State University, 1 Park Place, Suite 700, Atlanta, GA 30304, USA

Pedro Amaral
Cedeplar - Universidade Federal de Minas Gerais, Belo Horizonte, Brazil

Tzy-Mey Kuo
University of North Carolina, Chapel Hill, USA

Kristín Helga Birgisdóttir and Tinna Laufey Ásgeirsdóttir
Faculty of Economics, University of Iceland, Oddi v/ Sturlugotu, 101 Reykjavik, Iceland

Stefán Hrafn Jónsson
Faculty of Social and Human Sciences, University of Iceland, Oddi v/Sturlugotu, 101 Reykjavik, Iceland

Ebenezer Kwabena Tetteh, Steve Morris and Nigel Titcheneker-Hooker
University College London, Gower Street, London WC1E 6BT, UK

Wei Zhang, Huiying Sun and Aslam H. Anis
Centre for Health Evaluation and Outcome Sciences, St. Paul's Hospital, 588-1081 Burrard Street, Vancouver, BC V6Z1Y6, Canada

Wei Zhang and Aslam H. Anis
School of Population and Public Health, University of British Columbia, 2206 East Mall, Vancouver, BC V6T1Z3, Canada

Simon Woodcock
Department of Economics, Simon Fraser University, 8888 University Drive, Burnaby, BC V5A 1S6, Canada

Jamie O'Hara
Faculty of Health and Social Care, University of Chester, Chester, UK

Shaun Walsh and Charlotte Camp
HCD Economics, The Innovation Centre, Daresbury WA4 4FS, UK

Giuseppe Mazza
UCL Institute for Liver and Digestive Health, Royal Free Hospital, University College London, London, UK

Liz Carroll
The Haemophilia Society, London, UK

Christina Hoxer and Lars Wilkinson
Novo Nordisk A/S, Vandtårnsvej 114, -2860 Søborg, DK, Denmark

Piia Pekola and Hennamari Mikkola
Social Insurance Institution of Finland, PL 450, 00056 Helsinki, Finland

Ismo Linnosmaa
National Institute for Health and Welfare, PL 30, 00271 Helsinki, Finland

Carine Milcent
Paris-Jourdan Sciences Economiques, French National Center for Scientific Research, Paris, France

Saad Zbiri
EA 7285, Versailles Saint Quentin University, Montigny-le-Bretonneux, France

Steve Brito and Ana Corbacho
International Monetary Fund, 700 19th St NW, Washington, DC 20431, USA

Rene Osorio
Inter-American Development Bank, 1300 New York Avenue NW, Washington, DC 20577, USA

Tsuyoshi Takahara
Graduate School of Economics, Osaka University, 1-7, Machikaneyama, Toyonaka, Osaka 560-0043, Japan

Henrike Schulze and Christoph Gutenbrunner
Clinic of Rehabilitation Medicine, Hannover Medical School, Carl-Neuberg-Straße 1, 30625 Hannover, Germany

Marisa Nacke
Cancer Research UK, Beatson Institute, Glasgow, UK

Catarina Hadamitzky
Practice for Lympho-Vascular Diseases, Bahnhofstraße 12, Hannover, Germany

Jonas Minet Kinge
Norwegian Institute of Public Health, Pb 4404 Nydalen, 0403 Oslo, Norway
Department of Health Management and Health Economics, University of Oslo, Oslo, Norway

Beáta Gavurová, Viliam Kováč and Tatiana Vagašová
Technical University of Košice, Nêmcovej 32, Košice, Slovakia

Son Hong Nghiem
The Australian Research Centre for Health Services Innovation, Institute of Health and Biomedical Innovation, School of Public Health and Social Work, Queensland University of Technology, Kelvin Grove, Brisbane QLD 4059, Australia

Luke Brian Connelly
Centre for the Business and Economics of Health, Faculty of Health and Behavioural Sciences, The University of Queensland, Brisbane QLD 4072, Australia

W. Dominika Wranik
School of Public Administration, Department of Community Health and Epidemiology, Dalhousie University, Halifax, NS, Canada

Adam Muir
Department of Community Health and Epidemiology, Dalhousie University, Halifax, NS, Canada

Min Hu
Department of Economics, Dalhousie University, Halifax, NS, Canada

Johannes Clouth
Medical Affairs, Lilly Deutschland GmbH, Werner-Reimers-Str. 2-4, 61352 Bad Homburg, Germany

Astra M. Liepa
Eli Lilly and Company, Lilly Corporate Center, Indianapolis, IN 46285, USA

Guido Moeser
masem Research Institute GmbH, Unter den Eichen 5/G, D-65195 Wiesbaden, Germany

Heiko Friedel, Magdalena Bernzen and Elena Garal-Pantaler
Team Gesundheit GmbH, Rellinghauser Straße 93, 45128 Essen, Germany

Jörg Trojan
Universitätsklinikum Frankfurt, Medizinische Klinik 1, Theodor-Stern-Kai 7, 60590 Frankfurt, Germany

Thomas R. Staab
Roche Pharma AG, Grenzach-Wyhlen, Germany

Miriam Walter and Sonja Mariotti Nesurini
nspm ltd, Meggen, Switzerland

Charalabos-Markos Dintsios
Health Services Research and Health Economics, Heinrich Heine University, Düsseldorf, Germany

J.-Matthias Graf von der Schulenburg
Leibniz University Hanover, Hanover, Germany

Volker E. Amelung and Jörg Ruof
Medical School of Hanover, Hanover, Germany

Jörg Ruof
r-connect ltd, Hauensteinstr. 132, 4059 Basel, Switzerland

Index